Acupuncture in Pregnancy and Childbirth

Chapter 16 **Classical Five Element acupuncture and its use in postnatal depression** has been contributed by Gerad Kite Adv LicAc

Commissioning Editor: **Karen Morley, Claire Wilson**
Development Editor: **Kerry McGechie**
Project Manager: **Morven Dean**
Designer: **Charlotte Murray**
Illustration Manager: **Bruce Hogarth**
Illustrator: **Diane Mercer**

Acupuncture in Pregnancy and Childbirth

Second edition

Zita West SRN SCM LIC AC
Midwife and Acupuncturist, Banbury, UK

Consultant Editor
Lyndsey Isaacs RGN BSc(Hons) MBAcC
Acupuncturist specialising in Pregnancy,
London and Rickmansworth, UK

Foreword by
Giovanni Maciocia CAc (Nanjing)
Acupuncturist and Medical Herbalist, UK
Visiting Associate Professor at the Nanjing University of Traditional Chinese Medicine, Nanjing

CHURCHILL LIVINGSTONE
ELSEVIER

Edinburgh London New York Oxford Philadelphia St Louis Sydney Toronto 2008

CHURCHILL LIVINGSTONE ELSEVIER

Harcourt Health Sciences

First edition 2001
Second edition 2008

ISBN-13: 978-0-443-10371-1
ISBN-10: 0-443-10371-2

British Library Cataloguing in Publication Data
A catalogue record for this book is available from the British Library

Library of Congress Cataloging in Publication Data
A catalog record for this book is available from the Library of Congress

Note

Knowledge and best practice in this field are constantly changing. As new research and experience broaden our knowledge, changes in practice, treatment and drug therapy may become necessary or appropriate. Readers are advised to check the most current information provided (i) on procedures featured or (ii) by the manufacturer of each product to be administered, to verify the recommended dose or formula, the method and duration of administration, and contraindications. It is the responsibility of the practitioner, relying on their own experience and knowledge of the patient, to make diagnoses, to determine dosages and the best treatment for each individual patient, and to take all appropriate safety precautions. To the fullest extent of the law, neither the Publisher nor the Author assumes any liability for any injury and/or damage to persons or property arising out of or related to any use of the material contained in this book.

The Publisher

Printed and bound by CPI Group (UK) Ltd, Croydon, CR0 4YY
Transferred to digital print 2013

Contents

Foreword to the first edition

Like all branches of Chinese medicine, traditional gynaecology and obstetrics have a long history. The earliest records of gynaecological medical writings date from the Shang dynasty (1500–1000 BC): bones and tortoise shells have been found with inscriptions dealing with childbirth problems. The text 'Book of Mountains and Seas' from the Warring States period (476–221 BC) describes medicinal plants to treat infertility. The 'Yellow Emperor's Classic of Internal Medicine' (*Huang Di Nei Jing Su Wen*) has many references to women's physiology, anatomy, diagnosis and treatment of gynaecological problems.

Throughout the ancient Chinese medical literature, there are many references to obstetrics. The famous doctor Zhang Zhong Jing refers in his work 'Discussion on Cold-induced Diseases' (*Shang Han Lun*) to a previous book entitled 'Series of Herbs for Obstetrics' (*Tai Lu Yao Lu*) which proves that even before the Han dynasty there were books dealing exclusively with obstetrics; but all of these have been lost. 'Series of Herbs for Obstetrics' is the earliest recorded book on obstetrics in Chinese medicine. The 'Discussion of Prescriptions of the Golden Chest' (*Jin Gui Yao Lue Fang Lun*) by the same author has two chapters on pregnancy and post-partum problems.

The 'Pulse Classic' (*Mai Jing*, AD 280) by Wang Shu He, a famous doctor of the Jin dynasty, describes pulse pictures and differentiation of women's diseases in Volume 9. In this volume he discusses some pulse pictures found in pregnancy and labour. For example, he says that 'The Kidneys govern the Uterus, and its condition is reflected at the Rear position of the pulse. If the pulse at this region does not fade on pressure, it indicates pregnancy'. In another passage he says that 'A superficial pulse accompanied by abdominal pain referred to the midline of the lower back, indicates impending labour'. The book also describes the qualities of the pulse before an imminent miscarriage, normal and abnormal pulses during the postpartum stage, and pulses in women with abdominal masses in relation to prognosis.

The 'Thousand Golden Ducat Prescriptions' (*Qian Jin Yao Fang*, AD 652), written by Sun Si Miao during the Tang dynasty, has three volumes dealing with gynaecology and obstetrics. That author made the interesting observation that a metal knife should never be used to cut the umbilical cord; from a modern perspective, this was an important recommendation as, if dirty, a metal instrument could easily provoke a tetanus infection.

The 'Treasure of Obstetrics' (*Jing Xiao Chan Bao*) written during the Tang dynasty is the earliest surviving book dedicated entirely to obstetrics. The book contains

12 chapters on diseases of pregnancy, four on difficult labour and 25 on postpartum diseases. Problems in pregnancy discussed include morning sickness, bleeding, threatened miscarriage, miscarriage, urinary problems and oedema. The discussion on labour problems includes formulae for promoting labour, and on dealing with a dead fetus, prolonged labour or retention of placenta. The discussion on postpartum diseases includes tetanus, puerperal infections, abdominal pain, persistent bleeding, retention of urine, lactation insufficiency and mastitis.

Zhu Dan Xi (1281–1358) maintained that 'Yang is often in excess and Yin is often deficient' and therefore advocated nourishing Yin as one of the most important treatment principles. For example, for problems before childbirth he advised clearing Heat and nourishing Blood. He also indicated Huang Qin *Radix Scutellariae baicalensis* and Bai Zhu *Rhizoma atractylodis macrocephalae* as two important herbs to prevent miscarriage.

The doctors of the Ming dynasty (1368–1644) consolidated and integrated the theories of four great schools of medical thought. Many important gynaecological books were written during the Ming dynasty, for example 'Standards of Diagnosis and Treatment of Women's Diseases' (*Zheng Zhi Zhun Sheng-Nu Ke*, 1602) by Wang Ken Tang, which summarises the experience of doctors of previous generations in the treatment of gynaecological diseases and contains an extensive section on obstetrics. The 'Complete Works of Jing Yue' (*Jing Yue Quan Shu*, 1624) by Zhang Jing Yue has an extensive section on gynaecology and obstetrics, discussing the treatment of problems of pregnancy and labour amongst other gynaecological conditions.

The gynaecology volume of the 'Golden Mirror of Medicine' (*Yi Zong Jin Jian*) by Wu Qian discusses the pathology and treatment of labour, and postpartum diseases including postnatal depression. The 'Treatise on Obstetrics' (*Da Sheng Bian*) focuses on diseases of pregnancy, management of normal and difficult labour, and postpartum diseases.

During the late Qing dynasty, Western medicine was introduced to China and integrated with Chinese medicine. The two principal doctors who advocated the integration of Chinese and Western medicine were Tang Zong Hai (1862–1918) and Zhang Xi Chun (1860–1933). These doctors did not write specialised books on gynaecology but they did discuss gynaecological and obstetric problems in their works. For example, Zhang Xi Chun formulated several important prescriptions such as Regulating the Penetrating Vessel Decoction (*Li Chong Tang*), Calming the Penetrating Vessel Decoction (*An Chong Tang*), Consolidating the Penetrating Vessel Decoction (*Gu Chong Tang*) and Fetus Longevity Pill (*Shou Tai Wan*, to prevent miscarriage) in his book 'Records of Combined Chinese and Western Medicine' (*Yi Xue Zhong Zhong Can Xi Lu*, 1918).

Since 1949 the combination of Western and Chinese Medicine has been emphasised and many innovative treatments in obstetrics have been devised. For example, ectopic pregnancy is often treated with acupuncture and Chinese herbs without recourse to surgery; acupuncture is used in breech presentation of the fetus; Chinese herbs are used in the treatment of postnatal depression.

'Fetus education' was a feature of Chinese obstetrics in ancient times. This was based on the belief that various lifestyle influences from the mother (including diet, work, sexual activity and emotional state) could affect the fetus's forming constitution. This is of course borne out by modern research which shows that various lifestyle habits such as diet, smoking, alcohol consumption and so on do affect the constitution of the fetus deeply. The main difference from the ancient Chinese views on 'fetus education' is that modern Western views concentrate mostly on factors which affect the fetus adversely, while ancient Chinese gynaecologists believed that by manipulating her diet and environment and paying attention to her emotional life, the expectant mother could affect the fetus positively as well.

In particular, Dr Xu Zi Cai (493–572) gave detailed instructions on the nourishment of the fetus month by month. He said that in the first month of pregnancy the woman should eat nourishing and easily digestible cooked food; barley, which makes the fetus grow normally, is particularly beneficial at this time. During the second month of pregnancy the woman should not eat pungent, hot and drying foods and she should avoid sexual activity and excessive physical work. The fetus's body shape and sex are still changing during the third month under the influence of external stimuli (on the mother). During the fourth month the woman should eat rice, fish or wild goose; this makes the fetus's Qi and Blood strong, its ears and eyes sensitive and bright, and its channels free from obstructions. In the fifth month it is advisable for the expectant mother to sleep long hours, bathe and change her clothes often, stay away from strangers, wear enough clothes and be exposed to sunshine. She should eat wheat, beef and lamb. During the sixth month the fetus begins to receive from the mother the Qi of the Lungs which forms its sinews. The woman should take light exercise and not stay indoors all the time. During the seventh month the expectant mother should take enough exercise to encourage the circulation of Qi and Blood by flexing and extending her joints. She should avoid cold foods and eat rice which will nourish the fetus's bones and teeth. During the eighth month of pregnancy the mother should avoid emotional upsets and practise quiet breathing to maintain her Qi, which will promote a moist and lustrous skin in the fetus. During the ninth month the mother should eat sweet foods, wear loose clothes and not live in a damp house. During the tenth month the mother should concentrate her Qi at the Lower *Dan Tian* three *cun* below the umbilicus to promote the growth of the fetus's joints and its mental faculties.

In the process of transmitting the knowledge of Chinese medicine to the West, an increasing specialisation is taking place. Until a short time ago, only books dealing with the general theory of Chinese medicine were written, whereas now more and more specialised books are written on pediatrics, gynaecology, diet and so on. Zita West's book is the first to deal with the specialty of obstetrics only and it is a great pleasure to introduce this book to a Western audience.

Ms West is an acupuncturist and a midwife with 15 years' experience and therefore is uniquely placed to write about obstetrics. Her book is a lucid, coherent and practical guide to the care of pregnant women for acupuncturists. The book combines a comprehensive discussion of the acupuncture treatment of the pregnant mother before, during and after childbirth with possibly the most rigorous and detailed guidelines for administering acupuncture in childbirth ever published in the English language. The extensive chapters on the physiology and pathology of labour will give any acupuncturist complete confidence in assisting women during labour.

The book does more than this: it combines the acupuncture treatment with Western views and treatments, a knowledge of which is essential in this field. Ms West gives guidelines for the nutrition of the mother before and during pregnancy; this, combined with her guidelines according to Chinese nutrition, is truly a modern version of the ancient Chinese 'fetus education'. Her guidelines on how to adjust the needling technique during pregnancy are sensitive, sensible and very useful.

Ms West concludes her book with an interesting discussion of postnatal depression as seen from a Five Element School perspective, contributed by Gerad Kite; this adds another dimension to the traditional Chinese views of obstetrics and will be of interest to a broad range of acupuncturists.

In conclusion, I can highly recommend this book as an essential text for anyone who is interested not only in treating expectant mothers but also in preparing women for pregnancy and childbirth.

Giovanni Maciocia

Preface

Years of working as a midwife and acupuncturist have proved to me that the majority of pregnancy ailments can be treated successfully with acupuncture; yet these conditions are generally considered 'par for the course' because they are hard to alleviate conventionally. Pregnant women are understandably reluctant to take drugs unless it is absolutely essential and they therefore have no choice. Many would be happy to seek safe alternatives.

My first introduction to acupuncture came after the birth of my second child, when I was suffering from postnatal depression. The success of the treatment I received inspired me to study the subject further, and four years later I graduated from the College of Traditional Chinese Medicine in Leamington Spa. Having been a practising midwife for many years, and having had two children of my own, I understood the reluctance of pregnant women to take pharmaceutical remedies for their ailments. Acupuncture treatment, used in conjunction with conventional Western medicine, seemed to me the ideal solution.

In 1993 I set up an acupuncture clinic at Warwick Hospital, providing treatment on the NHS to pregnant women (only the second such clinic in the UK to be provided at a National Health hospital). The clinic offers acupuncture treatment to women from six weeks into their pregnancy until six weeks after birth. Women are referred by their consultant, GP, community midwife or hospital midwife, or they can come at their own request.

Treating between 40 and 60 pregnant women a week has given me a depth of experience that it would have taken a lifetime to acquire in private practice. When I first began to practise, I took many of the acupuncture points I used from texts and ancient prescriptions. Experience and the feedback of patients have extended my knowledge enormously. The points that I use now are the points that I know from experience to work, although the evidence for using them is largely anecdotal.

Acupuncture has gained a great reputation in the field of fertility and pregnancy and more and more evidence is available for its use and there is much more integration now between conventional medicine and acupuncture than when I first wrote this book.

As I began to teach and share my knowledge, I realized that many practitioners, particularly the newly qualified, are nervous about treating pregnant women because they lack a full understanding of pregnancy and fear harming the baby. This book is intended to fill in some of those gaps in knowledge. It is a practical rather than theoretical guide to what is happening to a woman's body during pregnancy, the development of the baby, the care provided within the NHS, the roles different professionals play in that care, the medical terms used and the possible danger signals. I have also included chapters on nutrition and diet, which are, of course, vital in a holistic approach to pregnancy.

My hope is that this newly revised copy of my book will give the practitioner more confidence in the treatment of pregnant women. This edition has information about IVF treatments as many more women who now get pregnant have undergone assisted fertility, and are a highly anxious group that need a lot of support. There is also more advances medically as to why some women have difficulty getting and staying pregnant and these advances medically involves women who have blood clotting disorders which as acupuncturists you should have a knowledge of.

More research into the use of acupuncture in pregnancy is still needed, but it is my hope that eventually every maternity unit in the country will have its own acupuncture clinic. In the meantime, I hope that this book will prove a valuable reference to readers, providing sufficient insight for them to feel confident in their practice and to be able to approach and work alongside mainstream health professionals.

Zita West
Banbury 2007

In 2002 I set up the zitawest clinic which specializes in fertility and pregnancy using an integrated approach. Zita West products are vitamins and minerals to support a woman's preconception and throughout the various stages of pregnancy. Available from www.zitawest.com

Acknowledgements

I would like to thank: Lyndsey Isaacs, Sharon Baylis and my husband, Robert, for their hard work and invaluable input; I could not have written the book without them; my teachers, Professor J R Worsley, Angela Hicks, Allegra Wint and Nikki Bilton; Sarah Budd, for her help in setting up the acupuncture clinic at Warwick Hospital; John Hughes, Hugh Begg, Robert Jackson, Karl Olah and Mike Pearson, consultants at Warwick Hospital, for their support in helping to provide an acupuncture service on the NHS; Nancy Hempstead, Chris Sidgwick, Annette Gough and Susan Ensor, for their help and support; Gerad Kite, for his invaluable contribution (Chapter 16); Gordon Gatesby, for his help in understanding electroacupuncture; all of my patients and the GPs and midwives who have supported me over the years.

1 Planning for a healthy baby

Chapter outline

Healthy parents produce healthy babies. And healthy babies, in general, have a better chance of growing into healthy children and healthy adults. All parents hope that their baby will be free of abnormality, 'bouncing' and strong, not sickly and weak.

Professor David Barker, head of the Environmental Epidemiology Unit of the Medical Research Council, has been conducting research into the effect of the mother's nutrition prior to conception and during pregnancy on the health of her children in later life. His early conclusion is that: 'it looks as though getting it right at the beginning may be a key to good health throughout life'. Ensuring optimum health in *both* partners in the period leading up to conception (as well as in the mother during pregnancy) can do a great deal to enhance fetal growth and minimise the risk of fetal abnormalities.

This chapter looks at the way in which parents can influence the health of their unborn child by optimising their own health before conception occurs. It examines the simple measures that can be taken to eliminate toxins, allergies and environmental pollutants from the body, along with all the other negative influences on prenatal health. It discusses methods of natural family planning and the vital role that nutrition plays, both preconceptually and throughout pregnancy. It explains conception from the viewpoint of traditional Chinese medicine (TCM) and details the acupuncture points that can be used prior to conception and at particular stages of the menstrual cycle. Finally, it gives pointers on exercise when planning a baby.

The Chinese viewpoint on preconceptual care

Eastern thinking has always maintained that a woman should take special care of herself during her periods and after childbirth. She should avoid heavy physical work and overexposure to cold and damp. This care extends not just to physical considerations but to her diet and emotional state as well:

- *worry* will inhibit Qi from flowing
- *anger* gives rise to Liver Qi stagnation (see Imbalance of the Liver in the next section)
- *fear* will cause Qi to sink, which may result in miscarriage
- *joy* may lead to irregular menstruation.

(The effects of emotions on pregnancy are considered in more detail in Ch. 5, p. 75.)

The ancient Chinese considered the uterus to be vulnerable during menstruation, during pregnancy and postnatally, susceptible to Cold, Damp and Heat. Certain rules were therefore advised. First, no alcohol should be consumed during periods as this may cause the Blood to be reckless. Second, sex during a period can cause stagnation of the Qi and Blood and so should be avoided. Third, the uterus should not be exposed to cold or dampness during menstruation, so swimming should be avoided and care should be taken to dry the body and especially the hair thoroughly after bathing. Finally, strenuous exercise during a period can deplete the Spleen Qi and so should be avoided.

The ancient Chinese considered that, at the age of 7, the Kidney Qi starts to flourish. Menstruation then usually starts around the age of 14 and continues at monthly intervals until the age of 50.

Having regular monthly periods depends on normal functioning of the Chong and Ren channels. As the Sea of Blood, the Chong Mai, or Penetrating (Thrusting) Vessel, is where the Qi and Blood of the 12 channels meet. It originates in the Uterus and emerges in the perineum. It then ascends centrally to the throat where it meets with the Ren Mai and then curves around the lips. The Ren Mai, or Conception (Directing) Vessel, is referred to as the Sea of all the Yin channels and presides over the Uterus and fetus. It originates from the Uterus, emerges in the perineum and then runs up the anterior midline and meets with the three Yin channels of the foot (the Liver, Spleen and Kidney channels) at the points CV-2, 3 and 4. It then ascends further to the lower jaw, where it penetrates internally to encircle the lips, with a branch to the eyes.

The Du Mai, or Governing Vessel, originates from the Uterus and emerges in the perineum. It then ascends along the posterior midline and meets with all the Yang channels at GV-14. It further ascends to the vertex of the head, then descends along the anterior midline to the lips and mouth. It ends inside the upper gum at GV-28, where it links with the Ren meridian.

The Ren and Du Mai circulate in endless cycles, maintaining a level of Yin and Yang balance in order for menstruation to occur.

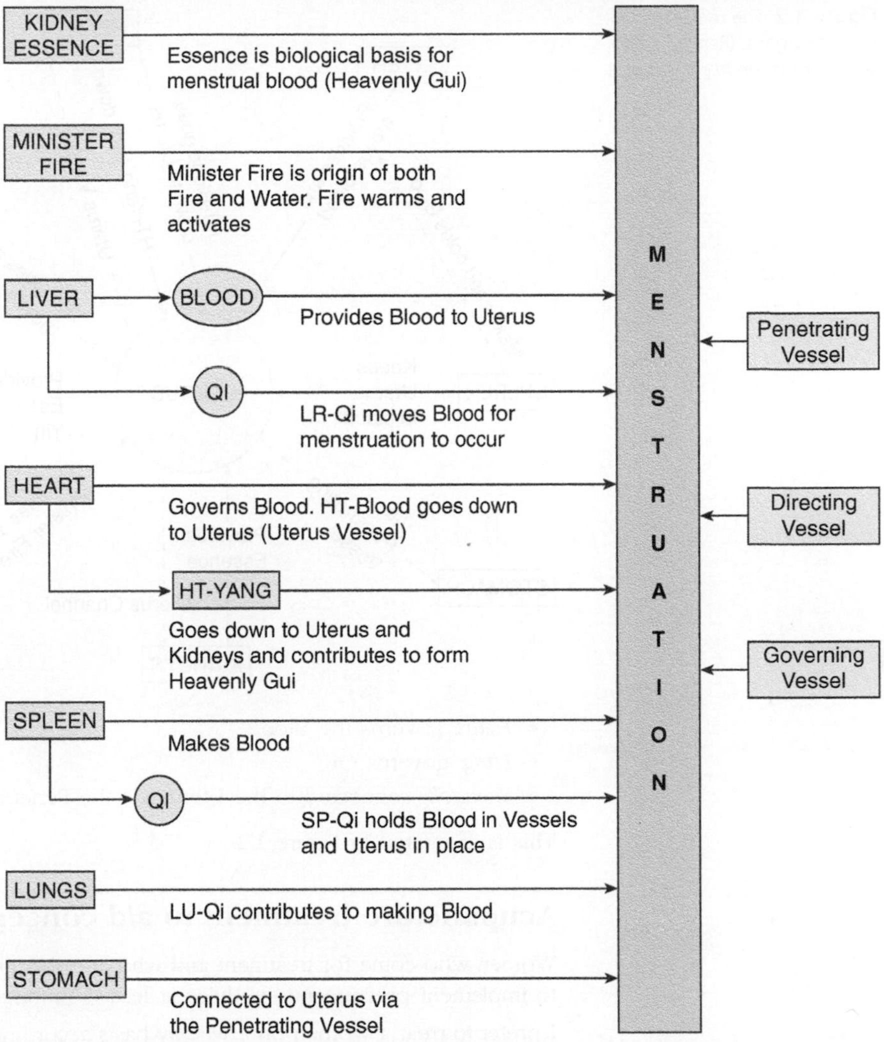

Figure 1.1 The internal organs and menstruation. (Reproduced with permission from Maciocia 1998, p. 16.)

The relationship between the three channels and the internal organs in menstruation is shown in Figure 1.1. The Liver stores the Blood and provides Blood for the Uterus. Either heavy or scanty periods may be signs of Liver Blood deficiency and therefore of possible fertility problems. Normal periods and good fertility also depend on the state of the Heart and Kidneys. If the Heart Blood is deficient, Heart Qi does not descend to the Uterus.

It is very common for women with infertility problems, with in vitro fertilisation (IVF) pregnancies or who habitually miscarry to have some form of Kidney deficiency. For conception to occur, the Governing Vessel, 'the Gate of Life', needs to be strong, to allow the Essence and the Blood to form.

The role of the different organs in relation to the Blood, Uterus and Qi is as follows.

- *Kidneys*: store the Essence and influence reproduction
- *Liver*: closely linked to the Blood
- *Spleen*: makes the Blood

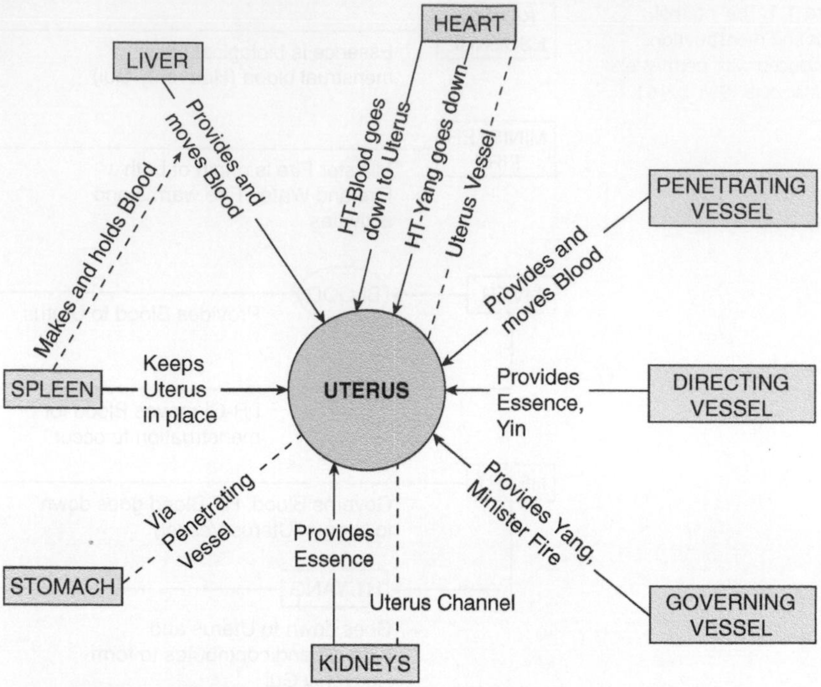

Figure 1.2 The uterus and internal organs. (Reproduced with permission from Maciocia 1998, p. 9.)

- *Heart*: governs the Blood
- *Lung*: governs Qi
- *Stomach*: connected to the Uterus via the Penetrating Vessel

This is illustrated in Figure 1.2.

Acupuncture treatment to aid conception

Women who come for treatment and who are planning for pregnancy should start to implement preconception advice at least 3 months before trying to conceive.

I prefer to treat a woman on a weekly basis according to her cycle. It is important to concentrate initially on correcting any imbalances the patient may have. A woman entering pregnancy with chronic imbalances is more likely to feel unwell during her pregnancy and certain conditions may arise as a result. I concentrate on any imbalances, using acupuncture points that will specifically help.

Imbalance of the Liver

Irregular periods and premenstrual tension can often be due to a Liver imbalance. Women with premenstrual symptoms often experience a great deal of nausea and vomiting of bile early in pregnancy. The Liver is responsible for the smooth flow of Qi so correction of these symptoms is very important.

Liver Qi stagnation

I know of very few women who do not suffer some form of premenstrual syndrome. The Liver plays a very important role in menstruation, especially in premenstrual syndrome, and Liver Qi stagnation is very common, giving rise to breast distension, irritability, depression and abdominal pain. Untreated Liver Qi stagnation can turn to Liver Heat or Liver Fire.

Liver Blood deficiency

The Liver stores the Blood and provides the Blood to the Uterus. A woman suffering from heavy periods or who has had heavy blood loss following her labour is likely to be Liver Blood deficient. Liver Blood deficiency can cause Liver Yang to rise, which results in throbbing headaches occurring around the time of the period.

Kidney

Women who have had a series of miscarriages very often show signs of Kidney deficiency. Common symptoms such as back ache around periods are indicative of this and strengthening the Kidneys is important.

Women who have had repeated IVF treatments very often show signs of Kidney Yin deficiency and need to nourish their Kidneys. High blood pressure may also be a symptom of Kidney Yin deficiency.

Oedema during pregnancy may be a sign of Kidney Yang deficiency.

Stomach

Vomiting during pregnancy can be a result of Stomach Qi deficiency, due to weak Stomach energy.

The menstrual cycle

During each cycle, approximately 100 millilitres of blood are lost. The blood flow will vary according to age, constitution, lifestyle, mental state and any drugs being taken. Each menstrual cycle usually lasts 3–5 days, though in some women it may last 7 days. Menstrual blood is usually light red at the beginning of a cycle, deep red in the middle and pinkish towards the end. A normal blood flow does not contain clots.

Questions about a woman's cycle are vitally important to establish where the imbalances are and the best way to correct them prior to conceiving.

- *Early periods* may be the result of Spleen Qi deficiency or of Heat in the Blood.
- *Late periods*, where the cycle lasts 40–50 days, may be caused by Blood deficiency, a cold Uterus, Kidney Yang deficiency or by Qi stagnation.
- *Irregular periods* may be due to Liver Qi stagnation, Kidney Yang deficiency or Kidney Yin deficiency.
- *Heavy periods* may signify Qi deficiency, Heat in the Blood or Blood stasis.
- *Pain* before, during or after a period is significant, depending on where it is felt:
  - pain in the mid to lower abdomen may mean Blood stagnation
  - pain on both sides of the abdomen suggests Qi stagnation
  - painful breasts suggest Liver Qi stagnation
  - lower back pain may mean Kidney deficiency.

Factors which affect periods

A woman's blood is vitally important; menstruation, pregnancy, labour and breast-feeding are all related to Blood. Blood relies on Qi for its control, circulation and adjustment. Qi relies on Blood for nourishment. Pathogenic factors such as Cold, Damp and Heat can cause disharmony.

- *Cold* coagulates the Qi, causing stagnation of the Blood. This can lead to a prolonged menstrual cycle, dysmenorrhoea or amenorrhoea.
- *Damp* affects the Chong and Ren channels and may cause scanty menstrual flow, ammenorrhea or dysmenorrhoea.
- *Heat* accelerates the Blood, causing profuse blood flow.

Emotional factors may also be significant, as follows.

- *Worry* will inhibit Qi from flowing, causing the Blood to stagnate and the Chong and Ren channels will not function well. Menstrual symptoms will include a prolonged cycle or scanty flow.
- *Anger* may lead to Liver Qi stagnation (see above: Imbalance of the Liver).
- *Fear* will cause the Qi to sink, which may result in miscarriage (see Ch. 5, p. 75).
- *Joy* may produce irregularities in the cycle.

Treatment with acupuncture during the cycle

The four phases of the menstrual cycle according to TCM are shown in Figure 1.3.

Postperiod – day 5 to day 11

After the period has finished, the Chong channel has emptied out and there is a need to build up the Blood again. The Blood and Yin are empty and the Penetrating and Directing Vessels are depleted. The Blood therefore needs to be tonified in order to nourish the Qi and Yin.

POINTS TO TREAT

- **CV-4, to tonify the Kidney and regulate the Chong and the Ren channels**
- **GV-4, to tonify the Kidney**
- **BL-20 and 21 to tonify the Blood**
- **BL-23 to tonify the Kidney**
- **SP-6 to nourish the Blood**

Ovulation – day 11 to day 15

Here there is a switch from Yin to Yang and the need to promote ovulation and the smooth flow of Qi.

POINTS TO TREAT

- **CV-3 benefits Qi and regulates the Chong and the Ren channels**
- **KI-15 promotes circulation of the Blood and regulates the period**
- **SP-6 regulates the function of the Spleen**

Postovulation, premenstrual – day 15 to day 28

Here the Yang phase of the cycle is increasing. If a woman is showing more signs of premenstrual tension (PMT), add more Liver points.

Figure 1.3 The four phases of the menstrual cycle. (Reproduced with permission from Maciocia 1998, p. 10.)

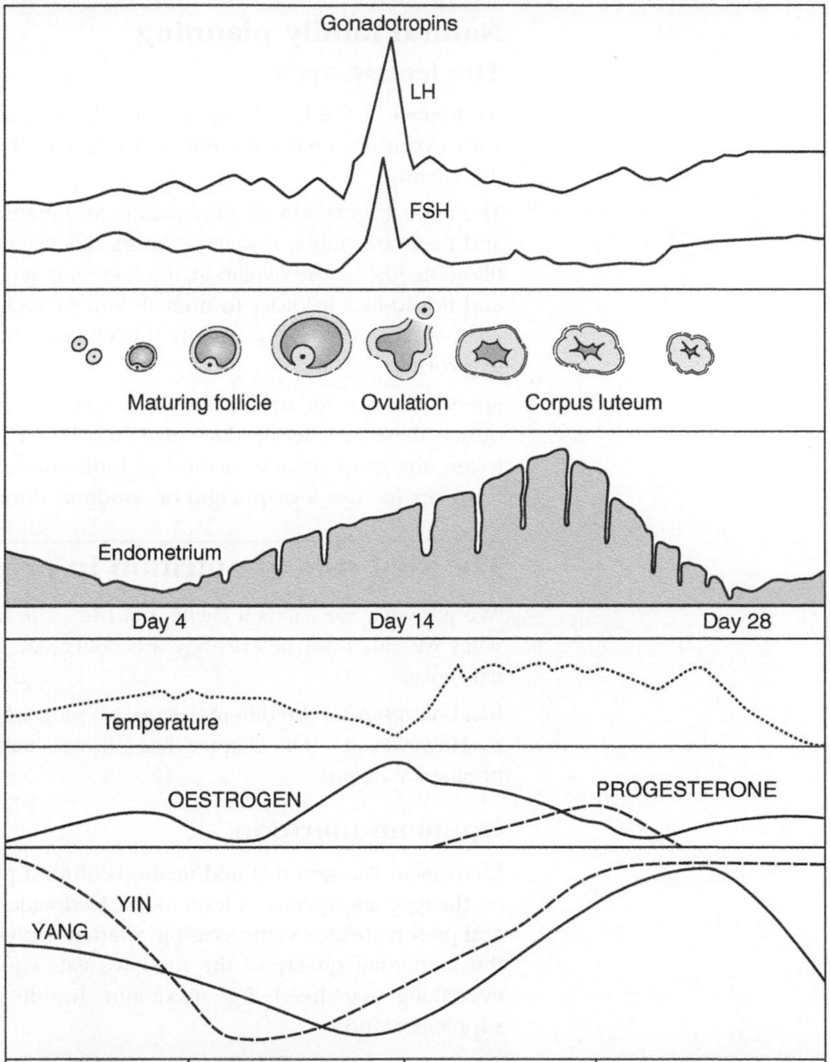

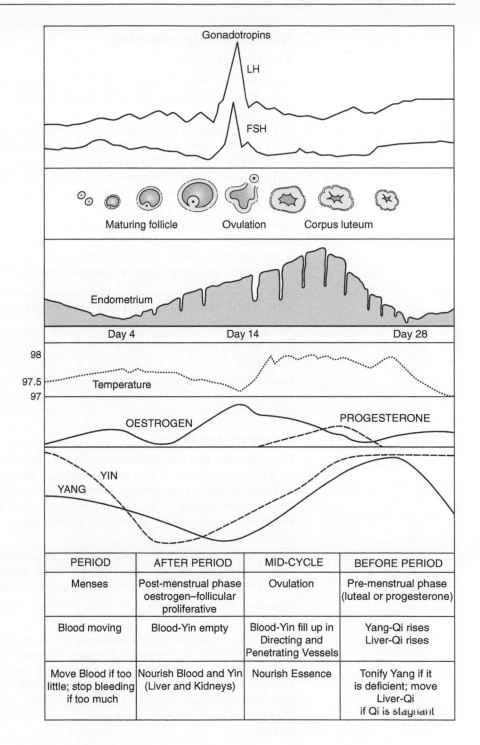

PERIOD	AFTER PERIOD	MID-CYCLE	BEFORE PERIOD
Menses	Post-menstrual phase oestrogen–follicular proliferative	Ovulation	Pre-menstrual phase (luteal or progesterone)
Blood moving	Blood-Yin empty	Blood-Yin fill up in Directing and Penetrating Vessels	Yang-Qi rises Liver-Qi rises
Move Blood if too little; stop bleeding if too much	Nourish Blood and Yin (Liver and Kidneys)	Nourish Essence	Tonify Yang if it is deficient; move Liver-Qi if Qi is stagnant

Natural family planning

The female cycle

Awareness of the female cycle can help a couple to time intercourse to coincide with ovulation, giving the released egg a far better chance of being fertilised by the sperm.

The natural female cycle of ovulation and menstruation varies from 23 to 35 days, and there are only a few days during this cycle when the egg is available for fertilisation. Just before ovulation, the secretion in the vagina changes, becoming sticky and thread-like in order to nourish and protect the sperm. With a little guidance, most women can easily identify this change and so recognise when they are due to ovulate.

Sperm can live for up to 5 days in optimum conditions, so frequent intercourse during these few fertile days gives the best chance of conception. By the same token, the most natural method of birth control without side-effects is to abstain from sex (or use a diaphragm or condom) during these few fertile days.

The vital role of nutrition in pregnancy

'We are what we eat' is a cliché, but true. The health of our offspring depends on what we eat, both before they are conceived and in the first 9 months of their existence.

Ideal nutrition for the different stages of pregnancy is examined in detail in Chapter 3. However, as this chapter has shown, eating properly has to start before pregnancy begins.

Optimum nutrition

Changes in Western diet and methods of food production have had a huge impact on the type and quality of food today. Herbicides and pesticides, chemical additives and preservatives, overprocessing, vitamin depletion and general pollution all affect the nutritional quality of the food we eat. Too often it simply does not contain everything we need for maximum health; hence the need for additional supplementation.

The government-set RDAs (recommended daily allowances – the figures on cereal and other packets) are designed to prevent people getting vitamin deficiencies, but these are only the basic requirements to prevent severe malnutrition.

Optimum nutritional levels vary from person to person and are designed to maximise health.

Recent research suggest that a woman needs only an extra 50 calories a day during the first 6 months of pregnancy – less than one extra apple. It is not how much a woman eats but the quality of what she eats that matters. Ensuring a healthy balanced diet and the right vitamin and mineral supplementation, before as well as after conception, is the most important thing parents can do for their unborn child. Table 1.1 lists the roles of different nutrients in the mother and baby, together with food sources.

Infertility

The average length of time that most couples take to conceive is around 6 months. However, figures suggest that around one in six couples suffers from infertility and is childless (Balen & Jacobs 2003).

Table 1.1 Effects of nutrients on the mother and baby

Mother	Baby	Food source
	Vitamins	
Vitamin A		
lactation placental membranes hormones	red blood cells fetal growth visual development hair, skin mucous membranes	milk, butter, fatty fish, yellow fruits and veg, dark green fruits and veg, liver, eggs
Vitamin B complex		
lactation, metabolism of fats and sugar	nerve function heart development protects against cleft palate development	wholegrains, nuts and seeds, leafy vegetables
Folic acid		
red blood cells bone marrow making antibodies	healthy bone marrow helps with spine formation division of cells	wheatgerm, nuts and seeds, milk, wholegrains, dark green leafy vegetables
Vitamin C		
connective tissue helps to protect baby against viruses helps with absorption of iron promotes healing after delivery	carries oxygen to every cell builds a strong infection system for the baby helps form good teeth, blood vessels	melon, citrus fruits, blackcurrants, strawberries, carrots, peas, spinach, broccoli, tomatoes, green peppers
Vitamin D		
good for teeth absorption of calcium and phosphorus	helps bones to harden skull development	sunlight on the skin, fatty fish, free-range eggs, organic meats
Vitamin E		
wound healing after birth protects against stretch marks protects against anaemia helps avoid varicose veins	protects against jaundice formation of blood cells heart development	wheatgerm, nuts, avocados, green leafy vegetables, eggs
Vitamin F (essential fatty acids)		
absorption of vitamins healthy skin	required for growth kidney and brain development sex and adrenal hormones	fatty fish, nuts, green leafy vegetables
Vitamin K		
good blood clotting	protects against haemorrhage	cauliflower, eggs, green leafy vegetables

Table 1.1 Effects of nutrients on the mother and baby (continued)

Mother	Baby	Food source
	Minerals	
Calcium		
healthy bones and teeth clotting mechanism nerves and muscles	formation of healthy bones and teeth	carob, Brazil nuts, green vegetables, cheese and milk, shellfish
Chromium		
regulation of blood sugar	regulation of blood sugar	wheatgerm, honey, grapes, raisins
Copper		
strong bones nervous system iron absorption	aids development of brain, connective tissue, nerves	meat, legumes, dates, nuts, raisins, seafood
Iron		
red blood cells respiratory functions protects against fatigue	blood cells bone growth	parsley, eggs, meat, almonds, apricots, green leafy vegetables
Magnesium		
energy muscles, especially labour contractions	heart development nervous system skeletal system	cashew and Brazil nuts, green leafy, vegetables, whole grains, seafood
Manganese		
enzymes metabolism of fats	bones and cartilage	leafy vegetables, onions, green beans, bananas, apples, wholegrains, nuts
Potassium		
fluid balance in the body regulation of acidity	fluid balance in the body regulation of acidity	lean meats, wholegrains, vegetables, dried fruits, sunflower seeds

In other words, it may take far longer to conceive, and 18 months is not unusual. Some couples never manage to conceive at all and will turn to assisted reproductive techniques (ART). These technologies include ovulation induction (OI), intrauterine insemination (IUI), in vitro fertilisation (IVF) and intracytoplasmic sperm injection (ICSI). Further techniques include the use of sperm and/or egg donation (see Ch. 8 for more details).

But failure to conceive, even after months or years of trying, does not automatically mean complete infertility. If and when a woman conceives depends on a whole range of factors, both physical and psychological. The nutritional status of *both* partners is almost certainly a key factor.

Recent studies have shown that there has been a marked increase in infertility related to both the man and woman. Male infertility is rising; in particular, sperm counts fell by 40% from 1938 to 1990, and more recent studies show a marked decline in semen quality. One reason for this is thought to be diet related, 'an increase in endogenous estrogen concentrations, which might affect the developing male fetus' (Balen & Jacobs 2003). So it is as important for the male partner as for the female to improve nutritional status prior to conception.

Male fertility

Nutrients that have been shown to improve male fertility include the following.

- *Vitamin C*: supplementation of this can increase both sperm count and sperm motility, and may decrease the risk of sperm damage. It is particularly important for people who do not eat ample amounts of fresh fruit and vegetables. The body cannot store vitamin C, which is why excess amounts are not a problem: the body simply excretes what it does not use. Very large amounts of vitamin C, however, may cause loose stools in some people, in which case the amount should be reduced until bowel tolerance is reached.
- *Vitamin E*: deficiency of this vitamin can cause damage to the reproductive tissues. Recent research showed a significant increase in both sperm motility and count with supplementation of organic selenium and vitamin E (Bleau et al 2006). Supplementation is important for this reason, and because it is difficult to get large enough amounts from dietary sources alone.
- *Zinc*: this is needed to make the outer layer and tail of the sperm and therefore is essential for healthy sperm. Deficiency can cause late sexual maturation, small sex organs, impotence and infertility. Zinc is generally found in high concentrations in male sex glands but if the diet is zinc deficient then concentrations fall radically. Zinc is also lost with each ejaculation, so an active sex life and a low zinc diet will put the male at risk.
- *Manganese*: this has been shown by research to be important for maintaining a high sperm count.
- *Potassium*: this has been shown to increase sperm motility.
- The trace element *selenium* and the amino acids *arginine* and *lysine* are also beneficial.

As a general rule, overall optimum nutrition is more beneficial than taking individual supplements, but where it is difficult to guarantee adequate quantities of the right sorts of food then supplementation is advisable.

Female fertility

Nutritional deficiencies have been found in the vast majority of women suffering from both unexplained infertility and known physical problems such as blocked fallopian tubes or amenorrhoea.

Nutrition to prevent defects

Important as it is to eat healthily during pregnancy, it is equally, if not more, important to start optimum nutrition *before* conception. Not only will this maximise fertility and ensure normal healthy sperm and ova, it can also help prevent birth defects in the crucial first few weeks after conception, before many women discover they are pregnant. The first 6 weeks are when the growing fetus is most at risk. Poor nutrition can slow down cell division and can have serious effects on birthweight.

Allergies

Food allergies are remarkably common, though in some people the obvious symptoms may be slight or masked. Allergies are linked to a range of conditions, including asthma, eczema, hayfever, migraine, hyperactivity and depression, any of which may require drug treatment.

For prospective parents there is particular reason to investigate and clear up any allergy. Many food allergies are the result of nutritional imbalance, and in particular of zinc deficiency. Any allergy is an impairment to good health and may well lead to poor absorption of vital nutrients.

Deficiencies

A number of crucial minerals are involved in the prevention of birth abnormalities, including the following.

Manganese

In tests, mothers who gave birth to babies with congenital malformations were found to have very low levels of manganese, as did their babies (Saner et al 1985). The best food sources are: nuts, green leafy vegetables, peas, beets, egg yolks and wholegrains.

Zinc

Zinc deficiency is linked to low birthweight, still births and male infertility, and to difficult births and poor weight gain in newborns. Zinc is probably the most important supplement to take in preparation for pregnancy (Caldwell 1969, Crawford & Connor 1975, Pfeiffer 1978); 15–20 mg a day should be adequate.

Zinc absorption is helped by vitamin B6 and by eating oranges (the citric acid increases absorption). Too much iron, on the other hand, depletes zinc. So does copper.

Good dietary sources for zinc are: meat, fish and shellfish, particularly oyster, sesame seeds, sunflower seeds, pumpkin seeds, almonds and other nuts, wheat and oat germ, sprouted seeds, ginger, fruit, leafy vegetables and watercress.

It is better to start supplementing zinc before conception – but it is never too late to start.

Folic acid

Folic acid deficiency has been linked to defects such as spina bifida, a condition where the spinal cord does not develop properly. Mothers who supplement folic acid and vitamin B12 before conception and during the first 3 months of pregnancy have a lower incidence of neural tube defects. A survey of 23000 women found that those who supplemented their diet in the first 6 weeks of pregnancy had a 75% lower incidence of neural tube defects than those who did not (DOH 1992).

Folic acid in food is destroyed by sunlight, heat and an acid environment, and the use of antibiotics also leads to deficiency. Supplementation of 400 μg a day is recommended from before conception up until the end of the first trimester (DOH 1992, Smithells 1983). This can be obtained on prescription but unless a woman qualifies for free prescriptions, it may be cheaper to buy it at a supermarket or pharmacy. Good food sources include: green leafy vegetables, brewer's yeast, wholegrains, wheatgerm, milk, salmon, root vegetables and nuts.

Negative influences on prenatal health

Stress

The medical world remains divided on the effect of stress on fertility although studies have shown it can affect both the man's and woman's ability to conceive (Berga et al 2003, Bethea et al 2005, Brkovich & Fisher 1998, Campagne 2006, Marcus et al 2001).

For women there is a link with the endocrine system and the hormones produced during stressful times. A recent pilot study from the USA showed that 85% women started to ovulate again following a 20-week course of cognitive behaviour therapy to reduce stress levels (Berga 2006).

Recent studies on sperm motility and morphology show a marked deterioration of both, when men are under stress (Eskiocak et al 2005).

The simple fact that many babies are conceived while their parents are on holiday suggests that stress plays an important role in fertility.

Smoking

It has long been accepted that a woman who smokes during pregnancy risks damaging her unborn baby (Himmerlberger et al 1978). Smoking may reduce birthweight, affect mental development, increase the risk of cancer to both mother and baby and increase the rate of spontaneous abortion (Chatenoud et al 1998). The incidence of low birthweight babies is higher among mothers who smoke because smoking reduces oxygen and food supply to the fetus, slowing down its growth rate and possibly causing damage to its DNA. The effects can remain with the baby for the rest of its life, as reduced resistance to infection, impaired intelligence, shorter attention span, hyperactive behaviour and an increased susceptibility to disorders of the nervous system, respiratory system, bladder, kidneys and skin.

The effects of preconceptual smoking in the father are less clear. However, if both partners smoke, there is a greater risk of having a low birthweight baby than if the mother alone smokes, and the risk of death in low birthweight babies is also increased.

Alcohol intake

Alcohol is a major factor in raised blood pressure. It badly affects the body's absorption of B6, iron and zinc. It also damages sperm, affecting fertility and increasing the risk of birth defects and miscarriage.

The effects of alcohol are probably greatest during the early stages of pregnancy, when cell division is at its highest. So it is best for a woman to avoid alcohol from the time that she decides she wants to conceive, and not wait until the pregnancy is confirmed. The first 20 weeks are regarded as the most crucial, but evidence shows that avoiding alcohol completely in the period leading up to conception and during pregnancy is preferable.

Research at Columbia University has found that a woman who drinks and also smokes has a four times higher risk of miscarriage (Plant 1987). Non-smokers who drink still have a risk two and a half times greater than that of an abstainer. Even a single alcoholic drink taken every other day increases the risk of miscarriage.

Babies born with fetal alcohol syndrome – that is, suffering the effects of maternal alcohol consumption – show a variety of different symptoms, ranging from low birthweight and mild facial deformity to heart murmurs, ear problems, congenital hip dislocations and hyperactivity (May & Himbaugh 1983). Even the children of mothers who drank only at 'socially acceptable levels' during pregnancy have been found to have poorer verbal skills, in speaking and understanding. All alcohol should be avoided prior to conception and during pregnancy.

There is also some evidence that spontaneous abortion, premature birth and still birth are more common if the father has a high coffee consumption (more than one or two cups a day).

Drugs

Drugs can be classified as substances that adversely affect the body's biochemistry. The myth that the placenta acts as a total barrier, preventing toxins from the mother from reaching the fetus, was destroyed at a stroke by the tragedy of thalidomide. Less commonly known is the fact that taking two or more substances together (such as alcohol and sleeping pills, alcohol and marijuana, cigarettes and coffee) can increase the danger to the fetus.

Most women who are pregnant are aware of the risk to their unborn child from both over-the-counter and prescription medications. Studies have shown that there is a marked reduction in the use of medications during pregnancy, even for illnesses such as asthma (Enriquez et al 2006, Schatz & Leibman 2005). In 1979 the FDA (Food and Drug Administration) in the United States set up a teratogenic classification system for prescription medicines that is now used throughout the Western world and is regularly updated. For those women who require medication, antenatal and postnatal advice from their GP should be followed (Briggs et al 2005).

One of the most detrimental effects of any drug – whether prescribed (for a medical condition), self-prescribed (such as aspirin), socially accepted (such as coffee, alcohol, tobacco) or recreational/illegal (such as marijuana, cocaine, heroin) – is that on the user's nutritional status. Some essential nutrients, vitamins and minerals are poorly absorbed, others are excreted. So this produces a double-bind effect. Although the potential danger of many drugs can be reduced by optimum nutrition, the deficiency that results from drug use means that less of the drug can be safely tolerated.

In particular, the use of marijuana, cocaine and heroin in pregnancy has been linked to low birthweight babies, anaemia, still birth, abruption placenta, premature delivery, congenital abnormalities and withdrawal symptoms in the newborn (Buehler 1995, Holzman & Paneth 1994, Kozer & Koren 2001, Thangappah 2000).

All this applies equally to both partners and is crucial in the period leading up to conception. Any nutritional deficiency can lead to abnormality or poor motility in the sperm, causing infertility, spontaneous abortion or miscarriage.

Toxic chemicals, metals and minerals

Every year, each one of us eats approximately 5 kilos of preservatives and additives, inhales 1 gram of heavy metals and has 4 litres of pesticides and herbicides sprayed on our fruit and vegetables. Pollution is more widespread than ever before.

The adverse effects of ingestion and inhalation of even low levels of toxic chemicals, metals and minerals can lead to a huge range of conditions, including cardiovascular disease, renal and metabolic disease, immune dysfunction, lethargy, depression, cancer, recurrent infections, behavioural and learning difficulties and developmental abnormalities. Some specific effects are as follows.

Lead

Lead is almost impossible to escape; it is absorbed from petrol and exhaust fumes in the atmosphere and from water that has passed through pipes containing lead.

High levels in men reduce sperm count and motility and increase the number of sperm abnormalities. In women, high levels can damage the ova, induce abortion and increase the number of congenital abnormalities, still births and neonatal deaths. There is a direct correlation between lead levels in the placenta and the baby's birthweight. Infants exposed to high levels of lead in utero have been found to suffer from developmental, behavioural and learning problems throughout childhood. It seems that low levels considered safe in adults cannot be regarded as safe for the fetus.

Nutritional status affects lead absorption. A diet low in calcium, zinc, iron and manganese (minerals often deficient in pregnant women) can actually increase lead uptake, making it more toxic. Optimum nutrition (particularly vitamin C supplementation) has been shown to remove lead from the body.

Cadmium

Cadmium is ingested from cigarette smoking and processed foods, and is also widely used in many manufacturing industries. Research links it to protein in the urine, low birthweight and small head circumference, and there is also a possible link to toxaemia.

Cadmium builds up in people deficient in vitamins C, D, B6, zinc, manganese, copper, selenium and calcium. Zinc is particularly effective in reducing the adverse effects of cadmium.

Mercury

Mercury enters the body from pesticides and fungicides, fish, industrial processes and dental fillings. Men exposed to mercury vapour report loss of libido and impotence, and organic mercury exposure has been linked to a whole range of psychological and physical disorders. The Japanese disaster in Minimata in the 1950s resulted in a number of children being born with disabilities after their mothers ate fish polluted with mercury from a local factory.

The danger from mercury fillings is very small, but it would be wise to avoid dental work involving fitting or removing mercury fillings during pregnancy.

Aluminium

Aluminium enters the body from saucepans, kettles and teapots, antacids, antiperspirants, food additives, tea and foil-wrapped foods.

Aluminium is easily absorbed and because it binds so readily with other substances, it destroys many vitamins and causes gradual long-term mineral loss. In babies it has been linked to kidney problems, behavioural problems and autism.

Copper

Copper is absorbed from water pipes, saucepans, jewellery, coins, the contraceptive pill and the copper intrauterine device (IUD).

Copper levels rise naturally during pregnancy and immediately after birth, so it is easy for a woman to reach toxic overload levels. This may be one of the causes of many premature births or miscarriages. Raised levels of copper can also lead to postnatal depression and they are usually accompanied by low levels of zinc and manganese, both of which deficiencies are known to cause birth defects. Zinc in combination with vitamin C can help to detoxify copper (Pfeiffer 1978).

How to protect yourself nutritionally

Good nutrition is undoubtedly the safest way to detoxify the body. If toxin levels are dangerously high, supplementation alone may not be sufficient, however.

- Zinc reduces lead and cadmium levels.
- Calcium removes lead and prevents absorption and acts against cadmium and aluminium.
- Selenium is antagonistic to mercury, arsenic and cadmium.
- Phosphorus is antagonistic to lead.
- Vitamin A helps activate detoxifying enzymes (diet only).
- Vitamins B1 and B complex protect against lead damage.
- Magnesium and B6 act against aluminium.
- Vitamin C helps reduce levels of lead, copper, cadmium and arsenic.
- Vitamin D aids calcium metabolism.
- Vitamin E may reduce lead.
- Peas, lentils and beans are good detoxifiers, as are garlic, onions and eggs, which have sulphur-containing amino acids.
- Pectin both detoxifies and reduces absorption (eat apples, bananas, pears, citrus fruit and carrots).
- Seaweed (from unpolluted waters) attracts lead and helps the body to excrete it.

Other pointers on protecting yourself from pollution

As well as good nutrition and supplementation, there are some general measures that can help minimise exposure to pollution.

- Wash all fruit and vegetables and remove the outer leaves of vegetables; buy organic whenever possible.
- Avoid copper or aluminium cookware and do not wrap food in aluminium foil.
- Avoid canned food, particularly from unlined tins.
- Use a water filter or drink bottled spring water and never drink hot tap water.
- Wash hands before eating.
- Avoid heavy traffic as far as possible and close car windows in tunnels.
- Refuse dental fillings containing mercury.
- Avoid deodorants and antiperspirants unless the ingredients are specified.
- Avoid antacids that contain aluminium salts.
- Natural sunlight (as opposed to artificial light) has many beneficial effects, including the elimination of toxic metals from the body and the metabolism of desirable minerals.
- Limit the use of chemical cleaning agents and garden pesticides.
- Do not stand near microwave ovens while they are in use.
- As far as possible, eat natural unprocessed foods that do not contain preservatives.

Exercise

Keeping fit and healthy in pregnancy means that a woman is less likely to suffer discomfort, she will have an easier labour and recover more quickly, get her figure back sooner after delivery and, most importantly, increase her chances of having a healthy baby.

The fitter she is *before* conception, the better; it is easier to stay fit than to get fit once pregnant. Aerobic fitness in particular ensures a healthy heart and arteries, both of which are good for the baby.

Summary

- The TCM viewpoint on preconceptual care includes avoiding: overwork, exposure to cold and damp, and excessive emotions (particularly worry, anger, fear and joy), alcohol, sex and strenuous exercise.
- Problems with conception may be due to: Liver Qi stagnation, Liver Blood deficiency, Kidney Yin or Yang deficiency, or Stomach Qi deficiency.
- Negative influences on prenatal health include: stress, smoking, and intake of alcohol, drugs and toxic chemicals, metals and minerals, including lead, cadmium, mercury, aluminium and copper.
- Nutritional influences in preconceptual care include:
  - *male fertility*: vitamins C and E, zinc, manganese and potassium, selenium, arginine and lysine
  - *female fertility*: copper (overload), zinc, magnesium, manganese and selenium
  - *to prevent birth defects*: allergy investigation, manganese, zinc and folic acid
  - *protection against toxic influences*: vitamins A, B (complex), C, D and E, zinc, calcium, selenium, phosphorus, magnesium, seaweed and foods containing soluble fibre.
- Acupuncture points to use during the period include:
  - *postperiod*: CV-4, GV-4, BL-20, 21, 23, SP-6
  - *ovulation* (days 11–15): CV-3, KI-15, SP-6
  - *postovulation, premenstrual* (days 15–28); tonify Liver yang, move Liver Qi if stagnant; use points such as LR-3 with even technique plus Liver points for PMT.

References

Balen AH, Jacobs HS 2003 Infertility in practice, 2nd edn. Churchill Livingstone, Edinburgh

Berga SL 2006 Stress, metabolism and reproductive compromise. Human Reproduction 21(1): i32

Berga SL, Marcus MD, Loucks TL, Hlastala S, Ringham R, Krohn MA 2003 Recovery of ovarian activity in women with functional hypothalamic amenorrhoea who were treated with cognitive behavior therapy. Fertility and Sterility 80: 976–981

Bethea C, Pau FK, Fox S, Hess DL, Berga SL, Cameron JL 2005 Sensitivity to stress-induced reproductive dysfunction linked to activicty of the serotonin system. Fertility and Sterility 83: 148–155

Bleau G, Boulanger K, Bissonette F 2006 Supplementation with a selenium/ vitamin E combination for the treatment of male infertility. Human Reproduction 21(1): i27–28

Briggs GG, Freeman RK, Yaffe SJ 2005 Drugs in pregancy and lactation, 7th edn. Lippincott, Williams and Wilkins, Philadelphia

Brkovich AM, Fisher WA 1998 Psychological distress and infertility: forty years of research. Journal of Psychosomatic Obstetrics and Gynaecology 19(4): 218–228

Buehler BA 1995 Drug and alcohol use effect on long term development. Nebraska Medical Journal 80(5): 116–117

Caldwell D F 1969 Effects of protein nutrition and zinc nutrition on behaviour in the rat. Perinatal Factors Affecting Human Development 185: 2–8

Campagne DM 2006 Should fertilization treatment start with reducing stress? Human Reproduction 21(7): 1651–1658

Chatenoud L, Parazzini F, di Cintio et al 1998 Paternal and maternal smoking habits before conception and during the first trimester: relation to spontaneous abortion. Annals of Epidemiology 8(8): 520–526

Crawford IL, Connor JD 1975 Zinc in hippocampal function. Journal of Orthomolecular Psychology 4(1): 39–52

DOH (Department of Health) 1992 Folic acid and the prevention of neural tube defects; report from the expert advisory group. DOH Health Publication Unit, Heywood

Enriquez R, Wu P, Griffin MR et al 2006 Cessation of asthma medication in early pregnancy. American Journal of Obstetrics and Gynecology 195(1): 149–153

Eskiocak S, Gozen AS, Yapar SB, Tavas F, Kilic AS, Eskioack M 2005 Glutathione and free sulphydryl content of seminal plasma in healthy medical students during and after exam stress. Human Reproduction 20: 2595–2600

Himmerlberger DU, Brown BW Jr, Cohen EN 1978 Cigarette smoking during pregnancy and the occurrence of spontaneous abortion and congenital abnormality. American Journal of Epidemiology 108(6): 470–479

Holzman C, Paneth N 1994 Maternal cocaine use during pregnancy and perinatal outcomes. Epidemiology Review 16: 3315–3334

Kozer E, Koren G 2001 Effects of prenatal exposure to marijuana. Canadian Family Physician 47: 236–234

Maciocia G 1998 Obstetrics and gynaecology in Chinese medicine. Churchill Livingstone, New York, pp 9, 10, 16

Marcus MD, Loucks TL, Berga SL 2001 Psychological correlates of functional hypothalamic amenorrhoea. Fertility and Sterility 76: 310–316

May P, Himbaugh KJ 1983 Epidemiology of fetal alcohol syndrome. Social Biology 30: 374–387

Pfeiffer C 1978 Zinc and other micronutrients. Institute of Optimum Nutrition, New Canaan, CT, p 102

Plant M 1987 Alcohol: safety in pregnancy? The Times, 4 November

Saner G, Dagoglu T, Ozden T 1985 Hair manganese concentrations in newborns and their mothers. American Journal of Clinical Nutrition 41: 1042–1044

Schatz M, Leibman C 2005 Inhaled corticosteroid use and outcomes in pregnancy. Annals of Allergy, Asthma and Immunology 95(3): 234–238

Smithells RW 1983 Further experience of vitamin supplementation for prevention of neural tube defects. Lancet i: 1027–1031

Thangappah R 2000 Maternal and perinatal outcome with drug abuse in pregnancy. Journal of Obstetrics and Gynaecology 20(6): 597–600

Further reading

Anonymous 1979 Environmental trace elements and their role in disorders of personality, intellect, behaviour and learning ability in children. University of Auckland Journal January: 22–26

Colgan M 1982 Your personal vitamin profile. Bloyar Briggs, London

Goujard J, Kaminski M, Roumeau-Rouquette C, Schwarz D 1978 Maternal smoking, alcohol consumption and abruptio placentae. American Journal of Obstetrics and Gynecology130(6): 738–739

Grant E 1986 The effects of smoking in pregnancy: guidelines for future parents. Witley, Surrey, pp 77, 85–86, 100

Hall M 1988 The agony and the ecstasy. Channel 4, 14 April

Lodge Rees E 1981 The concept of pre-conceptual care. Journal of Environmental Studies 17: 37–42

Varma TR 1987 Infertility. British Medical Journal 294: 853, 887–890

2 Pregnancy

Chapter outline

During pregnancy, more than at any other time in her life, a woman is likely to seek out natural remedies, non-invasive treatments and drug-free pain relief – things that will not cause any possible harm to her fetus. Though she may never have done so before, turning to alternative health care can offer a degree of choice and autonomy that orthodox medicine often denies, helping her to regain a feeling of control over her body.

Pregnancy is, after all, a natural physiological life event and not an illness. I find that women much prefer to be treated holistically, as a whole and individual person, rather than just a womb and a collection of symptoms. They appreciate the chance to get in tune with the changes happening within them and to work in harmony with their body's natural rhythms. Treatment with acupuncture is warmly welcomed by many women who may never previously have considered its benefits. And the benefits for the pregnant woman are many and great.

It is important for the acupuncturist to liaise closely with the woman's midwife or GP, particularly if there are any medical problems. Women should be encouraged to tell their midwives and GPs what they are being treated for, as most midwives and doctors are unaware of all the conditions that acupuncture can help with in pregnancy.

Safety in treatment is paramount and acupuncture practitioners must be fully aware of the contradicted acupuncture points, use of moxa and needling techniques in pregnancy. It is also essential to have a solid grasp of anatomy to needle the abdomen safely as the uterus grows (see below). Acupuncturists must also be aware that a large number of women, up to 40%, can miscarry within the first 12 weeks.

However, there are no significant data that show any adverse effects of acupuncture during the first trimester.

From a Chinese perspective, the Penetrating and Directing Vessels undergo many changes during pregnancy (Maciocia 1998). As there is no monthly period, Yin Blood accumulates in the Chong and Ren channels to nourish both fetus and mother. The whole body has an excess of Qi, resulting in an accumulation of Yin in the lower body and Yang in the upper body. In the first 12 weeks of pregnancy, there is excess Qi in the Chong channel, which is related to the Liver.

Physiological changes in pregnancy

The uterus

Western viewpoint

Before pregnancy the uterus (or womb) is a small pear-shaped organ, which then increases in weight and size to hold and protect the growing baby.

During the first 20 weeks of pregnancy, the uterine muscles are stimulated by oestrogen to grow, after which progesterone relaxes the muscles and allows them to stretch. At term, the uterus must be able to expel the baby. So the muscular coat of the uterus has to change, in order that contractions in labour can generate sufficient force.

After 20 weeks, the circulating blood volume also increases sharply, with a rise of 50% in plasma volume and 20% in red cell volume. Uterine blood flow in the pre-pregnant state is around 10 ml per minute. By term, this has increased to between 600 and 800 ml per minute, and the uterus receives nearly 20% of total cardiac output (Sweet 1997).

Chinese viewpoint

In TCM (traditional Chinese medicine), everything is considered to be created through the interaction of Yin and Yang. Conception occurs when the Yang sperm meets the Yin egg (Maciocia 1998). According to ancient Chinese texts, the best time for conception to take place is when the cock crows at 4 a.m., as this is considered the time when Yin and Yang are in balance.

The Uterus is one of the six extraordinary Yang organs. It is also known as the Envelope of Yin and is intimately related to the three Yin organs: the Liver, Spleen and Kidneys. The Uterus nourishes the fetus during pregnancy and is related to the Kidneys (via the Uterus Channel) and the Heart (via the Uterus Vessel). The state of both these two organs is vital. The fetus develops from the Yin and Blood of the mother.

The vagina

The vagina is the passage from the cervix at the neck of the womb to the outside of the body. It forms part of the birth canal, so must stretch during delivery to allow the baby through.

The breasts

Even before a women has missed a period, she may become aware of a tingling sensation in the nipples. This is due to the hormones oestrogen and progesterone, which make the breasts enlarge in preparation for producing milk after the birth. Blood flow starts to increase very soon after conception, and enlarged veins may become visible under the skin. The breasts may become tender and uncomfortable as ducts and glands prepare for breastfeeding. The nipples will become more prominent and the Montgomery's tubercles on the areola will become more obvious, owing to changes in the Directing Vessel.

The skin

During pregnancy, changes in hormone levels, particularly the hormone that stimulates melanin, may cause uneven patches of chloasma (pigmentation) on the skin and particularly on the face. Protection against full sunlight is recommended. The nipples, areola, vulva, perineum and perianal region will all darken considerably. And a brown line, known as the linea nigra, will develop from the navel to the pubic area, fading gradually after birth. The skin may sweat more owing to the increased metabolism and activity of the sweat glands.

The heart and lungs

The heart and lungs should be checked early in pregnancy to rule out the possibility of tuberculosis.

The blood

The number of red blood cells increases during pregnancy by 30% (Sweet 1997). Hence the importance of haemoglobin (Hb) testing to prevent iron deficiency. Blood is abundant and directed towards nourishing the mother and fetus.

Blood pressure

Blood pressure relates to the pressure exerted by the flow of blood against the walls of the arteries. The two figures measure the systolic beat (when the heart contracts) and the diastolic beat (when the heart is at rest). An increase in blood pressure during pregnancy could be an indication of pre-eclampsia.

The urinary tract

From around 8 weeks there may be an increase in the frequency of micturition, owing to pressure from the enlarging uterus and increased vascularity of the bladder. Urine will be checked regularly at antenatal visits for the presence of protein, glucose and ketones, which should not be present. Protein could indicate a possible infection (very common during pregnancy) or occasionally pre-eclampsia. Glucose could indicate diabetes, as could the presence of ketones, though this may just be the result of low blood sugar.

Hormonal changes

Hormones, the body's chemical messengers, are responsible for many of the physiological changes that occur during pregnancy. There is a complex interplay between maternal, placental and fetal hormones.

Progesterone is possibly the most important, preparing the lining of the womb for implantation of the fertilised egg, preparing the breasts for lactation and increasing the suppleness and expansion of ligaments and muscles ready for delivery.

Oxytocin causes the muscles of the uterus to contract during labour (see Ch. 11, pp. 173–174).

The placenta

The placenta is fully formed by the 12th week, and produces progesterone and oestrogen throughout pregnancy.

It transmits vital oxygen and nutrients from the mother's blood to the fetus via the umbilical cord, and removes carbon dioxide and waste matter from the baby to be processed by the mother's liver and kidneys. It provides a barrier to many infections, it provides an immune barrier so that the mother's body does not reject the fetus, and antibodies crossing from the mother give the baby passive immunity for the first 3 months of its life.

Changes in the fetus

The Western viewpoint

The development of the fetus from fertilised egg to baby in just 40 weeks is phenomenal (Fig. 2.1). During weeks 1–4 the following changes occur:

- the cells rapidly divide and grow
- the heart starts beating
- the central nervous system starts to develop
- the limb buds appear.

During weeks 4–8 (Fig. 2.1A):

- all the major organs appear in primitive form
- the facial features start to form
- the genitals form
- movements begin.

During weeks 8–12 (Fig. 2.1B):

- the fetal circulation begins functioning
- the eyelids fuse
- the fetus is able to swallow surrounding fluid
- the sex of the baby becomes apparent
- the kidneys start to function and urine is passed from 10 weeks.

During weeks 12–16:

- lanugo (fine downy hair) covers the baby's skin
- the skeleton rapidly develops
- the nasal septum and roof of mouth fuse
- the milk teeth buds are in place
- the fetal heart beats at 140–150 beats per minute, twice as fast as the mother's.

During weeks 16–20 (Fig. 2.1C):

- the vernix caseosa appears, a protective layer of creamy white covering the skin
- the fingernails appear
- 'quickening' movements are felt by the mother
- the lungs breathe amniotic fluid in and out.

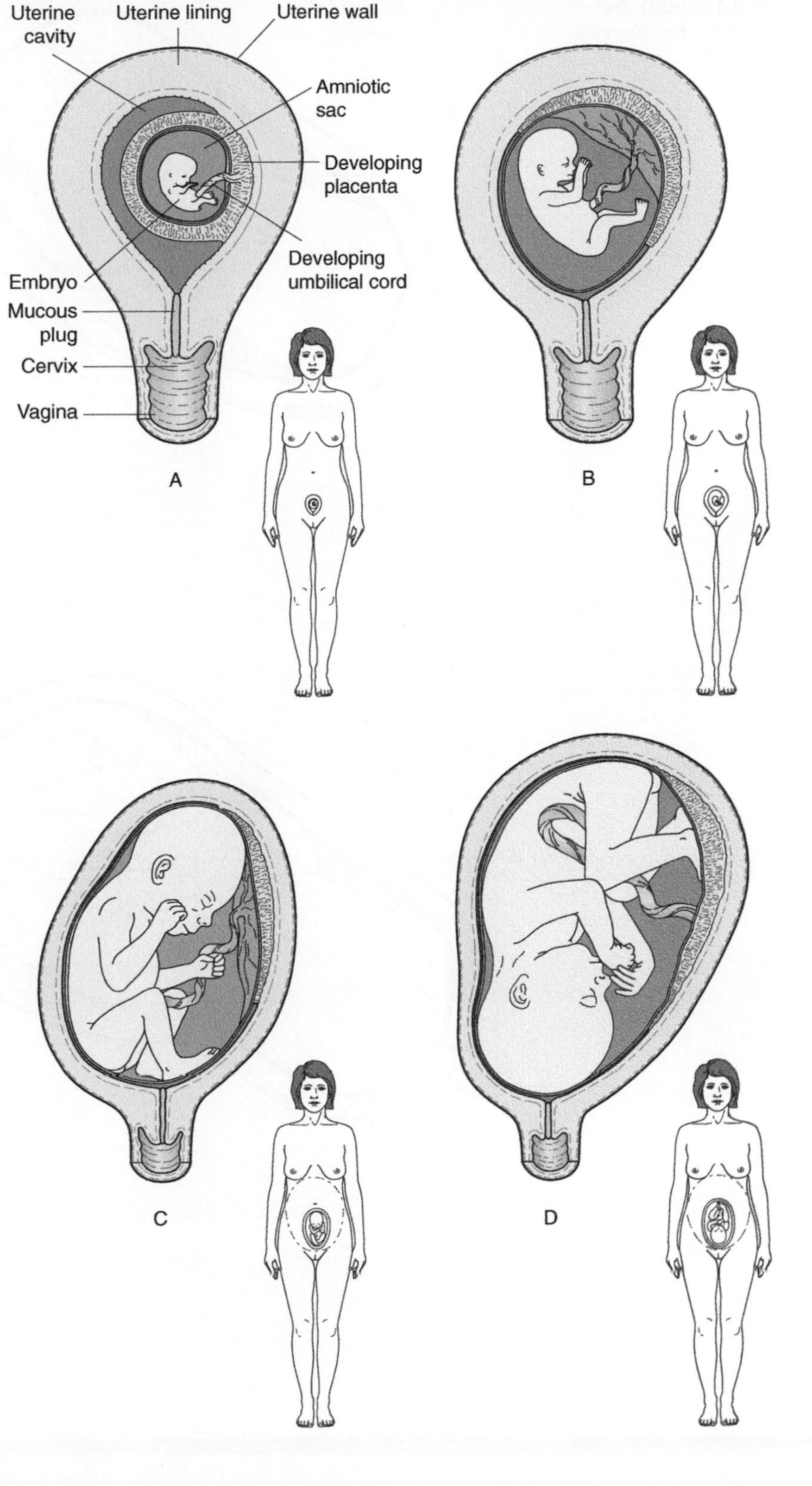

Figure 2.1 The growing fetus: **A** at 8 weeks; **B** at 12 weeks; **C** at 20 weeks; **D** at 24 weeks.

Figure 2.1 (contd) The growing fetus: **E** at 30 weeks; **F** at 40 weeks.

E

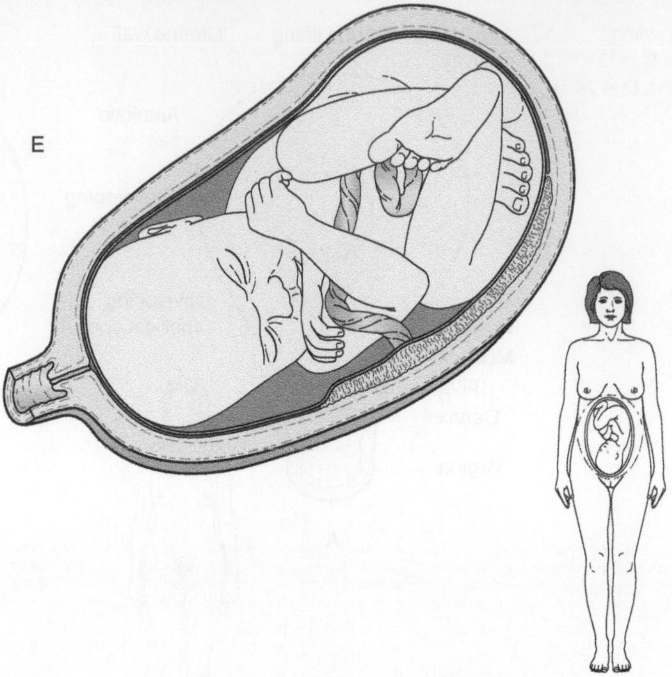

F

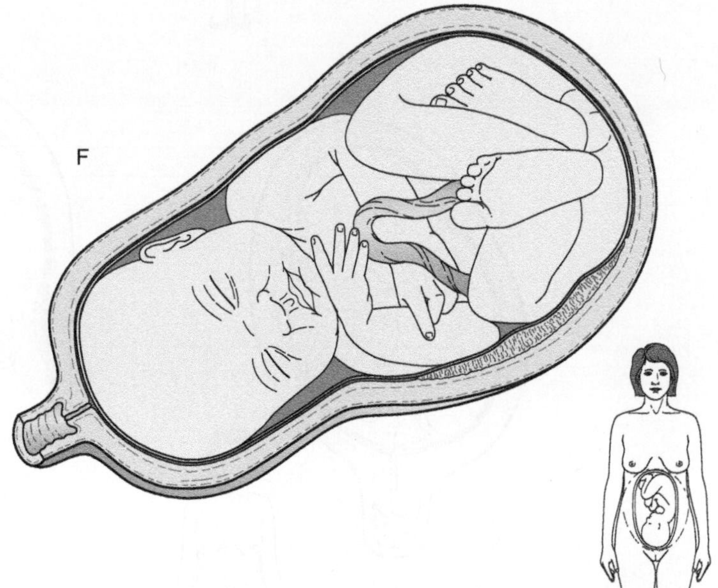

During weeks 20–24 (Fig. 2.1D):

- the eyebrows and eyelashes start to grow
- the skin is red and wrinkled
- most of the body systems are fully functional
- links between nerves and muscles are established and the fetus responds to sound and stimulation.

During weeks 24–28:

- the eyelids reopen
- the fetus is viable (i.e. could survive if born).

During weeks 28–32:

- a boy's testes descend
- stores of body fat and iron are laid down
- the taste buds form
- the body hair disappears from the face.

During weeks 32–36 (Fig. 2.1E):

- the body hair disappears
- the eyes blink and can focus
- fat stores increase and the body becomes more rounded.

At 40 weeks (Fig. 2.1F):

- the baby is now about eight times bigger than it was at 3 months, and has increased in weight approximately 600 times
- most of the lanugo has dropped off, although there may still be some down the centre of the back, in front of the ears and low on the forehead
- the fingernails extend beyond the fingers.

The Chinese viewpoint

According to Chinese texts written by a gynaecologist from the Qing dynasty known as Chen Jia Yuan, each developing organ in the fetus corresponds with a particular month, as follows:

- weeks 1–4: the Liver is formed
- weeks 4–8: the Gall Bladder
- weeks 8–12: the Pericardium
- weeks 12–16: the Triple Burner
- weeks 16–20: the Spleen
- weeks 20–24: the Stomach
- weeks 24–28: the Lungs
- weeks 28–32: the Large Intestines
- weeks 32–36: the Kidneys
- weeks 36–40: the Bladder.

As a basic rule of thumb, points on the corresponding channel each month should be avoided.

The Eastern philosophy of childbirth

The Yellow Emperor (1963) said: 'After the person's connection, the Jing is first composed. Then the Jing composes the brain and the bone marrow. The bones become the Stem, the vessels become the Ying, the muscles become firm. The flesh becomes a wall, the Jing is hard and then the hair and body grow'.

The chapter on preconception discusses the importance of getting healthy, regulating periods and correcting imbalances before becoming pregnant. In my experience, a woman's physical and emotional state when she enters pregnancy will have a huge effect on the outcome of that pregnancy.

The Chinese believe that if a pregnant woman pays attention to her diet, her environment and her emotional state, then the fetus will benefit. Sadness and grief are thought to deplete the Heart and Lungs, resulting in amenorrhoea. Worry knots the Qi, fear depletes the Kidneys. Anger, frustration and resentment are often to be seen in women suffering from morning sickness and excess bile. (This is discussed at more length in Ch. 5, p. 75.)

Pregnant women should eat nourishing foods that are easily digestible. They should avoid pungent and spicy foods, and excessively cold foods (such as ice cream) that can cause Cold in the Uterus (see Ch. 3).

Especially important are any persisting conditions such as Blood deficiency, Yin deficiency, Kidney deficiency or Qi stagnation.

A woman's physiology is dominated by Blood. Western medicine sees blood simply as a collection of cells with no emotional link, although it is recognised that a woman suffering from anaemia may be tearful and low in spirits. When menstruation stops as a result of pregnancy, changes occur in the Penetrating and Directing channels. An abundance of Yin Blood in the Chong and Ren channels nourishes the fetus. But the Blood in the body as a whole is Deficient and Qi is in Excess. This is the reason why many pregnant women feel warmer.

The kidneys

Kidney Essence is derived from both the mother and the father, so there is a hereditary influence determining a person's constitution. The Essence is stored in the Kidneys but has a fluid nature and circulates all around the body. Kidney Essence determines growth, sexual development, reproduction, conception and pregnancy. (See Ch. 14 for a discussion of Kidney Essence in relation to the baby.)

During pregnancy, a strain can be put on the Qi and Essence of the Kidneys, so the pre-existing state of the Kidneys is important.

Kidney Deficiency is at the root of many women's problems, and is often found in older mothers and women who have:

- recurrent miscarriages
- IVF (in vitro fertilisation) pregnancies (IVF drains the Kidneys)
- short intervals between pregnancies
- premature labour
- high blood pressure.

By improving the Qi, Yin and Yang of the Kidneys, the Jing (Essence) will also be improved. Factors that deplete Jing include stress, fear, anxiety and insecurity, overwork and many children. Foods that can help to build up Jing include chorella, spirulina, royal jelly, docosahexaenoic acid (DHA), fish and liver (these foods are rich in DNA and RNA, which protect the body from degeneration).

Another common pattern is that Liver Blood deficiency combines with Liver Qi stagnation. Prolonged Liver Qi stagnation causes Heat in the Blood, which may lead to miscarriage.

Forbidden points of pregnancy

There is much debate about the points that should be used in pregnancy. Some schools of thought say that you should not treat at all during the first 3 months of pregnancy, as acupuncture may cause miscarriage. I disagree with this view and have had some wonderful results in the treatment of severe morning sickness, which can be utterly debilitating for some women.

Women who have had recurrent miscarriages can also be helped greatly by acupuncture, if treatment is given to tonify Kidney weakness. The same applies to women with IVF pregnancies, who I often find suffer greatly from sickness in the first 3 months.

Other schools of thought warn against needling below the knee at certain times in pregnancy. When I first started to treat, there was so much conflicting advice that I often found it hard to work out what I could and could not do. I had a long list of points that I repeatedly referred to, and there was always a nagging anxiety at the end of the day if I had used an unfamiliar point. Soon I began to feel very restricted. But the more experienced I became, the less I worried.

The cardinal rules are:

1. treat the body with respect and always be careful and considered in what you are doing
2. do not use any strong needle stimulation during pregnancy, unless you are doing an induction of labour, in which case strong stimulation is necessary.

Points to avoid at all times during pregnancy include the following (Fig. 2.2).

- *LI-4 and SP-6*: these points are used for induction with strong stimulation and should be avoided throughout pregnancy. They should also not be used if a woman who comes for treatment is unsure whether or not she is pregnant.
- *GB-21*: this has a strong downward movement and must not be used before the second stage of labour.
- *BL-31 and* 32: these are in the first and second sacral foramina, very good for induction and not points that can easily be needled in error.
- *BL-67*: I would not needle this point during pregnancy but would heat it with moxa to turn a breech baby.
- *Abdominal points*: I will not needle lower abdominal points unless the patient is suffering a great deal of pubic pain.

Great care needs to be taken in treating pregnant women between 32 and 34 weeks. On no account should you give any strong treatments, especially in the back, as you do not want to do anything that might start contractions.

Position

Always sit a pregnant woman upright with a backrest so that she feels comfortable (Fig. 2.3). As the pregnancy progresses, it is a good idea for her to lie on her side.

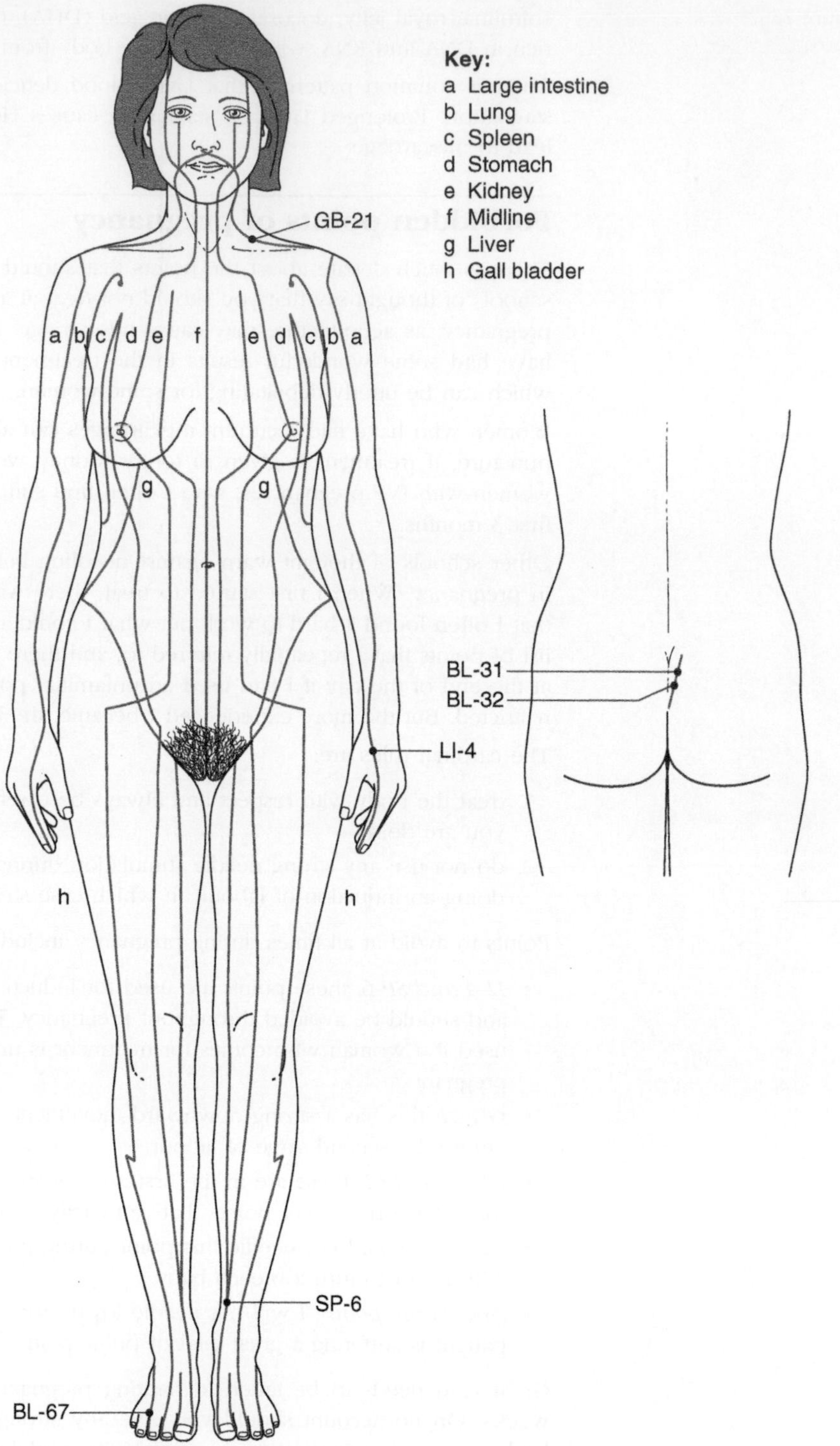

Figure 2.2 Forbidden points on the body.

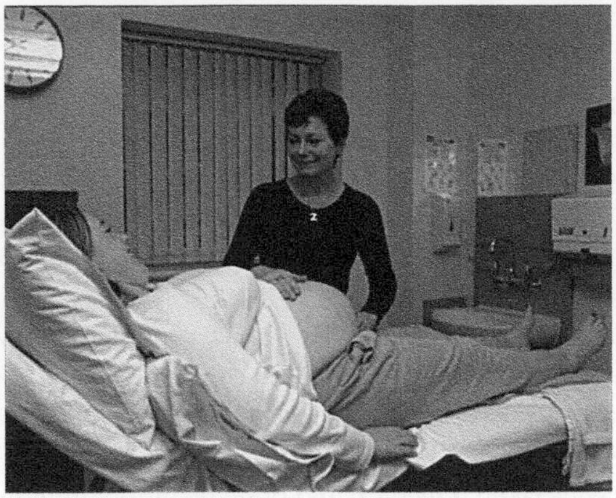

Figure 2.3 Position for a pregnant woman on the couch.

The pressure of the growing baby in the uterus can easily make her feel faint if she lies flat, as the weight of the baby inside presses on the vena cava, an important vein.

General recommendations for acupuncture use during pregnancy

Needle techniques

From personal experience, I believe the body adapts to whatever needle technique you use. Before my TCM training (at the College of Integrated Medicine), I studied Five Element acupuncture, so my techniques may be considered different from those of classically trained TCM practitioners. When I began training, I soon came to realise through observation that all practitioners develop their own personal needle technique. The following recommendations are therefore based on my own preferences.

1. One of the most important aspects when treating pregnant women is the initial assessment of their constitution. If they are weak or deficient, if they feel queasy or if they are anxious about needles, this will help me decide how long the needles should be left in, if they need to be.
2. Very gentle techniques need to be employed in pregnancy. The tonification I was taught was to insert the needle, get the Deqi, rotate the needle and then remove it. This follows the instruction in many ancient texts.
3. For deficient conditions, I tonify by leaving them in place for 15 to 20 minutes.
4. For a clearing treatment in pregnancy, such as Liver Qi stagnation or Heat, use even technique: insert the needle, get the Deqi, but use no movement to the needle at all.
5. In a full condition, use a reducing technique, leaving the needles in.
6. For certain other treatments such as induction of labour, I use strong stimulation of the needles (moving them in and out as I go) rather than tonification. The aim here is to really get things moving.
7. At the end of every treatment, I always tonify the underlying weakness, inserting the needle to get the Deqi, rotating the needle and then removing

it. I usually use points on the back or Source points, such as Stomach and Spleen (BL-20, 21), Liver (BL-19) and Kidney (BL-23).

My preferred needle technique is to insert the needle, get the Deqi and then leave the needle in – as a rule for no longer than 15 minutes at a first treatment – to see how the woman will react. Many women feel queasy anyway in pregnancy and this, combined with nervousness about the needles, can make them feel faint.

I would avoid needling oedematous areas in case of infection.

Many of the treatments I use in pregnancy are to help with relief of the patient's symptoms, backed up with treatment of the underlying condition.

Note: Some of the points you would normally use to treat similar symptoms in a patient who was not pregnant (such as abdominal points) cannot be used in pregnancy.

Having taken a medical and obstetric history from the woman, you will have some idea of her deficiencies and excesses, and the physical and emotional state she is in.

Finally, the same rules apply for pregnancy as for any other condition, whether it is a case of threatened miscarriage, skin problems, constipation, heartburn or indigestion – that is:

- tonify a deficiency
- clear Heat.

Common deficiences in pregnancy

The Kidneys will almost certainly be deficient, but try to ascertain from your case history whether the deficiency is predominately Yin or Yang. Treatment will centre on tonifying Kidney Yin and Yang conditions in women who have suffered recurrent miscarriages early on in pregnancy. They usually suffer from backache and are cold. Moxa cones can be used with care to tonify points such as BL-23, BL-20 and GV-4. If the woman suffers from constipation, use moxa and tonification. If there is oedema of the ankles, this is due to Kidney Yang deficiency; use BL-23 and GV-4 (Mingmen).

If the baby is not growing in the womb or seems small for its dates, there is usually a mixture of Spleen and Kidney deficiency. I tonify Kidney Yang, using BL-20, BL-23 and ST-36, and recommend plenty of rest. This condition is common in high-powered businesswomen who do not slow down or stop work during pregnancy, then wonder why at 34 weeks their baby is not growing.

To nourish Kidney Yin, I would use KI-6. To nourish the Liver, I would use LR-8.

If at the end of a treatment I want to boost the Blood or tonify an underlying condition, I will tonify certain points by putting the needle in and taking it out again.

Moxa

Women will feel hot and therefore need no extra heat. I use moxa:

- to turn breech babies
- for backache and sciatica where large areas of the back are cold
- for anaemia or Blood deficiency, placing small moxa cones on points such as BL-17 prior to needling.

CASE STUDY 2.1

A 40-year-old woman came to me with an irregular cycle and bleeding between periods. Her mother had died of cervical cancer and she was convinced that she herself was suffering from this disease. When I asked her about the possibility of being pregnant, she was adamant that she was not. I explained the points I could not use and gave her a first treatment. I also insisted that she have a pregnancy test prior to continuing treatment. She was not very pleased. The test proved positive – the bleeding was from a pregnancy. She went on to have a healthy baby boy.

Adverse effects of acupuncture

Although I have treated many pregnant women, there have been only a handful of occasions when the patient has had any negative reaction. This has usually been at a first treatment, when the woman was feeling frightened of the needles. Sometimes I think that as acupuncturists we forget how much people may worry before they come for a treatment!

There have been a couple of incidents when a woman felt faint, weak and clammy. I have immediately taken the needles out, given her a glass of water and encouraged her to lie down for a few minutes. On the next visit, she – and her baby – have both been fine.

On one occasion, a woman who was 33 weeks' pregnant told me that after her acupuncture treatment she had experienced strong contractions. When I questioned her about what she did after the treatment, I learnt that she had caught a train to London from Leamington, spent the whole day on her feet at an auctioneers and had not returned home until 8 p.m.

Another lady I treated had high blood pressure and was suffering from sickness in early pregnancy. I used PC-6 but the minute I put the needles in, she started to vomit. On questioning her, I learnt that she had had no breakfast and had taken her blood pressure tablets on an empty stomach (she was my first appointment of the day). She never returned for another treatment.

Factors to be aware of when using acupuncture in pregnancy

When treating a woman of child-bearing age for the first time with acupuncture, it is ***vital*** – and this point cannot be overstressed – never to assume or take for granted that she is not pregnant. It is far better to start with the assumption that the patient may be pregnant and try to establish the facts. For example, a woman may begin treatment because she is having problems conceiving. Her periods may be irregular or non-existent, or she may have bleeding between periods. *And yet she may be pregnant without knowing it.*

I try to establish at the outset of treatment the dates of her last three periods. I always stress on that first treatment that there are specific points that are forbidden before certain months of pregnancy and that I am therefore avoiding them. I also record this in her notes.

One case I treated is a good example of the importance of always carrying out this procedure (see Case study 2.1).

I must stress the importance of working closely with a woman's midwife and/or GP. It is also vital to take a thorough medical history prior to treatment, so that you are aware of any condition, such as diabetes or cardiac disease, for which Western medical intervention should be sought initially. You can also be alert to any exacerbation of the condition.

You should be particularly aware of the following signs.

First 12 weeks

- *Severe morning sickness, with vomiting up to 14 times a day*: this can be treated at a first appointment, but be aware that the patient may need hospitalising (see Ch. 4, Morning sickness).
- *Profuse bleeding*: treatment may be given but urge the patient to visit her GP at once.
- *Severe abdominal pain*: this could indicate an ectopic pregnancy and the patient should visit her GP.
- *Urinary tract infection*: this is not uncommon in pregnancy and the patient should visit her GP.
- *Epilepsy*: refer the patient to the GP.

12–28 weeks

- *Bleeding*: this should always be treated with caution and the patient referred to her GP.
- *Itching of the skin, particularly of the abdomen (obstetric cholestasis)*: this should be referred to the GP.

28–40 weeks

- *Frontal headaches and intolerance of bright lights*: this may be a sign of pre-eclampsia.
- *Swelling of the ankles and feet (oedema)*: this may indicate pre-eclampsia and needs to be treated with caution.

Trust your gut feelings and do not be afraid to admit if you are feeling unsure about how to proceed with the treatment. I have done this many times and always find that patients respect you more for admitting uncertainty.

An example is given in Case study 2.2. The moral of the story is: go by what you feel. Trust your instincts.

CASE STUDY 2.2

On one occasion, a lady who was 34 weeks' pregnant with breech presentation came to me to have her baby turned using moxa. There were no medical reasons to contraindicate treatment, but for some reason I did not feel happy about giving it and asked the woman to come back the following week. When she returned a week later, I asked the obstetric consultant to examine her. He confirmed that she was fine and that the baby was lying in the breech position. However, once again I was not happy about using the moxa, though the only explanation I could give was my gut feeling. The patient accepted this and left. On her way to the car park she began to bleed heavily, having suffered a placental abruption (where the placenta comes away). Both she and the baby were fine. But if I had used the moxa, I would never have convinced myself that it was not the treatment that had been responsible.

Summary

- During pregnancy, a strain is put on the Qi and Essence of the Kidney, so Kidney deficiencies are common.
- Factors that deplete the Jing include: stress, fear, anxiety and insecurity, overwork and many previous children.
- Acupuncture treatment in pregnancy aims to improve the Qi, Yin and Yang of the Kidneys, and hence improve the Jing.
- Another common pattern is Liver Blood deficiency combined with Liver Qi stagnation. Heat in the Blood from Liver Qi stagnation may lead to miscarriage.
- The acupuncturist needs to be particularly vigilant for adverse effects of acupuncture when treating pregnant women. Forbidden points must be noted (see list below).
- Factors to be aware of when using acupuncture include:
  - first 12 weeks: severe morning sickness, profuse bleeding, severe abdominal pain, urinary tract infection, epilepsy
  - 12–28 weeks: bleeding, skin itching
  - 28–40 weeks: frontal headaches and intolerance of bright lights, ankle and foot oedema.
- Acupuncture points during pregnancy generally include:
  - *backache and coldness*: moxa on BL-20 and 23, GV-4
  - *oedema of ankles*: BL-23, GV-4
  - *baby not growing in womb or small for dates*: tonify Kidney Yang using BL-20 and 23, and ST-36
  - *to nourish Kidney Yin*: KI-6
  - *to nourish the Liver*: LR-8
  - *moxa* to turn breech babies, for large cold areas on the back and for anaemia or Blood deficiency (BL-17).
- Points to avoid during pregnancy include: LI-4, SP-6, GB-21, BL-31, 32 and 67, and abdominal points.

References

Inner classic of the Yellow Emperor (Nei Jing): simple questions. 1963. People's Press, Beijing

Maciocia G 1998 Obstetrics and gynaecology in Chinese medicine. Churchill Livingstone, New York

Sweet BR (ed.) 1997 Mayes' midwifery, 12th edn. Baillière Tindall, New York, p 125

Further reading

Gasgoigne S 1994 Manual of aconventional medicine for alternative practitioners, vol. II. Jiansu Science and Technology, China

Kaptchuk T 1983 Chinese medicine: the web that has no weaver. Random House, London

Nanjing College of Traditional Chinese Medicine 1987 Concise traditional gynaecology. Jiangsu Science and Technology, China

Shou-Zhong Yang, Liu Da-Wei 1995 Fu Qi-Zhu's gynaecology. Blue Poppy Press, Boulder, CO

3 Nutrition in pregnancy

Chapter outline

What a woman eats during pregnancy affects not only her own state of health but that of her baby as well. Optimum nutrition greatly increases the chances of having a healthy, trouble-free pregnancy. More importantly still, it can have a profound effect on the health of children *for the rest of their lives,* helping to prevent problems such as coronary artery disease and stroke, bronchitis, obesity and diabetes. What's more, the size, and possibly even the function, of a child's brain depends on its mother's nutrition during pregnancy (Delisle 2002, Godfrey & Barker 2001, Harding 2003, Kind et al 2006).

The right nutrients from conception and onwards, throughout the first 5 years of life, provide the key to good health throughout life (Barker 1992).

The developing fetus

The developing fetus requires specific nutrients for healthy growth and development, so a well-balanced diet during pregnancy is essential to meet those needs.

Research carried out by Professor David Barker and his team at the Medical Research Council Environmental Epidemiology Unit in Southampton shows that, during life in the uterus and immediately after birth, particular organs undergo periods of rapid growth. This happens at certain brief, critical periods and is known as 'fetal programming'. For each organ, there is a particular window of opportunity. Getting the correct optimum nutrition at the right time is vitally important (Godfrey & Barker 2001). For example, a recent animal study has shown that a reduced intake of protein during pregnancy can cause elevated blood pressure and impaired glucose tolerance and increase the chance of obesity in offspring (Delisle 2002).

Why a well-balanced diet may still be inadequate

The type and quality of food that we eat have changed enormously in the last 50 years. Although there's a far bigger range of foods available on supermarket shelves today, methods of food production and preservation mean that very few products have been grown locally, and many are shipped in from the other side of the world.

Fruit and vegetables are only as good as the soil they grew in. Today's farming techniques rely on artificial fertilisers and pesticides, which rob the soil of nutrients without replacing them. So the plants keep on growing, but without their full complement of vitamins and minerals. So the people who eat them end up deficient too.

Chemical additives and preservatives mean that, although food may still look edible, it can be days or even weeks old. A fresh orange, for example, may provide around 115 mg of vitamin C. Or it may provide none at all.

Overprocessing and refining also rob food of vital vitamins and minerals. And what goodness is left is all too often destroyed by our methods of cooking. Heating destroys nutrients, destroys vitamins and destroys enzymes; 20–70% of the nutrient content of leafy vegetables is lost in cooking.

Guidelines for getting the most value out of food (from a Western nutritional viewpoint) include:

- eat raw organic food, as fresh as possible, as the first choice
- avoid processed and refined food containing additives and synthetic chemicals
- cook food as little as possible, and as whole as possible
- avoid frying: fats change their structure when heated to high temperatures, becoming 'trans' fats, which can cause harm to health
- steam in preference to boiling and do not overcook
- wash and, if necessary, peel fruit and veg
- drink filtered rather than tap water
- store food in cold dark conditions such as a fridge
- eat organic meat and game rather than the intensively produced variety, which may be contaminated with hormones and antibiotics
- supplement to ensure optimum levels of nutrients.

Western viewpoint of optimum nutrition in pregnancy

While in an ideal world everybody should eat a well-balanced diet, rich in essential nutrients, the expectant mother needs an even greater supply to accommodate the needs of her growing fetus. What may be an adequate diet for most people may not be adequate for a pregnant woman. Vitamins are responsible for maintaining normal growth; severe vitamin deficiency can cause birth abnormalities.

The mother's body becomes more energy efficient in pregnancy. Fat is deposited subcutaneously in the upper thigh and abdomen, to provide energy reserves for later pregnancy when the demand of the fetus is high, and for breastfeeding. This is an evolutionary design, to ensure survival of the baby in times of famine (Shein et al 1990). But the mother's body is also designed to divert essential nutrients to the baby during pregnancy. So her own health and energy levels can easily deteriorate if diet is inadequate, resulting in many of the common side-effects of pregnancy, such as morning sickness, high blood pressure, bloating and exhaustion.

Women at risk

Certain groups of pregnant women may find their diet particularly inadequate, and their babies therefore at risk of prematurity and low birthweight (Barker 1998). (Babies whose weight at birth is below 3.13 kg (6.9 lb) have been found to be at increased risk of cardiovascular disease in later life.) Certain congenital defects and high perinatal mortality are also linked to poor nutritional status.

Women at risk include those who:

- smoke
- consume alcohol
- take drugs such as marijuana, heroin or cocaine
- have a pre-existing medical condition, such as diabetes
- have food allergies or malabsorption syndromes
- are vegans
- are mothers with twins or multiple births
- are multigravidae with short gaps between babies
- are teenage mothers
- are recent immigrants, because they may have poor nutritional status.

A healthy diet

A well-balanced diet is made up of carbohydrates, protein and fats. All of these come in a variety of forms, and it is important to eat them in the correct form to ensure an adequate intake of vitamins and minerals (DOH 1991).

Carbohydrates

Carbohydrates, which include starches, sugars and fibres, are the main providers of energy. They are best eaten unrefined, with 'nothing added and nothing taken away', as processing removes many vital nutrients as well as much of the fibre that can help prevent constipation.

Foods to eat. These include complex carbohydrates, such as fresh fruit and vegetables, and wholegrains, such as wholemeal bread, brown rice and wholemeal pasta.
Foods to avoid. These include simple carbohydrates, such as white sugar, white flour and bread, white pasta and sweets. These simply add 'empty' calories without providing any goodness.

Proteins

Proteins are the body's building blocks, used for building and repairing cells, enzymes, muscles, organs, tissues and hair. Protein is utilised more efficiently during pregnancy, less being used for energy and more being stored for use by the baby. So the recommended intake goes up only slightly during pregnancy. It is important that the protein is of good quality, and that vitamin and mineral deficiency does not impede the body's utilisation of the protein.

Foods to eat. These include lean fresh (preferably organic) meat, poultry, offal, fish, milk, eggs and cheese. Excellent quality protein is obtained from combining vegetarian sources, such as nuts with pulses, nuts with seeds or pulses with seeds. This also avoids the high fat intake that comes with eating too much red meat.

Foods to avoid. These include processed meats and meat with a high fat content, such as pâté, sausage, salami and burgers.

Fats

Fats provide energy and build cell walls, but there are good and bad fats. The essential fats, linoleic and linolenic acid, are found in most of the body's cells, especially the brain, and play an important role in many of the body's mechanisms, including making healthy arteries, allergic reactions and making the sex hormones.

Foods to eat. Seeds and nuts, as well as sunflower, sesame and soya oil, are all good sources but heating causes oxidation (makes them rancid), so cooking with these should be avoided. It is important to buy cold-pressed oils and store them in the fridge. Oily fish such as mackerel and tuna are useful sources of eicosapentaenoic acid (EPA) and docosahexaenoic acid (DHA).

Chinese viewpoint of a balanced diet

Different foods correspond to different elements and may be Yang or Yin in nature (see Box 3.1). In the West, our food sources are a means of getting the right balance of vitamins and minerals. In Chinese medicine, the five flavours – sour, sweet, bitter, pungent and salty, corresponding to the different elements – are as important as the remedial action of the different foods: tonifying, sedating, moistening, cooling and dispersing. Also important is where the energies of foods are directed in the body and how they are used therapeutically.

In a healthy person, the five flavours should be balanced, although the sweet flavour tends to predominate. Sweetness is the Earth Element and the most central aspect of the body. Most carbohydrates are considered sweet.

Internal organs affected by taste

The other four tastes relate to the body organs as follows:

- sour flavour enters the Liver and Gall Bladder
- bitter flavour enters the Heart and Small Intestine
- sweet flavour enters the Spleen and Stomach
- pungent flavour enters the Lungs and Large Intestine
- salty flavour enters the Kidneys and Bladder.

Box 3.1 Food actions

Yang	Yin
Warming	Cooling
Sweet or pungent	Salty, bitter or sour
Energising	Building blood and fluids
Ascending energy	Descending energy

Food for conception and pregnancy

Ancient Chinese thinking says that the food that our parents ate prior to our conception and what our mothers ate while they were carrying us affects us throughout our lives. Likewise, what we eat will affect the health of our children throughout their lives. This is now being borne out by Western scientific research (Barker 1998).

Food cravings (the most common being for salty or sweet food) are usually a sign of nutritional deficiencies. In others words, the diet is not properly balanced and may have been out of balance for many years. This should be remedied before conception and pregnancy.

Chinese dietary therapy suggests that pregnant women should eat according to their intuition and be guided by what their body is telling them. Vegetarians will often find themselves drawn to dairy foods, eggs, fish and even chicken. They should try to eat a variety of foods, but bitter herbs should be avoided.

What is happening each month

If we look at the changes occurring trimester by trimester in fetus and mother, it is easier to see exactly what the nutritional requirements of both are.

First trimester

During the first 3 months of pregnancy all the organs of the baby's body, as well as its hands, feet and limbs, are formed. It is a period of incredibly rapid growth spurts and in many ways the most crucial stage of the baby's development. Specific nutrients are needed, though it should never be forgotten that nutrients do not work in isolation but interact with each other in a complex synergy. If the body is given nutrients in the right combination, lower doses may suffice. That is why, although supplements have an important role to play in optimum nutrition, there is no substitute for fresh wholefoods, which contain thousands of health-promoting substances, some of which we probably don't even know about yet.

Vitamin A

Vitamin A is vital for proper fetal growth and in particular the development of the eyes. It needs to work in balance with other nutrients, in particular zinc, B complex and vitamins C, D and E. It can be obtained from animal products in the form of retinol, or from vegetables in the form of beta-carotene, which the body changes with the help of zinc into proplasma vitamin A. (The long slow cooking of vegetables destroys beta-carotene, however.)

Good food sources. These include fish oils, egg yolk, butter, cheese and yoghurt, carrots, spinach, red peppers, tomatoes, broccoli, apples, apricots and mangoes.

B vitamins

B vitamins should always be taken as B complex (in conjunction with other B vitamins), as their functions are linked and dosing with one may lead to a deficiency of others. The body's need for all of them increases during pregnancy, and deficiencies have been linked with birth abnormalities such as cleft palate and shortened limbs.

Good food sources. These include brewer's yeast, molasses, egg yolks, wholegrains, wheatgerm, rice, legumes and green vegetables, bananas, papaya, dried peaches and prunes.

Folic acid

This was discussed in Chapter 1 (p. 12).

Vitamin C

Vitamin C helps to boost the immune system and increase resistance to viruses and toxins. It is needed to make healthy collagen (the body's connective tissue), and it aids the absorption of iron and so prevents anaemia. Deficiency has been linked to miscarriage.

Good food sources. These include citrus fruits, blackcurrants, melons, pineapples, bananas, raspberries, apples, pears, prunes, tomatoes, potatoes, green peppers, green vegetables such as Brussels sprouts, kale, broccoli, parsley, alfalfa and rose hips. Vitamin C is lost in storage.

Vitamin E

Vitamin E is important in the development of the heart, to help get oxygen to cells and to protect RNA and DNA from damage that could cause congenital defects in the baby. It also helps the utilisation of fatty acids and selenium.

Good food sources. These include unrefined cold pressed oils, wholegrains, wheatgerm, nuts, green leafy vegetables, avocados, molasses and eggs.

Iron

The volume of blood circulating round the body increases during pregnancy, to help get oxygen to the placenta. Iron is needed to make haemoglobin, the substance in the red blood cells that carries oxygen. Deficiency can lead to weakness, excessive tiredness, depression, headache, confusion and memory loss.

Iron supplementation on its own is not effective as it needs to work with other vitamins and minerals. Vitamin C in particular helps the body to absorb iron, as for example taking a glass of fresh orange with an egg yolk.

Good food sources. These include molasses, wholegrains, wheatgerm, lean red meat, poultry, almonds, egg yolk, wholegrains, avocados, dried fruit such as figs, currants and apricots, green leafy vegetables such as spinach, broccoli, watercress and parsley.

Zinc

In addition to its role in preventing defects and low birthweight in the newborn (see Ch. 1), zinc is needed for cell division and growth, for maintaining hormone levels and to keep the immune system healthy. Zinc deficiency inhibits metabolism of vitamin A and may also be one of the causes of morning sickness (Pfeiffer 1978) (see Ch. 5). The best dietary sources are meat and poultry, so vegetarians are likely to be zinc deficient.

Good food sources. These include meat and poultry, fish, shellfish (particularly oysters), ginger, sunflower, sesame, pumpkin and sprouted seeds, almonds and other nuts, soya beans, fruit, leafy vegetables, watercress, wheat- and oatgerm, wholegrains and brewer's yeast. The citric acid in oranges increases zinc absorption.

Foods to avoid. These include saturated fats (from animal sources) which provide energy but should only be eaten in small quantities or in low fat forms, such as skimmed milk, lean meat and low-fat cheese. Processed foods tend to be high in saturated fat.

Diet to prevent morning sickness

Nausea during pregnancy may be a sign of deficiencies, and supplementation of certain B vitamins, folic acid and the relevant minerals will help in most cases. Morning sickness and dietary changes to alleviate this are discussed in detail in Chapter 5.

Second trimester

Approaching the middle of pregnancy, the change in a woman's shape is becoming much more noticeable. The early feelings of nausea and tiredness should be passing and the appetite increasing, but the old adage about 'eating for two' is untrue. While it is vitally important to eat healthily, too much excess weight put on now will be difficult to shift later.

The baby is growing, its organs maturing, its bones hardening and its air passages developing.

Vitamin A

Vitamin A is needed for healthy eyes, hair, skin, teeth, mucous membranes and bone structure. It is linked to neural tube defects in still births. (For food sources see First trimester above.)

B vitamins

The body has an increased need for B complex during times of stress, infection, pregnancy and lactation. They can also help to improve utilisation of other vitamins and minerals, with deficiency causing lowered absorption. In pregnancy, deficiency may lead to loss of appetite and vomiting, which can in turn lead to low birthweight. B vitamins are needed for energy and the metabolism of carbohydrates and for the baby's developing nervous system. In particular, vitamin B3 helps to form serotonin, an important neurotransmitter that helps with sleep and mood. (For food sources see First trimester above.)

Vitamin C

The need for vitamin C goes up in pregnancy. Vitamin C aids absorption of both iron and zinc, it helps carry oxygen to all the cells, it nourishes the baby, helps to fight infection and keeps the mother healthy. It also helps make collagen, the connective tissue that keeps skin supple, so it plays an important role in preventing stretch marks. (For food sources see First trimester above.)

Vitamin D

Vitamin D is vital for healthy bones and teeth. It also aids the absorption of calcium and phosphorus. It is made in the skin in the presence of sunlight and is rarely deficient except in pregnant Asian women who produce less vitamin D.

Good food sources. These include whole milk, free-range eggs, fish oil and fatty fish.

Vitamin E

Vitamin E helps get oxygen to the cells and helps to keep skin supple. (For food sources see First trimester above.)

Vitamin F (essential fatty acids or EFAs)

These form a large part of the membranes of all cells and give rise to prostaglandins, which are used to make adrenal and sex hormones and which affect all the body's systems. They help in the absorption of nutrients and activate many enzymes. EFA deficiency may be a contributory factor in pre-eclampsia (Crawford & Doyle 1989).

Good food sources. These include nuts, unrefined oils, nuts such as Brazils, nut butters, green leafy vegetables, seeds such as sunflower and linseed, oily fish such as herring, mackerel, tuna, sardines and salmon.

Calcium

A woman's requirement for calcium goes up more than three times during pregnancy. It is needed to form strong bones and teeth in the baby, to help muscle growth, and to control nerve and muscle function. Deficiency is associated with low birthweight and low scores on developmental tests. Premature babies are often found to have low levels.

Good food sources. These include wholegrains, nuts, dairy products, carob, dolomite and green leafy vegetables.

Chromium

Chromium is needed to make GTF, the glucose tolerance factor, which lowers blood sugar levels by carrying blood glucose to the cells where it is either used or stored. It is not easily absorbed but is readily lost by the body, especially in those with a high intake of sugar.

Good food sources. These include brewer's yeast, molasses, wholegrains, wheatgerm, vegetables, butter.

Iron

Iron is in great demand from the growing baby and a woman's stores may be quickly used up. Iron is needed to make haemoglobin, the substance which carries oxygen in the blood, and the number of red blood cells increases by 30% during pregnancy. The expanding blood volume dilutes the concentration in the bloodstream. Deficiency can lead to poor memory, sluggishness and tiredness. In the fetus, iron deficiency can cause defects in the eye, bone and brain, and slow growth, as well as being a factor in neonatal mortality. (For food sources see First trimester above.)

Magnesium

Magnesium works with calcium and together they create strong bones and teeth and are both essential for the development of the baby's muscle and nervous system. Pregnancy will aggravate any deficiency, causing muscle cramps and twitching, insomnia and depression. Low levels are also associated with premature and low birthweight babies.

Good food sources. These include nuts, kelp, seafood, eggs, milk, wholegrains, green vegetables and dolomite.

Selenium

Selenium is a trace element that may be necessary for normal growth. It is a powerful antioxidant (hence its reputation as the anticancer element) and a vital ingredient of an enzyme that helps the body to fight infections. It is commonly deficient in the British diet.

Good food sources. These include tuna, herring, butter, wheatgerm, Brazil nuts, garlic and wholegrains. It is more effective when taken with vitamin E.

Zinc

Zinc and copper are antagonistic and, as copper levels rise naturally in pregnancy, zinc needs to be supplemented. Daily requirement in pregnancy is around 20 mg, although most women get less than half of this from their diet. The common use of phosphate fertilisers prevents plants from absorbing zinc from the soil – another good reason for eating organic vegetables and fruit. Deficiency is one of the major factors in low birthweight. Professor Bryce-Smith (1986) believes that any baby born weighing below 23.13 kg (6 lb 9 oz) should be suspected of have zinc deficiency. (For food sources see First trimester above.)

Third trimester

During the final 3 months of pregnancy a baby grows faster than ever, doubling in size, laying down fat stores and putting on around an ounce (28 g) of weight a day. Nerve cells increase, the lungs and immune system mature, the digestive tract develops, bones are strengthened, and stores of fat, iron and calcium are laid down. Bones both lengthen and harden and there are crucial growth spurts in the brain. The mother needs approximately 200 extra calories a day, and the need for protein is at an all-time high (Ford 1994). Her blood volume has by now increased by 40%, and she may be suffering from minor problems and discomforts such as breathlessness, insomnia, back ache, constipation, piles or heartburn.

Vitamin A

Vitamin A contributes to healthy appetite and digestion and the making of red and white blood cells. It also assists in preparing the body for making milk, as it helps to make the hormones connected with lactation. (For food sources see First trimester above.)

B vitamins

These help to prepare the body for making milk. (For food sources see First trimester above.)

Folic acid

The World Health Organization (WHO) reports that up to a half of pregnant women suffer from folic acid deficiency in the last 3 months of pregnancy (Foresight 1996). Folic acid is needed to manufacture DNA and, with vitamin B12, to make red blood cells. Deficiency can lead to pernicious anaemia. (For food sources see Ch. 1.)

Vitamin C

As well as helping the body to absorb iron (so preventing anaemia) and zinc and prepare for making milk, vitamin C is antiviral and so helps to fight infection and promote healing after delivery. (For food sources see First trimester above.)

Vitamin E

Vitamin E speeds up wound healing and helps to keep skin supple. It can help to ease labour by strengthening the muscles. It also helps the body to prepare for making milk. (For food sources see First trimester above.)

Vitamin F (essential fatty acids)

There are many fatty acids but research has identified two important ones for the development and functioning of the brain: arachidonic acid (AA) and DHA (Crawford 1992). During the third trimester, the brain of the fetus increases 4–5 times in weight, using two-thirds of the energy supplied by the mother. Large amounts of AA and DHA are needed during this 'brain growth spurt' that occurs in the baby just before and just after birth (Crawford & Doyle 1989). They are used as components of the brain cell membranes and to ensure that messages are transferred efficiently between brain cells. They are also found in high concentrations in the eyes and are essential for eye development; the eyes mature rapidly in the third trimester and during the first few months of life.

A lack of DHA supplied to the fetus and neonate via the mother can lead to a variety of long-term problems and conditions, such as hyperactivity, dyslexia, depression, alcoholism, drug addiction and schizophrenia. The decline in fish consumption has led to a reduction in the amount of DHA in the maternal diet. (For food sources see Second trimester above.)

Vitamin K

Vitamin K is involved in the manufacture of prothrombin, which is vital for blood clotting and so prevents haemorrhage in the mother and haemorrhagic disease in the newborn. It is made naturally by bacteria in the healthy gut, but a baby has a sterile gut so has to take what it needs from the mother. It is sometimes administered to women and to babies as an injection at the time of birth, in order to prevent haemorrhage. (See Ch. 14 for a more detailed discussion.)

Good food sources. These include cauliflower, cabbage, egg yolks, green leafy vegetables and soya beans.

Calcium

Stores of calcium are laid down by the baby as its bones and teeth harden, so the mother's supply needs to be plentiful. Calcium given in conjunction with vitamin D during labour may help to ease pain.

Good food sources. These include carob, Brazil nuts, yoghurt, rhubarb, green leafy vegetables and dairy produce.

Iron

Iron is needed for the manufacture of red blood cells and to help the body fight infection. The baby lays down its own stores by taking iron from the mother, so her supply needs to be plentiful. However, taking iron by itself can lead to malabsorption of other minerals, so it is best absorbed from food and taken with vitamin C. (For food sources see First trimester above.)

Zinc

Zinc is essential to help with milk production and for balancing hormones (Pfeiffer 1978). As well as helping the baby's growth, it has been found that zinc-deficient mothers have a greater incidence of complications at birth and of birth defects, and an increased risk of needing a caesarean section. Zinc deficiency is linked to undescended testicles in boys. Zinc also benefits in the immune system. (For food sources see First trimester above.)

Vegetarians

A well-balanced vegetarian diet offers excellent nutrition, and the protein derived from combining vegetarian sources (such as nuts with pulses, nuts with seeds or pulses with seeds) is just as adequate as that from animal sources, with the advantage that it contains complex carbohydrates and fibre rather than saturated fat.

However, there are a few areas where deficiencies may occur that need to be corrected during pregnancy and breastfeeding:

- B2, B6 and B12
- vitamin D
- zinc
- iron
- and calcium (in vegans).

The most common deficiency for vegetarians, especial if they are also vegan, is vitamin B12, which is required for fertility, red blood cells and immunity. It is essential for healthy growth during pregnancy. Enough vitamin B12 can be stored in the liver to last for several years so it may take a while for this deficiency to be spotted. Vegans would be well advised to get their level of B12 tested. Vegetarian food sources for B12 include fermented foods, algae and yeast sources. It can also be administered by injection.

Nutrition for labour

All the good work done throughout pregnancy, with optimum nutrition, the correct intake of foods and appropriate supplementation, needs to be followed up by the right diet for the finale of labour.

It is important for the mother to stock up on complex carbohydrates – the main energy source for the body – during the last 2 weeks of pregnancy. This means eating plenty of wholegrains, pulses and vegetables, to ensure that glycogen reserves stored in the muscles and liver tissues are filled to capacity. Labour can be compared in energy requirements to a marathon run. The last thing a woman wants to do is run out of energy and so risk a prolonged and difficult labour that may result in medical intervention and caesarean section, depriving her of a natural birth and increasing the baby's risk of birth-related trauma.

Postnatal nutrition

A healthy and well-balanced diet is just as important after delivery as before, because of the effects of blood loss, the risk of infection and the start of lactation. Sleepless nights and the stress of motherhood, combined with the extra nutritional needs of a breastfeeding baby, mean that an optimum diet and supplementation will really pay dividends.

- Iron helps healing and fights infection by making haemoglobin to carry oxygen in the blood. It is particularly important if there has been heavy blood loss.
- Zinc is needed for the production of hormones and to help combat postnatal depression, which may be related to an excess of copper. Supplementation with zinc and B6 will correct any imbalance.
- Vitamin C is good for the immune system; it helps wounds to heal and aids the absorption of iron.
- Essential fatty acids are vital for the baby's brain development.

Foods to avoid

Anyone wishing to maintain good health should steer clear of foods containing too much sugar or saturated fat, additives or preservatives and of drinks containing excess sugar and caffeine. This applies in particular to pregnant women. Generally this means avoiding processed and refined foods and many ready-cooked meals, including things like cakes, biscuits, pies, puddings and crisps and drinks such as cola and squash.

Pregnant women in particular should avoid: pâté, cooked chilled foods, under-cooked meat, uncooked eggs (as in home-made mayonnaise or soft-whipped ice cream) and soft, blue-veined or unpasteurised cheeses, such as brie, camembert and dolcelatte. These all carry the risk of infection from salmonella or listeria, both of which can have disastrous consequences for pregnant women.

Health risks

One in 10 pregnancies ends in miscarriage (the number may be far higher if the number of early miscarriages, when a woman may not even have realised that she is pregnant, is included). The risks of consuming alcohol and smoking during this period were discussed in Chapter 1.

Summary

- Nutrition for the first trimester includes: vitamins A, B, C and E, folic acid, zinc and iron.
- To prevent *morning sickness*: vitamins B6 and B12, folic acid, iron, magnesium, zinc, potassium, ginger, protein for breakfast, small frequent meals, plenty of water; avoid tea, coffee, concentrated sugar, fatty, strong-smelling and junk food.

- Nutrition for the second trimester includes: vitamins A, B, C, D, E and F (EFAs), calcium, magnesium, zinc, selenium, chromium and iron.
- Nutrition for the third trimester includes: vitamins A, B, C, E, F (EFAs) and K, folic acid, zinc, calcium and iron.
- Vegetarians need to be aware of possible shortages of vitamins B2, B6 and B12, zinc, iron and calcium (vegans).
- Postnatal nutrition includes: vitamins C and F (EFAs), iron and zinc.
- Pregnant women should avoid: foods and drinks containing excess sugar, saturated fat, preservatives or caffeine, pâté, cooked chilled foods, undercooked meat or eggs, soft, blue-veined or unpasteurised cheese, alcohol and smoking.

References

Barker DJP 1992 Diet for a lifetime. Mothers' and babies' health in later life. Churchill Livingstone, New York

Barker DJP 1998 Mothers' and babies' health in later life. Churchill Livingstone, New York

Bryce-Smith D 1986 The zinc solution. Century Arrow, London, pp 53–57

Crawford MA 1992 The role of dietary fatty acids in biology: their place in the evolution of the human brain. Nutritional Reviews 50: 3–11

Crawford M, Doyle A 1989 Fatty acids during early human development. Journal of Internal Medicine 225: 159–169

Delisle H 2002 Foetal programming of nutrion-related chronic disease. Sante 12: 56–63

DOH (Department of Health) 1991 Dietary references values for food energy and nutrients for the United Kingdom. HMSO, London

Ford F 1994 Healthy eating for your baby. Pan, New York

Foresight 1996 Planning for a healthy baby. Vermilion, London

Godfrey KM, Barker DJ 2001 Fetal programming and adult health. Public Health Nutrition 4(2B): 611–624

Harding JE 2003 Nutrition and growth before birth. Asia Pacific Journal of Clinical Nutrition 12 (suppl): S28

Kind KL, Moore VM, Davies MJ 2006 Diet around conception and during pregnancy – effects on fetal and neonatal outcomes. Reproductive Biomedicine Online 12(5): 532–541

Pfeiffer CC 1978 Zinc and other micronutrients. Institute of Optimum Nutrition, New Canaan, CT, p 102

Shein Z, Susset M, Saenger 1990 Famine and human development. The Dutch hunger winter. Oxford University Press, Oxford

4 Antenatal care explained

Chapter outline

The aims of antenatal care are, first and foremost, to look after the health and safety of the mother and to ensure delivery of a healthy baby. Monitoring the health of mother and baby throughout the pregnancy allows for the early detection and treatment of any problems.

A vital element in good antenatal care is the establishment of a good relationship between the woman and the professionals involved in looking after her, so that they are all working together in partnership. Communication and continuity of care are both important. If the woman is well supported, kept informed about all aspects of her care, and given whatever information and health education she needs, then she will feel empowered and able to make informed choices for herself and her baby.

The norm for most women who are not high risk is to have *shared care* – that is, shared between the GP practice and the hospital. But for some women this results in a lack of continuity of care, because they see a different midwife at every visit. This makes it difficult, if not impossible, to build up any kind of personal relationship and can leave a woman feeling that she has no one to confide in, that she is a 'case', not an individual, and that her pregnancy is a medical condition rather than a natural life stage. A more individualised, 'woman-centred' care is better for everyone involved.

Antenatal terms explained

Attitude. This is the relationship of the fetal head and limbs to its body (Fig. 4.1). When fully flexed, with arms crossed over the chest, the fetus forms a compact ovoid, able to move freely while fitting the uterus comfortably.

Br. Breech, as in a bottom-first presentation.

Ceph. Cephalic, as in a normal head-down presentation.

EDD. Estimated date of delivery.

Engagement. This is defined as how far the fetal head has passed through the 'brim' of the pelvis, the brim being at the level of the pubic bone (Fig. 4.2). It is usually measured in fifths. In first-time mothers, the baby's head usually engages at around 38 weeks and gives an indication that the pelvis is going to be large enough to accommodate a vaginal delivery. In multigravidae the head may not engage until delivery. With a breech presentation, it is hard to tell whether the pelvis will be adequate to deliver the head, which is why a caesarean section is sometimes advised for a breech baby.

FH. Fetal heart.

FMF. Fetal movements felt.

Fundus. This is the top of the uterus, the part furthest away from the cervix.

Geriatric or elderly primigravida. This describes a woman over 30 having her first baby.

Gestation. This is the length of time between conception and birth.

Hb. Haemoglobin; this is the pigment in red blood cells that enables them to carry oxygen round the body.

HCG. Human chorionic gonadotrophin, a placental hormone that tells the ovary to keep producing progesterone to suppress menstruation and prevent the lining of the womb from being shed.

Lie. This is the relationship of the long axis of the fetus to the long axis of the uterus (Fig. 4.3). Lie may be longitudinal, oblique or transverse, and should be longitudinal in the last few weeks of pregnancy.

LMP. Last menstrual period.

LOA, ROA. Left occipito-anterior, right occipito-anterior (this indicates the position of the back of the baby's head during its descent down the birth canal).

LOL, ROL. Left occipito-lateral, right occipito-lateral.

LOP, ROP. Left occipito-posterior, right occipito-posterior.

Multiparous. This is the term for a woman having her second or subsequent baby.

NAD. Indicates no abnormality detected.

Nullipara or primigravida. This is the term for a woman having her first baby.

Presentation. This is the part of the fetus that is lying in the lower pole of the uterus (Fig. 4.4). A cephalic presentation is most usual after about the 32nd week. Other possible presentations are breech, face, brow and shoulder.

Proteinuria. This is a condition of protein in the urine, when the sample is taken from the midstream flow and is not contaminated by vaginal discharge, amniotic fluid or blood. It is the last sign of pre-eclampsia and is always serious.

VX. Vertex, part of the fetal skull.

Calculating a pregnancy

It is possible to arrive at the estimated date of delivery by taking the date of the first day of the last menstrual period, counting forwards 9 months and adding 7 days. With a regular cycle of 28 days, this calculation is reasonably accurate. However, if the cycle is irregular, it is more difficult to estimate the due date.

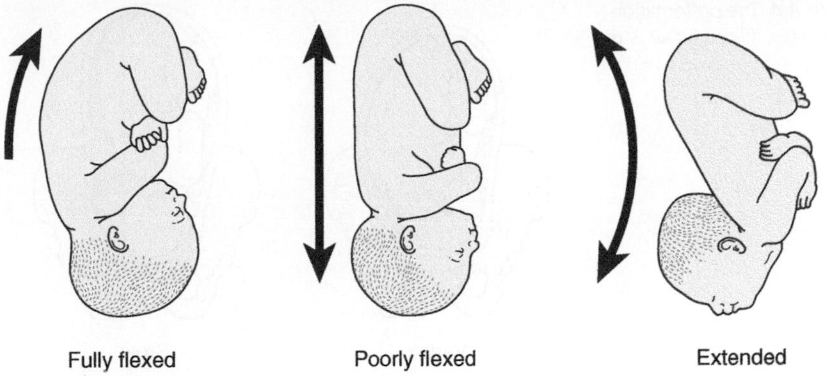

Figure 4.1 The attitude of the fetus. (Reproduced with permission from Sweet 1997, p. 224.)

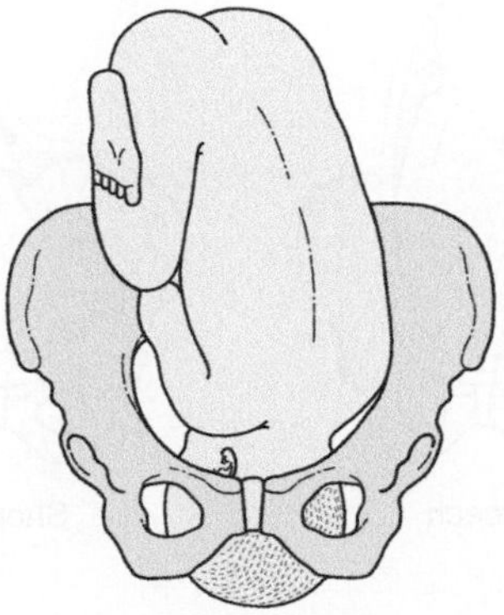

Figure 4.2 Engagement of the fetal head. (Reproduced with permission from Sweet 1997, p. 213.)

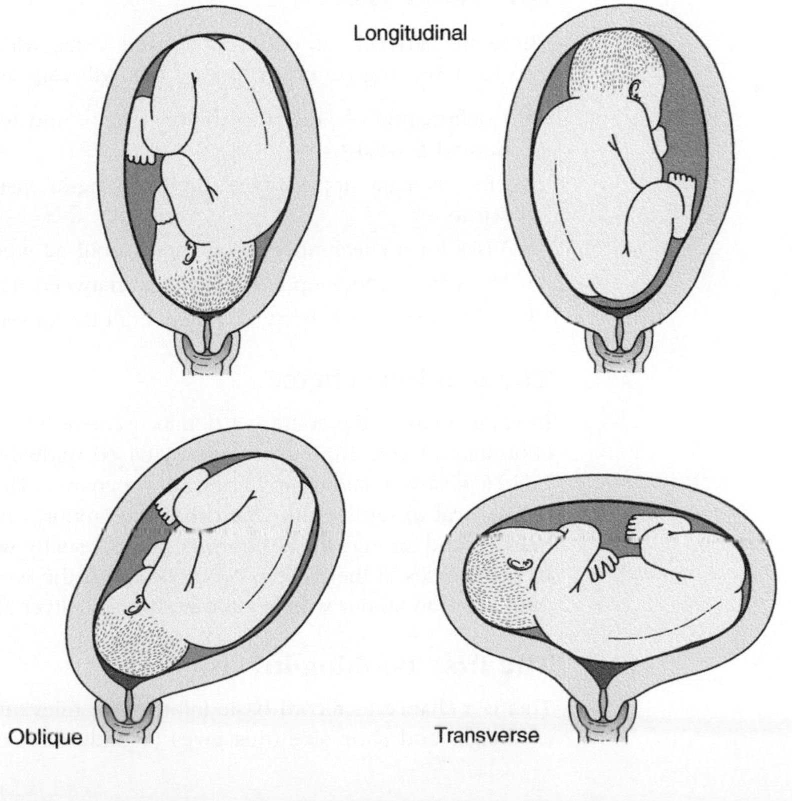

Figure 4.3 The lie of the fetus. (Reproduced with permission from Sweet 1997, p. 223.)

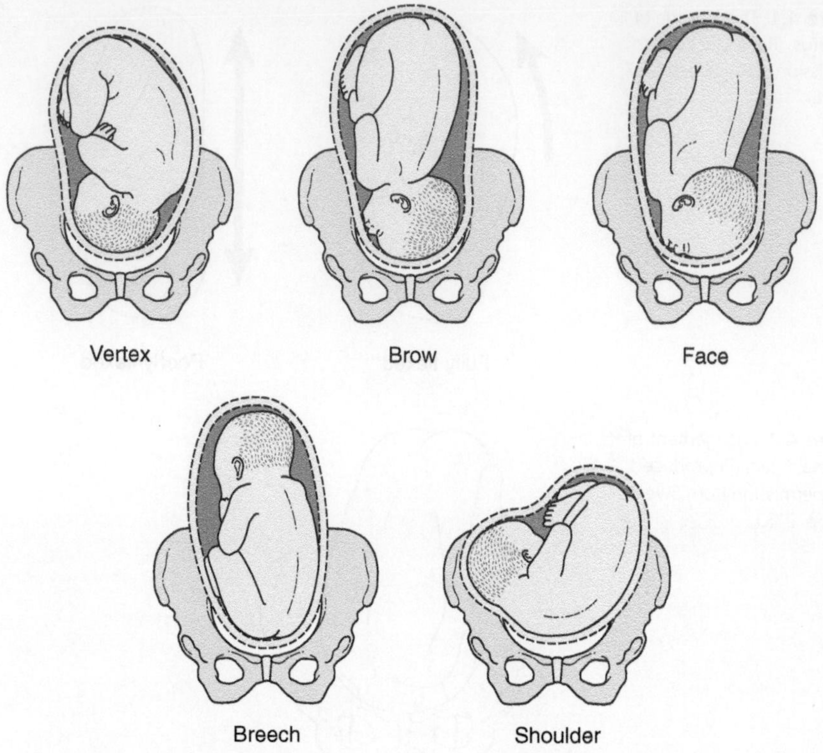

Figure 4.4 The presentation of the fetus. (Reproduced with permission from Sweet 1997, p. 224–225.)

Antenatal visits

There are generally around 10 antenatal visits, with the timetable usually falling into the following pattern. However this will vary around the country.

- Confirmation of pregnancy by the doctor and referral for antenatal care at around 6 weeks.
- First antenatal appointment, the 'booking-in' visit, at between 8 and 12 weeks.
- Visits for a check-up every 4 weeks until 32 weeks.
- Visits for a check-up every 2 weeks between 32 and 36 weeks.
- Visits every week from 36 weeks until the onset of labour.

The domino scheme

In some areas of the country a domino scheme is available. This offers far greater continuity of care from a community-based midwife with whom the woman can build a positive relationship during her pregnancy. This midwife will accompany her to the local maternity unit when she is in labour, care for her right through to the delivery and arrange for her transfer home, usually within a few hours of the birth. In some cases, if there are no complications, the woman does not have to decide until she is in labour whether she wishes to deliver at home or go into hospital.

The first 'booking-in' visit

This is a chance to record basic information relevant to the woman's health, such as: height and shoe size (this gives an indication of pelvic size), weight, blood pressure, personal health history, family health history (including that of the baby's father), and details of previous obstetric history.

Various tests will also be carried out:

- examination of the abdomen, to assess the height of the uterine fundus
- blood tests (for ABO blood group, Rhesus type and Hb value – see below)
- urine test, to detect the presence of protein, glucose and ketones.

The booking-in visit is an opportunity to discuss the various options for care that are available locally, things such as where the woman would like to give birth and how she would like the baby's birth to be. It is also a chance for the midwife to give information and offer advice on pregnancy matters, such as diet, alcohol, smoking, infections and so on.

Weight

The practice of routinely weighing women at every antenatal visit is increasingly being abandoned and is now considered of questionable value. Some women find being weighed distressing and demoralising and, unless there are other danger signs, nothing is done if somebody has put on a lot of weight. Maternal weight gain does not follow a predictable curve, so is not a reliable way of assessing fetal growth. Average total weight gain in pregnancy is 12–14 kg, with 3–4 kg going on in the first 20 weeks and then approximately 0.5 kg a week until term (Sweet 1997). But the range of weight gain is very wide. A sudden gain or loss of weight is important, as it could be a sign of pre-eclampsia or some other complication. Failure to gain weight could be the result of poor diet, vomiting or placental insufficiency, which could in turn lead to retarded fetal growth.

Blood pressure

The blood pressure (BP) reading in early pregnancy forms the baseline for subsequent readings. For a reliable reading, BP should be taken when the woman is relaxed and calm. Stress, anxiety or exertion (if a woman has been running late and had to hurry to the clinic, for example) can all affect the reading.

BP reading consists of two sets of figures: the top number is the *systolic* reading, the bottom number the *diastolic* reading. It is the systolic reading that is affected by stress or exertion and the diastolic reading that can give indication of problems.

There is no such thing as a 'normal' blood pressure – anything between 90/50 and 130/80 is acceptable. During the second trimester there is often a slight fall in BP, owing to the reduced viscosity of the blood and the rising level of progesterone (Sweet 1997). It will rise to its original level in the third trimester. BP of 140/90 or higher is a cause for concern, as is a diastolic rise of 20 or more (above the level recorded in early pregnancy).

Previous obstetric history

This can give an indication of the outcome for this pregnancy and will influence the care a woman receives from her midwife or consultant. A woman who has had a stillbirth in the past will be closely supervised throughout this pregnancy.

Blood tests

A sample of blood will be taken at the booking-in visit for various laboratory investigations (Marteau et al 1992). The blood group (ABO) will be identified and

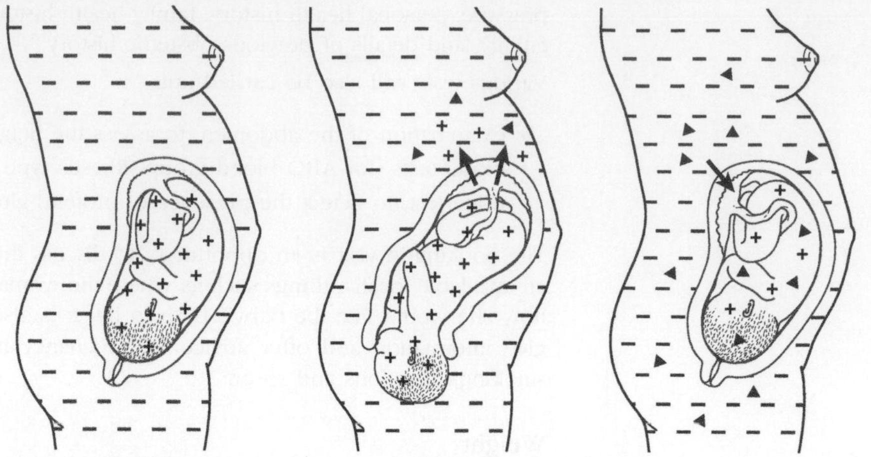

Figure 4.5 Rhesus status.

Rhesus status confirmed (Fig. 4.5). A Rhesus-negative mother with a Rhesus-positive baby will be offered an anti-D immunisation within 72 hours of giving birth, to make sure that subsequent children do not suffer from Rhesus disease, when antibodies produced by the mother attack the blood of Rhesus-positive babies.)

The haemoglobin level of the blood will also be tested, to check for anaemia.

Immunity to rubella (German measles) will be tested. Although rubella is a relatively mild disease for the mother, the effects on the fetus, particularly in the first trimester, can be devastating.

Tests will also be carried out for venereal disease, viral hepatitis (or hepatitis B) and diabetes. A test for HIV may be carried out on women at risk, such as drug abusers or those with a large number of sexual partners, and on request. Confidentiality is of key importance here; results will be kept separate from the notes and staff not informed until the woman is in labour (when there are implications for the health of the staff and of the baby).

Urine test

A sample of urine (taken from midstream and collected in a clean sample bottle) will be tested at every antenatal visit, to check for the presence of sugar, protein, ketones and blood. Protein may result from a vaginal discharge or, more seriously, a urinary tract infection or renal disease. In later pregnancy, when accompanied by raised BP and oedema, it is a serious sign of pre-eclampsia. A small amount of sugar in the urine is not uncommon in pregnancy, but if it recurs then further tests will be needed to check for diabetes. Ketones may be present if the woman is vomiting and may indicate that treatment is required.

A bacteriological examination will detect the presence of any urinary tract infections, such as cystitis or kidney infection, which may need treatment with appropriate antibiotics.

Subsequent antenatal visits

Subsequent visits can be used to assess the general health of the woman and to offer her support, information and advice. The following tests will be carried out regularly: fundus height, abdominal examination, BP, urine analysis and examination of any oedema. There should be an antenatal record chart to explain all these.

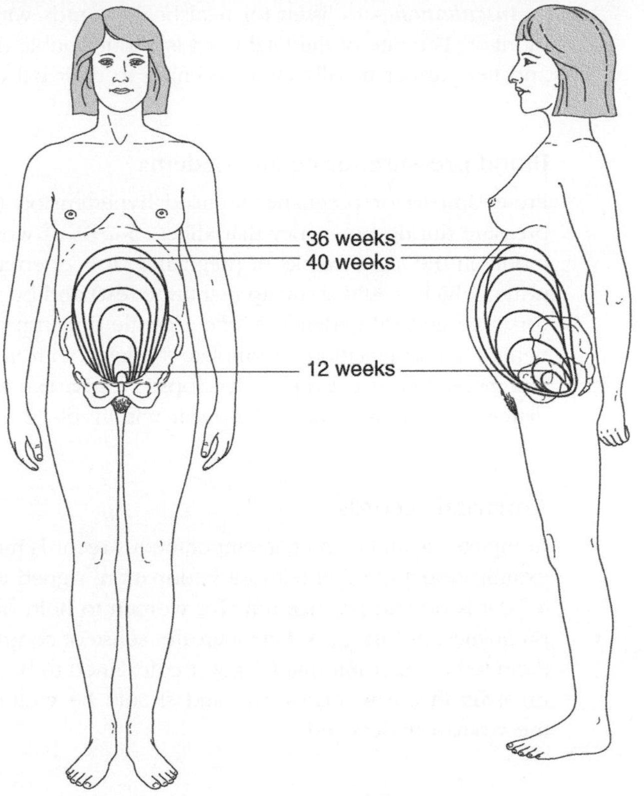

Figure 4.6 The growing fundus.

The growing fundus

The fundus is the top of the uterus, the part furthest away from the cervix. At antenatal visits the midwife will measure the fundal height, from the pubic bone to the top of the pregnant abdomen (Fig. 4.6). In relation to the number of weeks of pregnancy, this gives a very good indication of whether the baby is growing healthily and normally.

Palpation and position of the baby

As pregnancy advances, more information than just the fundal height will be needed and the midwife will carry out an abdominal examination at every visit. After emptying her bladder, the woman should lie flat, supported by pillows if necessary, with only her abdomen exposed. She should be as relaxed and at ease as possible. There are three stages to the examination.

1 *Inspection* – to note the size and shape of the uterus. The size should correspond with the estimated dates and period of gestation. The normal shape is a longitudinal ovoid. If the baby is lying obliquely or transversely, the unusual shape created will be unmistakable in late pregnancy. The dark line of pigmentation (the linea nigra), the quality of muscle of the abdominal wall, any abdominal scarring and any fetal movements should also be noted.

2 *Palpation* – to find out the lie, presentation and position of the fetus, and the relationship of the fetal head to the mother's pelvis. Palpation should be carried out gently with clean warm hands moving smoothly over the abdomen with the pads of the fingers palpating the fetal parts.

3 *Auscultation* – to listen for fetal heart sounds with a stethoscope or fetal heart monitor. The rate of the fetal heart is about double that of the mother. The mother and her partner usually enjoy listening to their baby's heartbeat.

Blood pressure, urine and oedema

Pre-eclampsia or pregnancy-induced hypertension (PIH) is an increase in blood pressure during pregnancy that affects 5–29% of women (Sweet 1997), most commonly in the last 8 weeks of pregnancy. It is often accompanied by protein in the urine (which would show up in a urine test) and by swelling of the feet and ankles (or more general oedema, where a gentle fingertip pressure briefly applied leaves behind an indentation). Complete bedrest with medical supervision is usually recommended. If eclampsia develops, a caesarean section may be needed immediately. Symptoms usually disappear within 48–72 hours of delivery.

Antenatal records

Complete, accurate and contemporaneous records must be made of every antenatal examination and of all relevant information, signed and dated by the midwife (Fig. 4.7). It is normal practice now for women to hold on to their own health notes in pregnancy, as this gives them a greater sense of control and involvement and allows them to be better informed. They are designed to be effectively shared by everyone involved in the woman's care and should be written in language and terms that the woman understands.

Detecting abnormalities of the fetus

The growth of various parts of the baby takes place at different rates (Fig. 4.8); hence harmful substances may affect a variety of organs, depending on the stage of pregnancy.

There are now a whole range of tests available for pregnant women, to assess the risks of the baby having an abnormality. While certain abnormalities can be diagnosed, there is always a margin of error. No test is 100% accurate. Nor does diagnosis in any way mean that a condition can be rectified. Often there is nothing a woman can do apart from use the option to terminate. For this reason, antenatal tests should perhaps be carried out only if the mother is sure she knows what she would do. If having a termination is not an option, there is little point in having the tests done.

For example, more women are opting to have the nuchal translucency test done to detect for Down's syndrome (see below; also Cuckle & Wold 1990). This is done early in pregnancy but is by no means 100% accurate. By the time a woman has had the AFP (alpha-fetoprotein) test done, she will be 15 weeks' pregnant. It takes a further 2 weeks for the results to come back and if these are abnormal, she is then faced with having an amniocentesis. Again she will have a 2–3-week wait, by which time she will be able to feel the baby moving inside her. By now she will undoubtedly be worried sick and very stressed. If she does decide to terminate the pregnancy, she will be between 18 and 22 weeks' pregnant. Termination at this stage means going through a mini labour.

Antenatal tests are not obligatory. If a woman does decide to have them, it is a good idea for her to explore all the possibilities and alternatives first.

Figure 4.7 Antenatal handheld records.

DATE	WEEKS	WEIGHT	URINE			BP	LIE & PRES	HEIGHT FUNDUS	REL PP TO BRIM	FETAL HEART	OEDEMA	HB	NEXT VISIT	REMARKS	SIGNATURE
			SUG	KET	PRO										
15/6/07	13	58 kg	nil	nil	nil	100/60	–	15		–	–	12.0	20/7	u/s arranged 17/7 to check maturity	JS
20/7/07	18	59.2 kg	nil	nil	nil	125/60	–	18-20		FMP	–		20/8		JS
20/8/07	22+	61 kg	nil	nil	nil	125/65	–	20-22		FHH	–		17/9	taking iron	JS
17/9/07	26+	64 kg	nil	nil	nil	125/75	–	24-26		H	–	11.2	17/10		JS

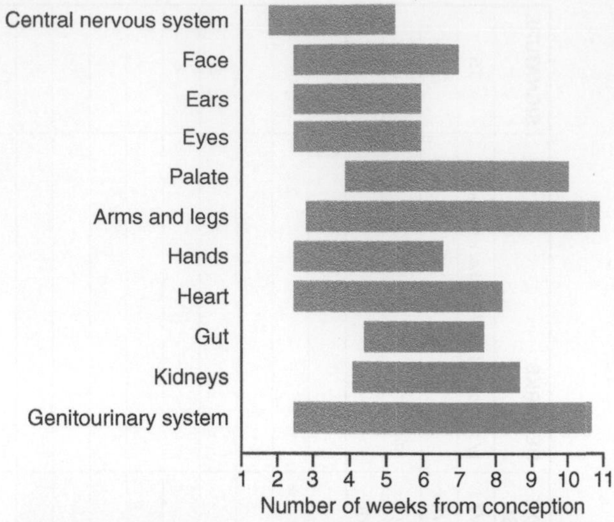

Figure 4.8 Embryonic and fetal development.

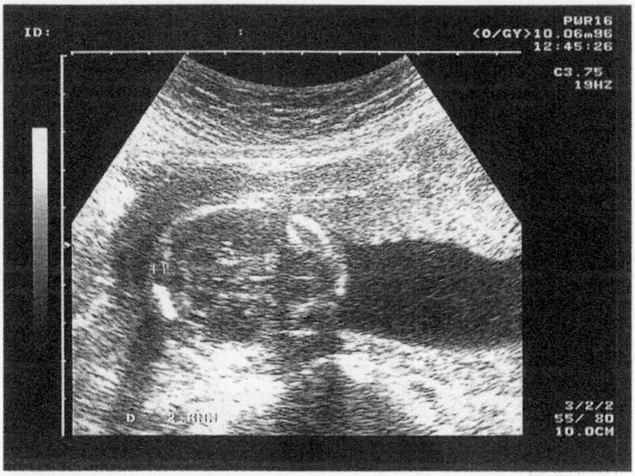

Figure 4.9 Measurement of the nuchal fold thickness and the appearance of the cerebellum dumbbell-shaped ventricles. (Reproduced with permission from Symonds & Symonds 1997.)

Dating ultrasound scan

This scan may be offered at 11–13 weeks and will identify if twins are present, and will also use fetal measurements to determine the exact stage of pregnancy. The fetal heartbeat will also be checked.

Nuchal translucency scan

This is also performed between 11 and 13 weeks. During the ultrasound scan, the fluid under the skin at the back of the baby's neck – the nuchal translucency – is measured (Fig. 4.9). The greater the depth of fluid, the higher the risk of Down's syndrome. At the same time a blood test can be combined to estimate the chances of a baby having Down's syndrome.

AFP (alpha-fetoprotein) test

This is one of several blood tests routinely offered in pregnancy. Concentration of AFP in the blood can be assessed most accurately between weeks 16 and 18, and

Figure 4.10 Amniocentesis.

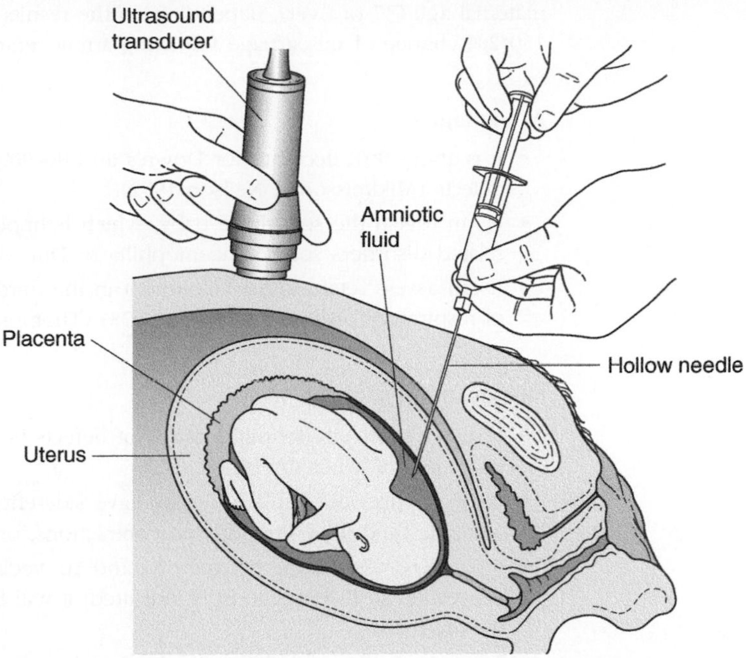

it is usually given in conjunction with an ultrasound scan (MacLachlan 1992). A high level of AFP in the blood might indicate that the pregnancy is more advanced than realised, a multiple pregnancy, a spinal tube defect such as spina bifida, Turner's syndrome (very rare) or death of the baby.

A low level of AFP might indicate that the pregnancy is less advanced than realised or possible Down's syndrome (Cuckle & Wold 1990).

Advantages

- The test is relatively non-invasive and has no physical side-effects.
- Results are available quickly (usually inside a week).

Disadvantages

- The test is only around 50% accurate.
- A false-positive rate of between 5% and 10% means some women will suffer anxiety and uncertainty about their baby for no reason.
- A negative result is no guarantee that the baby is without problems.
- There is not always enough counselling available about the accuracy and implications of a positive result.

Amniocentesis

This is a test (ideally performed between 16 and 18 weeks) in which a specially designed needle is inserted through the abdominal wall to take a sample of amniotic fluid (Fig. 4.10) (Assel et al 1992, MacLachlan 1992). Reasons for carrying out amniocentesis include: suspicion of abnormality following AFP or 'triple' testing or after ultrasound, a family history of congenital illness (such as muscular dystrophy) or of fetal abnormality, an illness in the mother that could affect the baby, or maternal age (37 or over), depending on the results of blood tests. There is a 1 in 150/200 chance of miscarriage following amniocentesis (Hanson et al 1992).

Advantages

- It is about 90% accurate for Down's and 80–90% accurate for neural tube defects (Mikkelsson & Neilson 1992).
- It can reveal the sex of the baby, which is important in the case of sex-related disorders such as haemophilia or Duchenne muscular dystrophy.
- It can assess fetal lung development in the third trimester and the chances of respiratory distress syndrome (RDS) (Thompson et al 1993).

Disadvantages

- It screens for only a limited range of defects (so a negative result is not a guarantee of a healthy baby).
- It can be uncomfortable and may have side-effects (such as leakage of amniotic fluid, bleeding, uterine contractions, or infection).
- It is safest when done between 14 and 16 weeks and it takes 2–6 weeks to get results so if termination is indicated, it will by this time be quite late in the pregnancy.
- In one out of every 1000 tests, the needle will miss the amniotic sac and the procedure will have to be restarted (Mikkelson & Neilson 1992).
- In one out of every 200 tests, the baby will have a low birthweight or neonatal respiratory problems (Mikkelson & Neilson 1992, Thompson et al 1993).
- In one out of every 50 tests, the culture will fail and the test have to be repeated (Mikkelson & Neilson 1992).
- The safety of the test depends on the operator's experience.

Cordocentesis

This is also known as fetal blood sampling. After 18 weeks, a sample of the baby's blood is removed from the umbilical cord under ultrasound guidance. This is the quickest method of detecting chromosomal abnormalities. It is also used to test for rubella or toxoplasmosis infection in later pregnancy. The risk of miscarriage is 1–2%, so the test is only used in specialist centres.

Bart's test/triple test

This is a blood test, usually taken around 16 weeks, which checks levels of AFP and the hormones oestriol and human chorionic gonadotrophin. It can show if there is an increased risk of spina bifida or Down's syndrome.

Chorionic villus sampling (CVS)

This is an antenatal diagnostic test for chromosomal and/or genetic disorders, usually given between 8 and 12 weeks (Fig. 4.11) (Hogge et al 1986). It is often recommended for women over 35 or if there is a family history of genetic disorder. It carries a 2% risk of spontaneous miscarriage (Thomas 1996). It is an invasive technique via the vagina or through the abdominal wall, under ultrasound guidance. A sample of the chorionic villi is taken from the placenta.

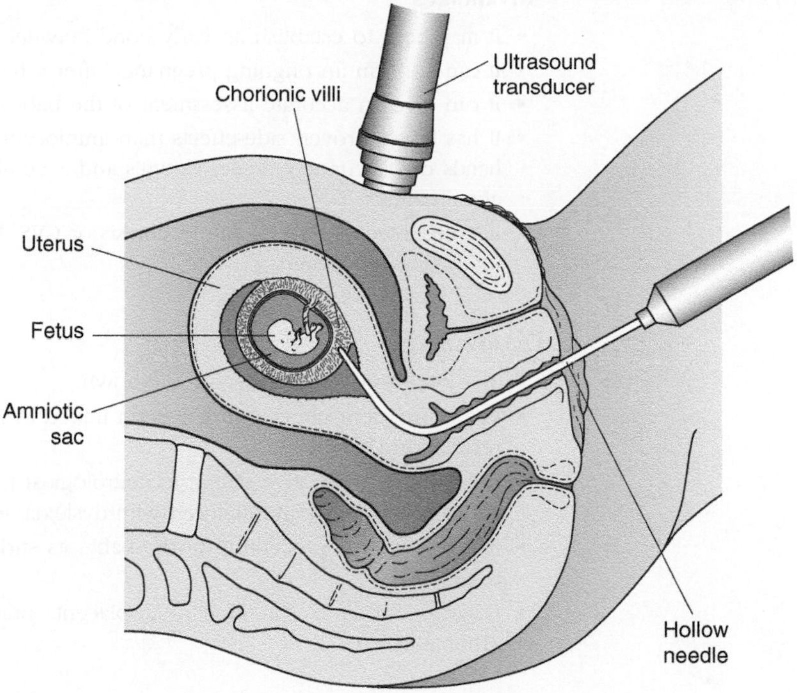

Figure 4.11 Chorionic villus sampling.

Advantages

- Speedy results (preliminary results available with 48 hours, full results within a week).
- Early testing can give reassurance to mothers with a high risk.

Disadvantages

- A 2–4% of miscarriage (about double that of amniocentesis), plus there is evidence that CVS can cause abnormalities if done before 9 weeks (Firth et al 1991).
- The effects on the child of removing placental tissue are unknown.
- There is up to a 6% chance the test will be inconclusive because of culture failure or mixing with the mother's cells (Thomas 1996).

Ultrasound scan

This has been routinely used for more than 25 years in the UK and is given to most pregnant women at least once, usually between 16 and 18 weeks. High-pitched sound waves are reflected back from internal organs, and can be electronically reproduced on screen as a recognisable image of the baby. It is used to confirm dates, to diagnose multiple pregnancy, to assess risk of spina bifida or Down's syndrome and to check the position of the placenta. An experienced operator may well be able to see what sex the baby is, especially on a scan done late in pregnancy. This information will be revealed only at the express wish of the parents.

Advantages

- It may help to establish an early bond between parent and baby.
- It can confirm an ongoing pregnancy after a heavy bleed.
- It can give an accurate assessment of the baby's age in the first trimester.
- It has fewer proven side-effects than amniocentesis or CVS and in skilled hands can accurately detect Down's and a number ofcongenital abnormalities.
- It is an essential part of amniocentesis or CVS, helping to guide the needle safely into the womb.

Disadvantages

- The long term side-effects are unknown.
- Use of frequent ultrasound has been linked to intrauterine growth retardation (IUGR).
- It may have a negative effect on neurological function, producing more left-handed babies and children with dyslexia and delayed speech.
- It is an invasive procedure for the baby; its shrill sound can cause pain and distress.
- Diagnosis of some conditions (e.g. placenta praevia) is 95% inaccurate (Thomas 1996).

Getting off the conveyor belt

The whole area of antenatal testing raises complex and emotive issues, and the decision for parents to test or not to test is fraught and often irrational. The concepts of risk, normality and imperfection will be viewed differently by different mothers in different situations. Support and counselling are vital to help a mother and her partner make the right choice for their own circumstances, especially if they choose to resist medical pressure and say 'no' to taking routine tests. After all, no test is 100% accurate. If a termination is not an option, then the best way of getting off the conveyor belt of antenatal testing with all its attendant risks is not to get on it in the first place.

Antenatal maternal infections

The baby is generally protected from infection by the sac surrounding it and by the placenta. However, certain micro-organisms can cross the placenta from the mother's blood. The most common of these are intrauterine infections: rubella, cytomegalovirus, toxoplasmosis and syphilis. The acronym 'TORCH' has been devised to list some of them.

T – toxoplasmosis
O – other, e.g. listeriosis, *Chlamydia*, chicken pox, parvovirus
R – rubella
C – cytomegalovirus
H – herpes

These infections can present in several ways. First, if severe, they can cause still birth or malformation. Second, if they are systemic they can cause anaemia, jaundice, purpura or enlarged liver or spleen. Third, they can affect the central nervous system, as in encephalitis or meningitis. Fourth, there may be mild skin and bone involvement. Finally, they may lead to intrauterine growth retardation.

Toxoplasmosis

This is the most serious infection in pregnancy. Toxoplasmosis is caused by a parasite called *Toxoplasma gondii.* It is contracted by eating or handling raw or undercooked meat or contact with infected cat faeces. The infection is passed across to the fetus from the placenta and the risk of infection to the developing fetus has been estimated at between 10% and 76% (RCOG 1992), increasing as the pregnancy progresses. The most serious consequences are seen in women between 10 and 24 weeks of pregnancy. Spontaneous abortion may occur in early pregnancy and the infection is also associated with miscarriage and stillbirth. Treatment of toxoplasmosis in pregnancy is complicated as the drugs used can also affect the fetus.

Rubella

This is very serious in the first trimester (Wang & Smaill 1989), with an 80% rate of infection in babies. Fetuses infected in the first 8 weeks run a high risk of abnormality, including eye defects and deafness. Spontaneous abortion may occur. Deafness can also occur with infection after 14 weeks. Intrauterine growth retardation is common and the baby may be born with abnormalities. It is important to note that a baby born with infection can excrete rubella in its urine for up to 10 years, and so can continue to be a risk to pregnant women.

Women are screened antenatally for rubella and are offered rubella vaccination if they do not have immunity.

Cytomegalovirus

Cytomegalovirus is caused by the herpes virus and is a common infection to acquire prenatally. Infection can occur at any time during pregnancy and may produce mild influenza-type symptoms. Over 50% of pregnant women are immune and of those who are not, only a small proportion will pass the infection to their baby. A blood test can confirm whether the infection is past or present.

Cytomegalovirus can lead to serious problems and in very severe cases will lead to still birth. It is a known risk factor associated with miscarriage and is implicated in causing mental retardation in infants.

Herpes

Herpes is caused by the herpes simplex virus type 2 and is transmitted through sexual intercourse. (Type 1 virus can cause genital infection but is usually associated with lesions of the face, lips and eyes.)

Herpes simplex infection of the newborn (neonate) is a serious disease, which may result from passage of the virus across the placenta or from direct contact with infectious lesions during delivery. The major risk to the fetus occurs after the first or primary infection. Recurrent disease is associated with a low risk to the fetus, even when genital lesions are present.

Symptoms of the type 2 virus include itching followed by a crop of blisters, which quickly become moist and ulcerated. The glands in the groin may swell and a slight fever may develop. The first infection presents with painful genital ulcers. Recurrences tend to be milder and shorter.

Routine screening for the virus during pregnancy is no longer recommended for those women who have had a primary infection in the past. In women who have a primary infection during pregnancy, screening to establish the diagnosis will be necessary. Diagnosis is confirmed by taking a swab from the area and having it cultured.

If the lesions are active or there is an outbreak of the infection prior to delivery, the baby may have to be delivered by caesarean section. However, this may not be necessary for recurrent herpes if there are no lesions or positive swabs at delivery.

Treatment includes painkillers to help relieve pain and drug therapy (generally a 5–7-day course of aciclovir). Aciclovir helps to reduce excretion of the virus, symptomatic recurrence and so the likelihood of a caesarean section.

Alternative remedies for herpes

- Ulcers can be bathed in homeopathic solutions such as Hypericum and Calendula. Use five drops of each in half a pint of boiled water 4–5 times a day to help to soothe the area. You can also buy Calendula in ointment form from most healthfood stores.
- Other homeopathic remedies, such as Natrum muriaticum 6c or Capsicum 6c, can be used but it is advisable to visit a homeopath to get the right help and remedy for you.
- Essential oils such as tea tree (5–15 drops) may be added directly to a bidet or bath.
- Acupuncture can be used to help boost the immune system, but it will not get rid of the underlying condition.

Listeriosis

Listeriosis usually results from the mother having eaten soft cheese or contaminated chicken. Infection in the first trimester often results in spontaneous abortion.

Chlamydia

Chlamydia trachomatis is now the most common sexually transmitted disease organism. It is particularly common amongst teenage girls. Treatment consists of antibiotic therapy. However, most people experience no symptoms, which makes it particularly insidious.

Stage 1 of the infection occurs between 1 and 3 weeks after sexual intercourse with an infected person, when an abnormal discharge and a burning sensation on passing urine may be experienced.

Stage 2 can occur several weeks or months after infection. In women it can cause pelvic inflammatory disease and it may result in infertility problems in both men and women. In pregnancy, infection is linked to premature birth, miscarriage and still birth. Babies born with clamydia may have low birthweight and suffer from conjunctivitis or pneumonia.

Chicken pox

Chicken pox in pregnancy is rare (one case in 2000 pregnancies). Most people in developed countries have had chicken pox at some time during childhood and have developed immunity. Where there is doubt or where there is concern about recent contact by a pregnant woman with someone infected by the virus, a blood test may be performed to check for past (immunoglobulin G level) or recent (immunoglobulin XI level) infection with the virus. Where immunity is in doubt, contact should be avoided.

The virus is spread from person to person. The carrier is highly infectious 2 days before the rash appears until 1 week after.

Generally, if a woman develops chicken pox in the middle part of pregnancy, there is little risk to the fetus. However, infection in the first trimester, and particularly the first 8 weeks of pregnancy, may cause birth defects in a minority of babies. During this time, the fetus is developing rapidly and by the end of the first 8 weeks all the baby's organs are fully formed. Any attack during this period is thus more likely to result in a problem. There is a recognised syndrome, the 'varicella syndrome', which consists of limb shortening, scarring, possible brain development problems and eye defects.

Primary infection in the mother in late pregnancy is associated with infection in newborns that is usually mild, but if infection occurs within 5 days of delivery then it may be severe. Giving immune therapy (immunoglobulin) to an infected mother or an infected baby reduces the risk.

Parvovirus

In childhood, human parvovirus causes erythema infectiosum or fifth disease, which is sometimes mistaken for rubella or German measles. It may also be called 'slapped face syndrome' because of the reddened appearance of a child's face.

Infection is commonly asymptomatic. In pregnancy, if the fetus is infected this causes anaemia and fluid retention or hydrops. In approximately half of all cases of fetal infection, miscarriage or still birth occurs but in the remainder the anaemia and hydrops resolve with no long-term adverse effects. There has been only one case report of a human fetus with a congenital abnormality after parvovirus infection.

Screening for parvovirus is not thought to be justified. However, the placenta from an unexplained still birth or late miscarriage should be checked for possible infection. In addition, where there is clinical suspicion (e.g. contact with an infected child), a blood test will demonstrate a past infection (and thus immunity) or a recent infection, with potential problems to the developing fetus.

Strengthening the immune system and building up immunity

Foods rich in vitamin C or a vitamin C supplement will boost the immune system and help to fight viruses.

Acupuncture treatment to strengthen the immune system

The model of the immune system in Western medicine is a complicated one. In Chinese medicine, the immune system depends on whether the protective Qi is strong and able to ward off viruses and climatic influences such as colds and flu (on an exterior level) and more serious disease (on a deeper level).

POINTS TO TREAT

- **ST-36 has been shown in animal studies to raise the white cell count.**
- **GV-14 has been shown to enhance phagocytic activity.**

If a patient has any concerns about infections, she should contact her midwife or doctor.

Summary

- Antenatal visits include: confirmation of pregnancy and referral by GP (about 6 weeks), 'booking-in' visit (8–12 weeks), then visits every 4 weeks to 32 weeks, every 2 weeks between 32 and 36 weeks, and finally every week from 36 weeks.
- At the booking-in visit, the following are recorded: weight, blood pressure, previous obstetric history, and blood and urine tests.
- At subsequent visits the following are recorded: blood pressure, abdominal examination, urine analysis and oedema (to check for PIH).
- Tests for fetal abnormalities include: nuchal scan, AFP test, amniocentesis, Bart's test/triple test, CVS and ultrasound scan.
- Techniques to palpate the uterus and baby include: inspection, palpation and auscultation.
- Possible maternal infections to be aware of ('TORCH') include: **t**oxoplasmosis, **o**ther (e.g. syphilis, listeriosis, *Chlamydia*, chicken pox, parvovirus), **r**ubella, **c**ytomegalovirus and **h**erpes.
- Acupuncture points in the antenatal period generally include ST-36, GV-14 to boost the immune system.

References

Assel B, Lewis SM, Dickerman LH 1992 Single operator comparison of early and mid trimester amniocentesis. Obstetrics and Gynecology 79(6): 940–944

Cuckle HS, Wold NJ 1990 Screening for Down's syndrome prenatal diagnosis and prognosis. Butterworth, London.

Firth H, Boyd PA, Chamberlain P et al 1991 Severe limb abnormalities after chorionic villus sampling at 56–66 days' gestation. Lancet 337: 762–763

Hanson FW, Tennant F, Hune S, Brookhyser K 1992 Early amniocentesis outcome risks and technical problems at <12.8 weeks. American Journal of Obstetrics and Gynecology 166(6, pt1): 1707–1711

Hogge JS, Hogge WA, Golbus MS 1986 Chorionic villus sampling. Journal of Obstetrics, Gynaecology and Neonatal Nursing Jan/Feb: 24–28

MacLachlan NA 1992 Amniocentesis. In: Brock DJH (ed.) Alphafetoprotein and acetylcholinesterase prenatal diagnosis and screening. Churchill Livingstone, New York

Marteau TM, Slack J, Kidd J 1992 Presenting a routine screening test in antenatal care. Public Health 106: 131–141

Mikkelsson M, Neilson KB 1992 Prenatal diagnosis and screening. Churchill Livingstone, New York

RCOG (Royal College of Gynaecologists) 1992 Pre-natal screening for toxoplasmosis in the UK. RCOG, London

Sweet BR (ed.) 1997 Mayes' midwifery, 12th edn. Baillière Tindall, New York, pp 2–3, 218, 223, 224–225, 227

Symonds EM, Symonds IM 1997 Essential obstetrics and gynaecology. Churchill Livingstone, Edinburgh

Thomas P 1996 Every woman's birth rights. Thorsons, London

Thompson PJ, Greenough A, Nicolaides KH 1993 Lung volume measured by functional residual capacity in infants following first trimester amniocentesis or chorionic villus sampling. British Journal of Obstetrics and Gynaecology 99: 479–482

Wang F, Smaill F 1989 Infection in pregnancy. Oxford University Press, Oxford

Further reading

Kitzinger S 1974 The experience of childbirth. Penguin, London, pp 102, 227, 228

5 First trimester: 1 to 12 weeks

Chapter outline

During the first trimester of her pregnancy, a woman very often feels, well, downright lousy! Symptoms are many and various, including an overwhelming tiredness, a constant hunger, a craving for odd things to eat, an aversion to foods previously enjoyed, a mouth full of saliva or an unpleasant metallic taste, and nausea and sickness, often just in the morning but in some cases lasting all day.

Anatomy and physiology

Within 7 days of implantation of the fertilised egg in the lining of the uterus, human chorionic gonadotrophin (HCG) will start to be produced. The blastocyst now develops into an embryo and begins to form a placenta.

By week 4, the fetus is just visible to the naked eye. It is about 4 mm long and weighs less than 1 gram.

By week 8, the fetus is the size of a small strawberry and all its systems have developed, ready to mature over the next 7 months.

By week 12, the fetus will be recognisably human although only about 6.5 cm. The placenta will be fully formed.

Morning sickness

Common causes

The causes of morning sickness are unknown. It is thought it may be due to high levels of HCG, which is secreted by the placenta, and to progesterone released by the ovaries. In some women, the problem is so severe that it causes a condition called hyperemesis or excess vomiting (Weigel & Weigel 1989, Whitehead et al 1992). Seventy to ninety percent of all pregnant women experience some form of nausea (Sweet 1997). Although there is a great deal of research on the subject, no firm conclusions can be drawn as to what causes it.

If a patient suffers from any of the symptoms listed below, she should take advice from her GP or midwife. Practitioners should enquire whether a patient suffers such symptoms and be cautious if she does.

If the patient is being sick several times a day there is a danger of dehydration and she should always seek help. The clinical findings of dehydration are: weight loss, a rising pulse rate (above 120 bpm), low blood pressure, loss of skin elasticity as a result of dehydration, a dry, furry tongue, infrequent passing of urine, and ketotic breath, smelling like nail varnish or pear drops.

Other causes of sickness

There are certain conditions of pregnancy that can make the nausea and vomiting worse. None is particularly common but their diagnosis should be considered in severe cases. They include: hydatidiform mole, multiple pregnancies, which make greater physical demands on the mother, pregnancy-induced hypertension (PIH), hydramnios and placental abruption.

Hydatidiform mole

A hydatidiform mole is very rare and is found in only about one per 2000 pregnancies (Sweet 1997). Placental tissue develops in the same way as in a potential miscarriage, as a 'blighted ovum', where part of the pregnancy cells grow in the absence of the fetus. In this case, the chorionic villi do not develop normally so that large quantities of the hormone HCG can be produced, which gives a very positive pregnancy test. The mole is usually described as looking like a tiny bunch of grapes, which are in fact cysts.

The extremely high levels of HCG cause considerable pregnancy sickness and abdominal swelling. A molar pregnancy should therefore be considered if a patient has severe sickness, is much bigger than expected for her dates and suffers intermittent bleeding.

Treatment involves hospitalisation to remove the mole and careful monitoring of blood and urine samples for the following 2 years or so, in order to check that no malignancy has developed.

Symptoms associated with morning sickness

Morning sickness is linked to the digestive system and can affect the other senses of smell, taste and touch. Some women feel nausea just from the stimulus of things they see and handle. Others find that altering position, for example between sitting and standing, can make them feel sick.

There is a strong link between sickness and the dreadful fatigue that a woman gets in early pregnancy. Symptoms associated with morning sickness (Whitehead et al 1992) include: cravings, food aversions, pica, metallic taste, intense hunger, heartburn, belching, excess salivation or ptyalism, smell and tiredness.

Craving

This is the desire to eat particular foods. It is sometimes overwhelming, and may be for something which the patient does not usually like but which her body is demanding. The craving may indicate that she is lacking something nutritionally.

Food aversion

As well as craving certain foods, many women feel an aversion to foods they have previously enjoyed, such as tea, coffee or toast. This is often put down to the action of hormones in part of the brain known as the chemoreceptor trigger zone (Whitehead et al 1992), which is associated with vomiting and with taste aversion.

Pica

This is the desire to eat something inedible, traditionally a frequently recognised symptom of pregnancy.

Metallic taste

This is typically a very unpleasant, copper-like taste that occurs in the early weeks of pregnancy. It can range from moderate to severe, spoiling the sense of taste, giving rise to nausea and making all food taste unpleasant.

Intense hunger

Responding immediately to urges to eat may keep nausea at bay for a while, or may make the sufferer feel sick straight away.

Heartburn

This is one of the standard miseries of pregnancy and is often associated with the later stages. It can, however, be present in the early stages as a burning sensation associated with sickness.

Burping or belching

This is caused by excess gas from the stomach, which gives an unpleasant sensation of fullness and nausea.

Excess salivation or ptyalism

This occurs when saliva output increases to the extent that it becomes difficult to swallow.

Smell

As well as suffering changes in taste, the sense of smell can also be impaired. Most distressingly, foods that previously smelled pleasant to the sufferer, such as toast, can now smell abhorrent.

Tiredness and fatigue

These are sometimes extreme and are very common in early pregnancy. This can be overwhelming, particularly in a first pregnancy, and especially when the sufferer is still having to work or to look after young children. There is a link between pregnancy sickness and tiredness.

Western medical treatment of morning sickness

Women are reluctant to take drugs in pregnancy, especially in early pregnancy, because of possible effects on the baby. It is important for you as an acupuncturist to know what doctors may be advising your patients.

Drug treatments

Antihistamines such as promethazine, hydrochloride, Phenergan, promethazine theoclate and Avomine are recommended in doses of 20–50 mg orally, with or without 10–20 mg of pyridoxine. The usual dose for oral metoclopramide and Maxolon is 10 mg three times a day.

If a woman has hyperemesis, diagnosed by the presence of ketones, weight loss or dehydration, she is usually admitted to hospital for correction of her fluid and electrolyte imbalance. She will often be administered vitamins via a drip, will be put on bedrest and will sometimes be given sedation. These sedatives might include Phenergan 25 mg, promazine (Sparine) 50 mg, chloromazine, and Largactil 25–50 mg, all of which may be administered via a drip. Stemitil 25 mg can also be given, as an injection three times a day or rectally as a suppository.

Side-effects

The British Medical Journal and others recommend treating nausea and vomiting in pregnancy with Valoid, which is widely used and appears to be safe. However, GPs are often reluctant to treat sickness occurring during pregnancy (Gadsby 2004). There has been concern about the association of the use of drugs with congenital malformations such as cleft lip or palate, although this has never been substantiated. There may, however, be a weak association between meclozine and congenital eye defects. Promazine may be associated with an increase in congenital hip dislocation.

The mother might as a side-effect experience dry mouth, blurred vision and drowsiness. Side-effects of metoclopramide might include drowsiness, restlessness, diarrhoea and depression, but at low dosages these are described as unusual. Phenothiazines have similar side-effects for the mother; studies into effects on the baby are inconclusive (Howden 1986).

Chinese viewpoint of morning sickness

During pregnancy, huge changes take place in the Directing and Penetrating Vessels. The Blood Essence and Kidney energy of the mother are required to nourish the fetus, which leads to a deficiency of Blood and a hyperactivity of Yang in the mother, and the circulation of Qi, both ascending and descending, is disturbed by the growing fetus. Most women adapt to these changes but where there is a constitutional weakness, or emotional or lifestyle problems prior to the pregnancy, sickness may develop. The three organs that most commonly affect the flow of Qi in pregnancy are the Spleen, the Liver and the Kidneys (see below, The common patterns of disharmony, pp. 79–82).

The Penetrating Vessel is linked to the Stomach, and in my experience nausea is always associated with some sort of Stomach disharmony. The Stomach and Spleen are the root of the postnatal Qi and Blood production. In pregnancy, Blood accumulates in the Chong and Ren channels to nourish the fetus. The Chong channel sends Blood down to the Uterus but until the fetus is more developed, it cannot make use of it all, so that the Blood accumulates. The Chong channel is connected to the Yang Ming, which helps the Stomach Qi to descend. The Chong and Yang Ming channels are connected at ST-30. If the Stomach and Spleen are weak to begin with, Blood and Qi will counterflow upwards, resulting in nausea.

Emotions

Emotions strongly affect morning sickness because of their links to particular organs.

Anger. Anger causes Liver Qi stagnation. When the cause of anger is repressed frustration and resentment, it leads to Liver Qi stagnation which affects the Spleen, causing diarrhoea. The Stomach is also affected, as Stomach Qi is prevented from descending, causing obstruction, epigastric pain, belching and nausea. The influence of the Liver on the Stomach is frequently seen in patterns of disharmony of the Stomach.

Worry. Worry affects the Spleen and the Stomach and causes stagnation of Qi and retention of food. The Stomach and the Spleen are also adversely affected by overexertion, which leads to dull pain, tiredness and weak muscles. Overwork, both when it is mentally taxing and when it involves long hours, can cause deficiency of Stomach Yin. Irregular eating habits over several years can have a similar effect. Constitutional weakness is also a potential cause of stomach disorders, and is often an inherited trait.

Fear. Fear can cause sinking of Qi, which inhibits the Kidney's ability to control the Chong and Ren channels. Because these are vital in nourishing the fetus, there is a strong risk of miscarriage.

These effects are summarised in Box 5.1.

Box 5.1 Effect of emotions on organs

- **Worry affects the Stomach and Spleen: if the Spleen cannot transform or transport, Damp occurs. Long-term Dampness leads to turbid Phlegm.**
- **Anger affects the Liver: Liver Qi stagnation accumulates, turns to Fire, leading to Heat signs, and eventually to Yin deficiency.**
- **Fear affects the Kidney: Kidneys nourish the fetus with Jing. If deficient, Yin is deficient and Yang rises, causing a counterflow of Stomach Qi.**

Other factors

Other factors that the practitioner should be aware of that cause some women to be sicker than others include the following.

- *IVF (in vitro fertilisation) pregnancies*: many women enter pregnancy with Kidney deficiency problems, and the drugs used in IVF treatments can weaken the system further in this respect.
- *Older mothers*: in older women the Jing is becoming weakened because of their age.
- *Too short a gap between pregnancies*: this gives insufficient time to recover, leaving Blood Qi deficiency and weakened Essence Jing.
- *Heavy periods prior to pregnancy*: these are likely to cause Blood deficiency.
- *Long-standing chronic conditions*: these may cause Kidney deficiency.

These subjects are discussed in more detail in other chapters.

Acupuncture for early pregnancy

Morning sickness

Diagnosis

In diagnosing morning sickness there are important questions to ask, as follows.

1. At what time of day does the sickness occur?
   - If it is in the morning, Deficiency is indicated.
   - If it is in the afternoon, Stagnation is indicated.
2. Are any pains or dull aches present?
   - Severe pain indicates Excess.
   - Dull pain indicates Deficiency.
   - Distending pain indicates stagnation and any burning pain indicates Heat.
   - Any feeling of fullness indicates Dampness.
3. How does eating affect the sickness?
   - I would want to know whether the sickness is better after eating, as this indicates Deficiency.
   - If it was worse after eating, it would indicate Excess.
4. How does activity affect the sickness?
   - If it is better with rest, Deficiency is indicated.
   - If it is better with slight exercise, Stagnation of Qi is indicated.
   - If it is better after vomiting, Excess is indicated.
   - If it is worse after vomiting, Deficiency is indicated.
5. What is the nausea like?
   - If the nausea is slight it may indicate Deficiency.
   - Vomiting soon after eating indicates Excess.
   - Vomiting a little while after eating indicates Deficiency.
   - Vomiting of food indicates Excess.
   - Vomiting of thin fluids indicates Deficiency.
   - Sour vomiting indicates an invasion of the Stomach by the Liver.
6. What is being vomited?
   - What a patient is regurgitating is important. Undigested food indicates Excess.
   - Watery fluids indicate Deficiency.
   - A sour regurgitation indicates Liver Qi in the Stomach.
   - Retention of food indicates Stagnation of Qi.
7. Is there any thirst?
   - If a patient was intensely thirsty and wanted to drink cold fluids, Heat would be indicated.
   - If a patient has a dry mouth and desires to sip fluids, Empty-Heat would be indicated.
   - Absence of thirst indicates Cold.
   - Thirst without desire to drink indicates Damp-Heat.
8. What is the sense of taste like?
   - A sticky taste can be Damp.
   - Bitter taste can be Heat.
   - Sweet taste can be Damp-Heat.

- Sour taste can be retention of food.
- Absence of taste can be Spleen deficiency.

Treatment and treatment planning

The main aims of treatment are to subdue rebellious Qi, to harmonise the Stomach, and to stop the vomiting. At the same time, any other patterns of disharmony that the mother may have should be treated: the severity of sickness will depend on any pre-existing patterns of disharmony.

Depending on the severity of the sickness, 4–6 treatments should be enough to get the patient stable. Ideally three treatments should be given in the first week, two in the second, and then weekly as necessary, though a practitioner's schedule may make this difficult. The aim of treatment is to pacify the Stomach and stop the vomiting. Use no more than 4–6 needles and no moxa, because to do so can increase uterine Qi.

When I first started treating morning sickness, the only points I used were taken from prescriptions in various texts, and from observations of other practitioners. Little tends to be said about needling technique, except to tonify for a deficiency and reduce for an excess condition. However, I feel that pregnancy requires a gentler technique: putting in the needle, finding the Deqi and leaving it in for about 10 minutes. This will help me to gauge the constitution of my patient, and her reaction to needles. In subsequent treatments I would then be happier to leave needles in longer.

In this sense needling is more to do with the patient's comfort and reaction than with the treatment itself, and for me the key is to gain a very clear concept of the changes I want to achieve in my patient and to guide the treatment accordingly. As long as the right points are needled, the body will generally use the stimulus to draw what it needs from the treatment.

Treating morning sickness can be difficult because of the very varying manifestations of symptoms between individuals, and the variations in each patient's past health. For this reason you should use the prescriptive treatments that you may read in the texts with careful thought for the specific circumstances of your patient. I have had most success by making my treatments as simple as possible and by not looking for complicated syndromes. The points that I list here are commonly used ones that I have found to be beneficial.

Moxa

I am wary of using moxa in pregnancy because it can increase body Heat, when pregnancy is a condition that is likely to be generating internal Heat in any case. However, in a deficient/cold conjoint, such as Stomach Qi deficiency with Empty-Cold, moxa would be appropriate. If the patient is very weak, deficient or needle phobic, moxa cones are very useful alternatives to needles, applied to the needling points; CV-12 is especially effective.

Recent research

In 2002, Smith et al presented two papers on the outcome of a randomised controlled trial on 593 pregnant women who were less than 14 weeks pregnant and complaining of morning sickness. One article (Smith et al 2002a) reviewed the efficacy of acupuncture and the other the safety of acupuncture as a treatment for morning sickness (Smith et al 2002b). The women were split into four groups.

- Traditional acupuncture treatments: pattern differentiations used were Liver Qi stagnation, Stomach or Spleen deficiency, Stomach Heat, Phlegm, Heart Qi deficiency and Heart Fire.
- Acupuncture at PC-6 only.
- Sham acupuncture: points needled close to but not on acupuncture points.
- No acupuncture.

Results

The outcome was that all the treatment groups showed less nausea than those women who had no treatment. The traditional acupuncture groups showed less nausea in the first week of treatment, and the PC-6 only group from the second week of treatment. By the third week the sham acupuncture group showed less nausea. Perinatal outcome showed no difference in all four study groups so it was deemed that acupuncture in early pregnancy was thought to be a safe and effective treatment for nausea.

A more recent pilot study on acupuncture and acupressure at PC-6 in the treatment of hyperemesis gravidarum (HG) showed positive results (Habek et al 2004). However, this was a small study and HG is a serious complication and care must be taken in the treatment of these women.

POINTS TO TREAT

- ***PC-6*: this is the point that has been most researched for its use in relieving nausea, not only for pregnancy but also for postoperative sickness. It helps to relax the chest and diaphragm and to ease the sickness by removing stagnant Qi in the Upper and Middle Jiao. It is the mainstay of morning sickness treatments, and is a good point to combine with other points according to the patient's history.**
- ***ST-36*: this point works very well in deficient conditions and for patterns of rebellious Stomach Qi. It is good combined with PC-6 and CV-12.**
- ***CV-10*: this is the crossing point of the Conception and Spleen channels. One of its functions is to control the cardiac sphincter at the entrance to the stomach, so that it is an effective point to use to help retention of food in the Stomach, in combination with PC-6.**
- ***CV-12*: this corresponds to the centre of energy for the Spleen, and is good for nausea caused by deficient Spleen and Stomach conditions. Use moxa if the deficiency is accompanied by Cold. The point is good for rebellious Stomach Qi.**
- ***CV-14*: this helps the Qi to descend from the Collecting point of the Heart. It is good to use if there are a lot of emotional problems.**
- ***ST-19 or 20*: I use this in combination with KI-21, especially for patterns of the Stomach where the patient feels fullness or blockage in the epigastrium that is relieved by vomiting.**
- ***ST-21*: this, combined with ST-44 for Stomach Heat, is beneficial.**
- ***ST-34*: this is the Accumulation point of the Stomach, which I use if there are excess Stomach conditions. It is especially good in combination with PC-6 for excess vomiting in pregnancy.**
- ***ST-40*: this is used in combination with PC-6, especially where there is a lot of Phlegm.**
- ***KI-21*: I find this excellent in an emergency combined with ST-19.**
- ***SP-4 on the right and PC-6 on the left*: this is a prescription (Maciocia 1998) that I have used very effectively for women with very persistent conditions, where other points have not been making any significant improvement. I would use it as a last resort because I feel that it is a strong treatment.**

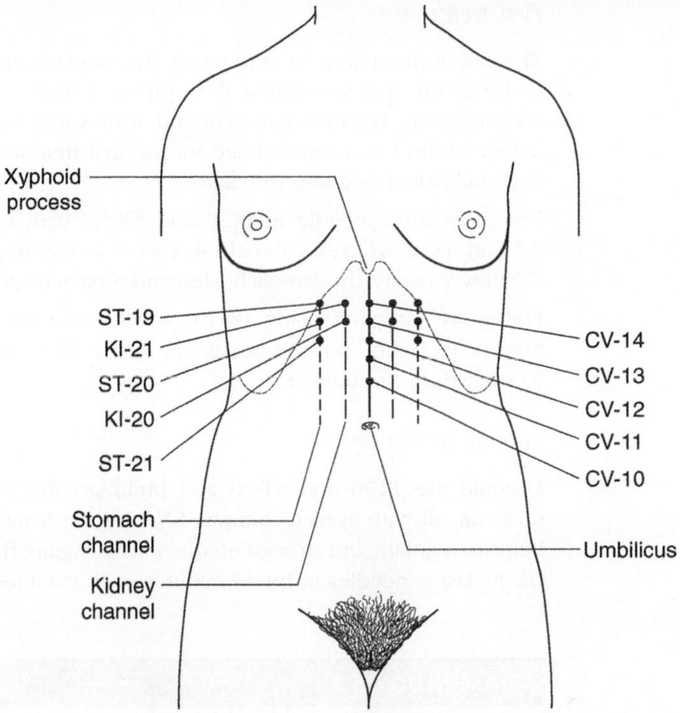

Figure 5.1 Main abdominal points used for morning sickness. (Reproduced with permission from Maciocia 1998, p. 453.)

Some of these points are illustrated in Figure 5.1.

The common patterns of disharmony

Main pattern - Stomach and Spleen deficiency

If the Stomach and Spleen are weak to begin with, Qi and Blood accumulate in the Chong and counterflow upwards, causing nausea. The Spleen generates and transforms the Blood after conception when there is an increased demand for Blood to nourish the fetus. When the Stomach and Spleen are weak they are unable to do this, causing a counterflow upwards. If there is an existing weakness prior to conception then poor diet, worry and fatigue will aggravate the condition in pregnancy.

The clinical manifestations of Stomach and Spleen disharmony may include nausea, vomiting, poor appetite, abdominal distension and fatigue. Weakness and lethargy are signs of Stomach/Spleen deficiency. Characteristically the patient will report feeling better after eating and with rest, but her sickness is likely to feel worse in the morning. Typically she looks weak and miserable, and moves slowly; her tongue will be pale with a white coating, and she will have a loose, rolling pulse.

With deficiency, the needle technique seeks to reinforce the points used. For a pattern of Stomach and Spleen weakness, I will end a treatment by tonifying or reinforcing points such as BL-20 or 21 to treat the underlying Stomach or Spleen weakness. I put the needle in, reach the Deqi, rotate the needle and remove it. I may also moxa the point before removing the needle; I find that this achieves very good pulse changes.

First treatment

The aim of the treatment is to pacify the Stomach and descend the flow of Qi, and to boost Qi and strengthen the Spleen. I leave the needle in no longer than 10 minutes for the first treatment and always use even technique with no manipulation. Caution is recommended for the first treatment as you cannot be sure how each individual is going to react.

Use a 34-gauge needle in PC-6 and ST-36, with even technique, to a depth of 0.5 cun. PC-6 will relax the chest, ease the diaphragm and help with the nausea. ST-36 will pacify the Stomach, descend Stomach Qi, and strengthen the spleen.

Follow by tonifying using BL-20, which treats the underlying weakness of the Spleen. To tonify, put the needle in, turn it 180°, then remove it. The intention is to strengthen the Spleen.

Second treatment

I would use PC-6 and ST-36 and build up the treatment, with CV-12 inserted 0.75 cun, all with even technique. CV-12 is the front low point of the Stomach and helps to regulate and strengthen the Spleen. Again, finish the treatment by tonifying BL-20. Leave needles in for 30 minutes, with even technique and no manipulation.

CASE STUDY 5.1

Kate, now 13 weeks' pregnant, started to be sick even before she had missed her period. She would be sick on waking, would force down a bowl of cereal and bring that back an hour and a half later. She suffered the same routine at lunchtime and felt nauseated all the time. She was terribly lethargic and was not sleeping well because she had a 2-year-old child who was waking at night. The nausea felt better when she was lying down, and after rest. She looked pale, weak and miserable, and clearly felt wretched. She was tearful and couldn't be bothered to talk.

These symptoms indicated to me a deficiency of Stomach and Spleen, so that her treatment was aimed at pacifying the Stomach and strengthening the Spleen. I treated her twice weekly, leaving the needless in after the initial treatment for 30–45 minutes.

- Treatment 1: PC-6, ST-36, even technique; BL-17 and 20, tonify
- Treatment 2: PC-6, ST-36, CV-12, even technique; BL-17 and 20, tonify
- Treatment 3: PC-6, ST-36, CV-12, even technique; BL-17 and 20, tonify
- Treatment 4: PC-6, SP-4, even technique; BL-17, and 20, tonify

After her fourth treatment, Kate was visibly different, even actually smiling! Between treatments, Kate used a TENS machine, stimulating PC-6.

Third treatment

I would expect there to be an improvement after treatment, but if you feel that this is insufficient, add Penetrating Vessel points PC-6 and SP-4. I find this combination excellent in cases of rebellious Qi. It moves Blood and Qi and is the link between Preheaven and Postnatal Qi. It is very good used for weak constitution, digestive symptoms and poor appetite. The eight meridians will relax the chest, ease the diaphragm and stop vomiting.

Finish by tonifying BL-20.

Further treatments

Continue to pacify the Stomach and strengthen the Spleen.

Disharmony of the Liver and Stomach

The second most common disharmony related to morning sickness is that of the Liver and Stomach. It is generally believed that there has to be some sort of Liver Qi stagnation to prevent the energy moving and affecting the fetus. The Liver stores the Blood, the smooth flow of Qi, and this is the most important part of all the Liver functions. Liver Qi moves upwards and outwards in all directions and can affect all the other organs, which explains the importance of its function. The Liver helps the Spleen to transform and the Stomach to rot and ripen food. Liver Qi also helps the Spleen Qi to ascend and the Stomach Qi to descend.

Causes of Liver and Stomach disharmony can be due to long-term emotional problems.

Clinical manifestations may include nausea, a bitter taste in the mouth, the bringing up of bile, fullness in the chest, abdominal and hypochondrial pain, restlessness and thirst. Of these, the bitter taste and hypochondrial pain are the clearest clue to Liver/Stomach disharmony. The aim of the treatment is to regulate the Qi, harmonise the Middle Jiao and stop the vomiting.

CASE STUDY 5.2

Sarah was 7 weeks' pregnant and suffering from severe morning sickness. This had been a much longed for pregnancy, she had tried naturally to conceive for 3 years. Sarah had IVF treatment and conceived in the first treatment. She had had regular acupuncture through her IVF cycle and always showed signs of Liver Qi stagnation.

She presented with vomiting of bitter-tasting fluids, and was very thirsty, restless and irritable. She also stated that she had 'great waves of sadness' and felt terrible because her husband was so excited over the pregnancy and she could not share his joy.

Her sickness was due to Liver Qi invading the Stomach, but there was also some Liver Fire causing her thirst. Her restlessness and irritability came from stagnant Liver Qi interrupting Stomach Qi from descending. The stagnation of her Liver Qi was causing her to vomit bitter fluids.The heat from all the stagnation was having an effect on her Heart Qi, causing the depression.

The following points helped to quell her sickness.

- PC-6 bilaterally with even technique, to stop the vomiting and pacify the stomach
- GB-34 with even technique, to move the stagnant Liver Qi
- CV-12 with even technique, to help the Stomach Qi descend
- ST-36 tonified
- GV-20 tonified to raise the Qi and lift her mood
- CV-14 tonified to nourish the Heart Qi

By the time Sarah was 12 weeks' pregnant the nausea had lifted but she remained sad with very low mood swings. I recommended that she speak with her midwife and doctor. She was referred to a psychiatrist and continued her acupuncture treatment weekly. Sarah is now 20 weeks' pregnant. The counselling has helped her realise that not all pregnant women are in a state of joy and although her moods are not as high as before pregnancy, she is content.

First treatment

Use PC-6 to remove the obstruction, and LR-3 to soothe the Liver, using even technique. Tonify BL-17 and 19. Use a 1-inch (2.5 cm) 34-gauge needle, inserted to 0.5 cun for 10 minutes.

Second treatment

Use PC-6, LR-3 and ST-36, using even technique and leaving the needles in for 30–45 minutes. In severe cases, I have left the needles in for up to an hour. Tonify BL-17.

Third treatment

Continue using the same points until you see an improvement in the sickness.

These are the two patterns of disharmony in pregnancy that I most frequently treat. Every patient is an individual, and will enter pregnancy in a different state of health. I have found that keeping the points simple has produced the most effective results.

POINTS TO TREAT

Use the basic points, PC-6, ST-36 and LR-3, and add points only where particular syndromes suggest, as listed below.

- **ST-40 if there are signs of Phlegm and Damp**
- **ST-44 and 21 if there is a lot of Stomach Heat**
- **LI-11: combine with ST-44 for general Heat**
- **CV-13 for acute excess Stomach conditions**
- **GB-34 if there is a lot of Liver Qi stagnation**
- **CV-12 with KI-21: an emergency treatment if the patient cannot stop vomiting**
- **ST-34 if there is retention of food (this is the Accumulation point of the Stomach)**
- **ST-21 and CV-13 is a good combination**

Disharmony of the Liver and Gall Bladder

A third pattern of disharmony is that between the Liver and Gall Bladder. The clinical manifestations of a disharmony of the Liver and the Gall Bladder vary in severity. The most common symptoms are nausea and bile, which may be accompanied by depression and irritability. Sometimes there is a fullness or heavy feeling in the chest, or hypochondriac pain. Needles are left in, with reducing technique and with the intention of clearing the stagnation.

First treatment

As for Liver/Stomach disharmony, use PC-6 to remove the obstruction and LR-3 to soothe the Liver, using even technique.

Second treatment

Again as for Liver/Stomach disharmony, use PC-6, LR-3 and ST-36, using even technique.

Third treatment

Depending on any improvement, use points such as:

- LR-14 with even technique for hypochondrial pain
- ST-34 Accumulation point for acute patterns of sickness
- GB-34 to move Liver Qi stagnation.

Again, I would end a treatment by tonifying and removing the needles on points such as BL-19 to strengthen the Liver and underlying weakness.

Hyperemesis gravidarum

This is a severe form of vomiting, which usually begins in the first 10 weeks of pregnancy and is thought to affect 5–10 women in every thousand. Mothers who suffer from it in one pregnancy are very likely to suffer again in following pregnancies. However, there are many measures that can be taken preconceptually to help avoid it (see Ch. 3).

Hyperemesis is defined as persistent vomiting, which interferes with nutrient fluid and causes electrolyte imbalance. It can be very serious and may require the woman to be hospitalised and to receive intravenous fluids. (See Signs of clinical dehydration on p. 72.) A woman who has suffered from it is often very nervous about the potential effects from another pregnancy, especially on the baby itself. It is important that she understands that the baby will continue to get all the nutrients it needs from her, and that this in part is why the condition can be so debilitating for her.

There is very little written about the long-term effects of hyperemesis on the mother although, on the positive side, studies have shown that women suffering hyperemesis have less chance of miscarriage.

CASE STUDY 5.3

Lauren was 28. Most of her first pregnancy had been spent in hospital with hyperemesis; she was admitted eight times between week 5 and week 18. An abiding memory of her first pregnancy was that at 12 weeks she had felt so ill that she had wanted a termination. Such thoughts are certainly not uncommon for women suffering from hyperemesis. Although she wanted to have a second child, she was desperately worried that the same thing would happen again.

She came to see me because she had heard acupuncture could help and she wanted treatment before she got pregnant again. Though I told her I could offer no guarantees, she was only too happy to give it a try.

She was Kidney Yang deficient so I needled points on the Chong Mai and also lots of warming Kidney points:

- BL 23 with moxa
- GV-4
- CV-4
- BL-17.

I also encouraged her to take vitamin B6 and zinc.

I gave her weekly treatments for 3 months before she conceived. The pregnancy followed the same pattern of feeling nauseated.

The points I concentrated on were PC-6 and ST-36, and BL-17 and 23, giving twice-weekly treatments. She also continued to supplement her diet with vitamin B6 and zinc.

Lauren felt terrible and was admitted to hospital twice in the first 12 weeks. But compared with her first pregnancy there was a vast improvement and, importantly, she felt that she was coping. She carried on with weekly acupuncture treatments throughout the 9 months – a good example of preventive medicine.

As well as severe vomiting,12 times a day or more, a patient with hyperemesis may find it impossible to keep down any food at all, and may become dehydrated. Most of the women with hyperemesis that I see on the ward are really dehydrated, vomiting excessively and with a drip up.

POINTS TO TREAT

In cases like this, a good treatment would be PC-6, although you will probably be able to get the needle into only one arm, as the drip will be in the other one. If the patient is bringing up a lot of bile, add LR-3, CV-12 and KI-21 and leave the needles in for up to 60 minutes. This can really help to relieve them.

Other treatment

According to the ancient texts, the acupuncture point KI-9 is said to block adverse hereditary patterns and produce a child who will sleep through the night. Treatment should be by needling once at 3 months of pregnancy and once at 6 months.

Diet and nutrition

Most women suffering from sickness in pregnancy find that bland carbohydrates, such as rice, baked potatoes, pasta, scones, bananas, rusks, porridge and dry toast, are foods that they can tolerate. 'Little and often' is the rule, and such foods should be taken every hour or two, for instance snacks of fruit and seeds. This way they can avoid the daunting prospect of a full meal, while maintaining a reasonably steady blood sugar level. It has also been suggested that taking drinks separately from meals is likely to make a sufferer feel less sick.

It is quite acceptable to indulge cravings, even though women may feel guilty that some of the food they are eating is unhealthy. It is important to carry on eating adequately, and it is much worse if a patient chooses to eat nothing rather than the 'wrong' thing.

A list of foods to avoid is given in Box 5.2. Other dietary pointers that can help include the following.

- Ginger has been used for centuries to ease nausea in early pregnancy, probably because it is a rich source of zinc. It can be used in cooking or in drinks, teas or biscuits.
- Drink plenty of water and avoid tea and coffee.
- Concentrated sugar (even in the form of dried fruit or concentrated fruit juice) should be avoided.
- Avoid fatty and strong-smelling food, high-fat junk food and anything containing lots of preservatives and additives.

- Always eat breakfast, preferably containing some protein such as eggs or yoghurt.

Box 5.2 Things to avoid if you are feeling sick

- Greasy or fried food
- Cooking: some women cannot bear the smell but are happy to eat if food is cooked for them
- Bad smells
- Coffee and caffeine, coke or tea: all of these can make people feel unwell
- Routine iron preparations: some iron tablets, prescribed routinely for pregnant women, can add to the nausea and constipation
- Brushing teeth: this can often be problematic, making some women gag. It may be advisable to clean teeth at a time of day when the nausea has abated. Dental hygiene is important in pregnancy as gum disease is more prevalent

Supplements

It is thought that morning sickness may be indicative of marginal nutritional deficiency in vitamins and minerals. Vomiting will further deplete reserves, and a vicious circle of cause and effect can set in. The following nutrients are especially important (Czeizel et al 1992).

Vitamin B6

Vitamin B deficiency is associated with anxiety, malaise and depression. There has been controversy about B6 (Tuormaa 1998). Even so, for women who have suffered from hyperemesis in the past, it is a good idea to boost intake of vitamin B6 before attempting another pregnancy. If taken in doses of 25 mg orally, every 8 hours for 72 hours, this has been shown to have a significant effect, reducing nausea and vomiting in women with severe pregnancy sickness symptoms. A double-blind randomised controlled trial of 59 women showed that it helped those whose nausea and vomiting symptoms rated more than 7 on a scale of 0–10, but it was no more effective than a placebo for those who were not badly affected (Sahakian et al 1991).

The maximum recommended dosage in pregnancy is 100 mg daily but it is preferable to take B6 as part of a B complex, because B6 taken in isolation can upset the balance of the other B vitamins (Czeizel et al 1992). Good food sources to maintain B6 levels are sesame seeds, chick peas, bananas, sweetcorn, raisins and hazelnuts.

Magnesium

Magnesium stores are diminished by vomiting, and magnesium deficiency can exacerbate nausea so that magnesium-rich foods such as nuts, pumpkin seeds, beans, wheatgerm, avocado and broccoli can be important in the diet.

Potassium

In the same way, potassium can be diminished, and potassium-rich foods include dried apricots, bananas, melons, figs and fruit juices such as orange and pineapple.

Zinc

Zinc requirements increase during pregnancy, and zinc deficiency is also associated with nausea. Zinc is required during pregnancy for the growing tissues of both mother and baby, so there are extra demands on the mother's supply. If a woman goes into pregnancy deficient in zinc, she is more likely to experience nausea, especially if she has been using a contraceptive pill prior to getting pregnant (see Ch. 1). The best dietary sources of zinc are given in Chapter 3 (p. 12). In particular, ginger is a rich source of zinc. It improves motility in the gastrointestinal tract so that food passes more rapidly, and is considered to have absorbent properties which may reduce stimuli to the chemoreceptor area of the brain which sends messages to the emetic centre. I advise patients to take a ginger capsule four times a day.

General advice

There are several simple self-help measures that can help to relieve pregnancy sickness.

First, encourage patients to rest as much as possible. Overwhelming tiredness is a symptom of early pregnancy, but it often comes as a great surprise to some women, who find it hard to believe they can feel so exhausted. They will also find it difficult to get rest or extra sleep if they are working or are at home with young children. Many of my patients find it necessary to go to bed well before their normal bedtime, as early as 8.00 p.m., just to be able to cope with the next day.

Second, encourage patients to take time getting up and preparing in the morning.

Finally, encourage patients to get out and take plenty of fresh air, even though they feel tired.

Summary

- Possible causes of morning sickness include: elevated HCG and progesterone levels, hydatidiform mole, multiple pregnancy, PIH, hydramnios, placental abruption and hyperemesis gravidarum.
- Other factors include: IVF, age, multiple pregnancy, gap between pregnancies, heavy periods and long-standing chronic conditions.
- Symptoms associated with morning sickness include: cravings, food aversions, pica, metallic taste, intense hunger, heartburn, belching, excess salivation, smell and tiredness.
- Drug treatments for morning sickness include: antihistamines, pyridoxine, Stemetil, Valoid, meclozine, metoclopramide, phenothiazines and electrolyte solutions to correct fluid balance.
- Emotions strongly affect morning sickness, particularly anger, worry and fear.
- Acupuncture points during the first trimester include:
  - for *morning sickness*: PC-6, ST-36 with PC-6 and CV-12, CV-10 with PC-6, CV-12 (with moxa for very weak, deficient or needle-phobic women), CV-14, ST-19 (or 20) with KI-21, ST-21 with ST-44, ST-34 (or ST-40) with PC-6, or SP-4 (on right) and PC-6 (on left)
  - *Stomach and Spleen deficiency*: BL-20 or 21, PC-6 and ST-36, CV-12, PC-6 and SP-4

- *disharmony of Liver and Stomach*: PC-6, LR-3, BL-17 and 19, ST-36; plus ST-40 (Phlegm and Damp), ST-44 and 21 (Stomach Heat), LI-11 with ST-44 (general Heat), CV-13 (excess Stomach conditions), GB-34 (Liver Qi stagnation), CV-12 with KI-21 (unstoppable vomiting), ST-34 (food retention), ST-21 and CV-13 (a good combination)
- *disharmony of Liver and Gall Bladder*: PC-6, LR-3, ST-36; plus LR-14 (hypochondrial pain), ST-4 (acute sickness), GB-34 (to move Liver Qi stagnation).

References

Czeizel AE, Dudas I, Fritz G, Tecsoi A, Hanck A, Kunovits G 1992 The effect of periconceptional multivitamin-mineral supplementation on vertigo, nausea and vomiting in the first trimester of pregnancy. Archives of Gynecology and Obstetrics 251(4): 181–185

Gadsby R 2004 General practitioners are wary of treating sickness in pregnancy. British Medical Journal 328: 505–506

Habek D, Barbir A, Habek J, Januliak D, Bobi-Vukovi M 2004 Success of acupuncture and acupressure of the PC6 acupoint in the treatment of hyperemesis gravidarum. Research in Complementary and Classical Natural Medicine 11: 20–23

Howden C 1986 Prescribing in pregnancy: treatment of common ailments. British Medical Journal 293: 1549–1550

Maciocia G 1998 Obstetrics and gynaecology in Chinese medicine. Churchill Livingstone, New York, p 453

Sahakian V, Rouse S, Spier D 1991 Vit B6 is effective therapy of nausea and vomiting: a randomised double blind placebo control trial. Obstetrics and Gynaecology 78: 33–36

Smith C, Crowther C, Beilby J 2002a Acupuncture to treat nausea and vomiting in early pregnancy: a randomized trial. Birth 29(1): 1–9

Smith C, Crowther C, Beilby J 2002b Pregnancy outcome following women's participation in a randomized controlled trial of acupuncture to treat nausea and vomiting in early pregnancy. Complementary Therapies in Medicine 10(2): 78–83

Sweet B R (ed.) 1997 Mayes' midwifery, 12th edn. Baillière Tindall, New York, pp 2–3, 223, 224–225, 227

Tuormaa T 1998 The vitamin B6 controversy. Foresight newsletter, spring

Weigel RM, Weigel MM 1989 Nausea and vomiting of early pregnancy and pregnancy outcome: an epidemiological study. British Journal of Obstetrics and Gynaecology 96: 1304–1311

Whitehead SA, Anders DLR, Chamberlain GUP 1992 Characterisation of nausea and vomiting in early pregnancy: a survey. Journal of Obstetrics and Gynaecology 12(6): 364–369

6 Second trimester: 13 to 28 weeks

Chapter outline

During the second trimester of her pregnancy, a woman usually starts to feel better. Feelings of exhaustion generally diminish and the traditional 'bloom' of pregnancy takes over. There are, however, a number of minor ailments that may be experienced. Although these are rarely life threatening, they can cause varying degrees of discomfort and anxiety and spoil a woman's enjoyment of her pregnancy.

Anatomy and physiology

By week 12, the uterus is around the symphysis pubis and is enlarging. According to Chinese embryology, the fetus is nourished through the Heart channels. There should be no needling of this particular meridian at this time.

By week 16, the uterus has risen out of the pelvis. The fundus is half way between the pubic bone and the umbilicus. At this stage the fetus is nourished through the Triple Burner channel. While the Yang organs of the fetus are being formed, the mother is advised to keep herself calm and away from any emotional disturbance.

By week 17, the first movements are felt by multiparous women and by around week 19 by the first-time mother.

By week 24, the fundus is level with the umbilicus (Fig. 6.1). The fetus is nourished through the Spleen channel.

Skin changes in pregnancy

Increased pigmentation of the skin is very common in pregnancy and found in 90% of expectant women (Fitzpatrick et al 1979). The exact causes are uncertain but are almost certainly linked to hormonal changes. The nipples and areola generally darken, as may the face, vulva, perineum and perianal region, and the linea alba on the anterior abdominal wall becomes the linea nigra. Stretch marks may also appear on the breasts, abdomen, thighs and buttocks. These will fade to silver after pregnancy.

Figure 6.1 The growing fetus and abdominal growth of the mother in the second trimester.

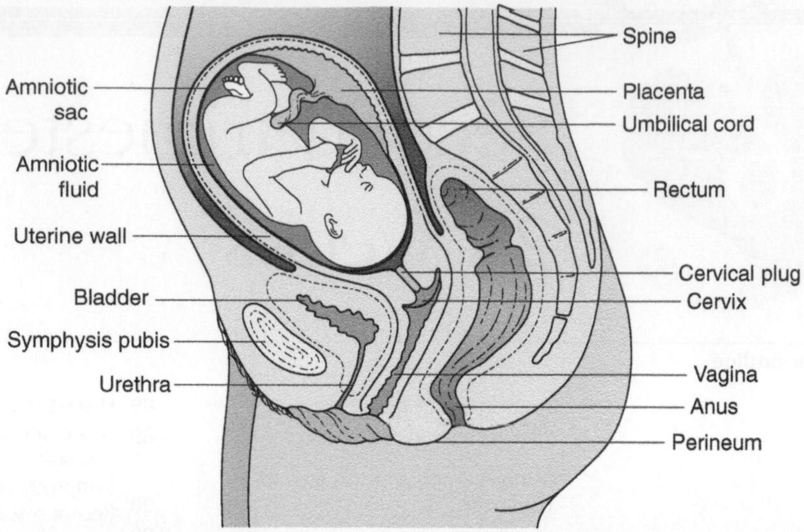

Minor ailments in the second trimester

Heartburn

Heartburn commonly occurs in women during pregnancy.

Causes

The hormones oestrogen and progesterone decrease the tone and motility of the smooth muscles that line the digestive tract, relaxing pressure on the cardiac sphincter, which usually blocks the stomach contents from moving up into the oesophagus. This results in regurgitation and decreased emptying. The pressure of the enlarging uterus on the stomach adds to the problem.

Western remedies

The antacid Gaviscon is often prescribed, but overuse can result in imbalance and poor iron absorption.

Chinese perspective on diet

As the Stomach rots food and the Spleen transforms and transports it, the downward movement of the Stomach Qi co-ordinates with the upward movement of the Spleen Qi. The two working together are vital to the balance of the Middle Jiao.

The nature of the food eaten is also important, both its quality and quantity. In Chinese dietary therapies, foods are classified according to their nature: hot, cold, cool or neutral.

Hot spicy foods include curries, spices, alcohol and meat. An excess of these tends to produce Stomach Heat. Cold foods include ice creams, cold drinks, raw vegetables and salads and these create Cold.

Excessive consumption of sugar can produce Damp and Heat in the Stomach.

Cooling foods that reduce Heat and are therefore good for heartburn include fruits such as watermelon, apples and bananas, vegetables such as spinach, cabbage, courgettes, cucumber, celery, broccoli and cauliflower, legumes, barley, tofu and soya milk. Peppermint, nettles and lemon balm are also helpful.

Acupuncture treatment of heartburn

Acupuncture can give temporary relief to the symptoms of heartburn, but a further treatment may be needed after a few days. Even a couple of days' respite, however, can be a huge relief to a patient who has been suffering constantly.

There are various syndromes that equate with heartburn, including Stomach Heat and retention of food in the Stomach. If the Stomach Qi is weak, the symptoms are likely to be more severe.

When giving a treatment for heartburn, my main aim is to:

- strengthen the Stomach and Spleen
- eliminate stagnation in the Middle Burner
- clear Heat if necessary.

POINTS TO TREAT

Different acupuncture points are used depending on which week of her pregnancy the patient is in. (Note: I *never* use abdominal points on the abdomen of a pregnant woman.) For example, at 24 weeks the fetus is at the level of the umbilicus and by 32 weeks it is between the umbilicus and the xiphisternum (see Fig. 4.6). Useful points to use prior to 32 weeks would be CV-12, 13 and 14.

- **CV-12 is very good for Heat in the Middle Jiao and is a good point for retention of food in the Stomach. I would recommend leaving the needle in place for 20 minutes.**
- **CV-13 is the best point to subdue rebellious Qi and for Excess Stomach patterns.**
- **CV-14 helps to clear Heart Fire.**
- **ST-44 clears Heat in the Stomach.**
- **ST-45 clears Heat in the Stomach but it also dissolves the accumulation of food and can help with insomnia due to retention of food.**
- **LI-11 to clear Heat, especially if the heartburn is accompanied by constipation.**

At a first treatment for severe heartburn, depending on the pattern and how many weeks pregnant the woman is, I would use LR-11 and ST-44, using an even technique and leaving the needles in place for up to 30 minutes. The aim of treatment is to clear Heat.

General advice

Some general pointers include:

- heartburn is aggravated by large meals and by eating foods that produce gas
- fatty and spicy foods should be avoided
- several small meals should be eaten in preference to one large one
- coffee, alcohol and chocolate should be avoided
- walking or sitting upright after eating is recommended
- keep the head elevated when in bed and sleep propped up with extra pillows
- limit fluid intake at meal times.

Varicose veins

Varicose veins are enlarged and twisted veins just beneath the skin. In Western terms, veins contain valves that aid the return of blood to the heart. When their function is impaired, blood circulation also becomes impaired. Varicose veins tend to be hereditary in women. Varicosities can occur during pregnancy because increased progesterone dilates and relaxes the veins, and because of the extra weight a woman carries. They usually improve after pregnancy but tend to get progressively worse with subsequent pregnancies.

Varicose veins are found most frequently in the back and inside of the legs but can also occur in other parts of the body, in particular the vulva and the anus (haemorrhoids).

Cause

The two principal venous systems in the body are the deep veins, which lie among the muscles and carry 90% of the blood, and the superficial veins, which are visible just below the skin. Valves in the veins prevent the backward flow of blood but these can become defective in pregnancy owing to hormonal changes and additional pressure on the pelvic veins.

Symptoms

Some people have no symptoms at all whereas others have a severe ache in the backs of their legs. This can become progressively worse throughout the day and can be accompanied by swelling of the ankles and itching. There may also be the appearance of large dilated veins. The patient may complain of heaviness and tiredness in the legs. This can be relieved by elevating the legs.

Diagnosis

Diagnosis is by physical examination.

Western treatment

This is aimed at aiding the return of blood. Rest is advised along with the wearing of support stockings.

Nutritionally women should be encouraged to take vitamin C (to make collagen, which keeps the arteries supple), vitamin E and essential fatty acids (to help transport oxygen).

Chinese treatment

In Chinese terms, the syndrome that usually corresponds to varicose veins is stagnant Qi and Blood with deficient Spleen and Qi sinking. The success of acupuncture depends on the severity of the varicose veins. In many cases improvement is minimal and treatment may seem ineffectual, but some women feel that it helps with the throbbing sensation and opt to continue with treatment, regardless of the success.

Acupuncture in combination with a TENS (transcutaneous electrical nerve stimulation) machine appears to be the most effective in relieving the heaviness and pain. Needling will depend on where the veins are and whether or not it is possible to needle. Some women have very bad veins around the site of the acupuncture points, making it impossible to needle.

POINTS TO TREAT

- **LR-5 Connecting point, which is good for moving stagnant Qi in the lower legs; use an even technique and leave the needles in.**
- **LR-8 tonify, to normalise Qi and Blood.**
- **SP-5 Empirical point for vessels.**
- **GV-20 for sinking Qi and holding up.**

If the veins are very swollen and throbbing, I insert needles very superficially in a circle around the veins. A 30-minute session very often takes the redness out of the veins and helps to relieve the throbbing.

Using a TENS or an Acu-TENS machine between acupuncture treatments can be very effective and women can be encouraged to do this for themselves, especially after 36 weeks of pregnancy. Simply place the pads near the most troublesome veins.

Deep vein thrombosis

This is a potentially serious condition which can result from varicose veins or from any condition which causes a reduced blood flow, such as the increased clotting tendency in pregnancy.

Symptoms include pain, tenderness and swelling of the affected leg, usually in the calf. If in doubt, the patient should contact her GP for treatment with anticoagulants.

Vulval varicose veins

These can be very debilitating and painful. Sufferers will also have varicose veins elsewhere on their bodies. The same syndromes apply but these are much harder to treat with acupuncture.

POINTS TO TREAT

The points I have used are:

- **GV-20, associated with sinking of Spleen Qi**
- **LR-3 with even technique.**

Improvement in pain has frequently been noted.

Bowel problems

Constipation can be very debilitating for a pregnant woman. It is common during pregnancy because of the relaxation of plain muscle by progesterone. This causes general sluggishness and decreased peristalsis of the colon.

The Chinese viewpoint is that constipation is due to a Blood deficiency, especially if this is a pre-existing blood deficiency. It may also be due to Qi stagnation, which is common in the first 3 months because of the growing fetus. Another contributory factor may be if the mother is suffering from morning sickness and is not drinking the amount she should.

Treating constipation during pregnancy is difficult because no abdominal points should be used.

Chinese dietary therapy

- Excess cold foods block the function of the Spleen.
- Excess hot foods dry up the Stomach fluids.
- Foods that promote bowel movement include peas, cabbage, figs, bran and asparagus.
- Foods that lubricate the intestines include bananas, spinach, honey, prunes, apples, pine nuts and carrots.
- Acidophilus puts the flora back into the intestines and can help with bowel movements.

Diagnosis will depend on the individual and the pattern she is displaying. The points to use would depend on the syndrome. For example, if the woman is generally deficient, pale and tired, with dry stools, Blood deficiency would be suggested.

POINTS TO TREAT

- **Bl-17, an influential point, to tonify the Blood.**
- **ST-36 to tonify the Qi and the Blood.**
- **LR-8 to nourish the Liver Blood.**

If the woman is irritable and her stools are pebble shaped, Liver Qi stagnation would be suggested.

POINTS TO TREAT

- **GB-34 with even technique to move Qi and increase the flow of Qi in the Lower Jiao.**
- **LR-3 with even technique to move stagnant Qi.**
- **LI-11 with even technique if there are a lot of Heat signs.**
- **LR-2 with even technique to clear Heat in the Lower Jiao and harmonise the Liver.**

Some women who are having IVF (in vitro fertilisation) treatment present with Kidney Yin deficiency.

POINTS TO TREAT

- **Bl-23 to tonify the Kidneys.**
- **KI-3 and 6 to nourish the Kidney Yin.**

Haemorrhoids

Haemorrhoids are swollen veins in the lining of the anus. If they occur close to the anal opening they are called external haemorrhoids. If they occur higher up in the anal canal they are called internal haemorrhoids. If they protrude outside the anus they are called prolapsing haemorrhoids.

Causes

Some people have a congenital weakness that predisposes them to haemorrhoids. In pregnancy, they can also result from hormonal changes affecting the veins, constipation or straining to pass hard faeces.

They are common after delivery as a result of a prolonged labour, pelvic pressure and straining during a lengthy second stage, delivery of a large baby or the use of instruments. In most cases the haemorrhoids will regress of their own accord within a few days of the birth, although recent studies have shown that they can continue to be a problem for up to 2 months after the birth and may become chronic.

Symptoms

Symptoms include increasing discomfort and pain on passing a bowel motion, and rectal bleeding. Itching, mucus and increased pain may accompany prolapsed haemorrhoids; strangulation and thrombosis may be a further complication.

Chinese viewpoint

According to TCM (traditional Chinese medicine), haemorrhoids can be due to:

- Blood deficiency
- Heat in the Blood
- Blood stasis
- Damp-Heat
- Qi stagnation.

Treatment with acupuncture depends on the severity of the patient's pain and also the background and causes of the haemorrhoids.

Bleeding haemorrhoids

Usually the woman will feel discomfort and pain.

POINTS TO TREAT

- **LI-11 with SP-10 to clear Heat and cool the Blood; LR-2 could also be added, using even technique and the needles left in.**
- **BL-17 to tonify the Blood.**

With Blood stasis, the pain is usually intense and the haemorrhoids are swollen and bleeding.

- **If the pain is very bad, you could add GV-1, leaving the needle in for 20–40 minutes as well as the points above LI-11 and 2; treat the woman lying on her side.**
- **BL-57 and 58 are the empirical points for haemorrhoids located on the back of the calf.**
- **GV-20 if the haemorrhoids are due to sinking Qi.**

Acute and chronic back ache and sciatica

I really enjoy treating women with back ache in pregnancy because I find treatment to be so successful. And in fact, back ache and sciatica are the most common problems I am asked to treat in pregnancy.

CASE STUDY 6.1

Sasha came to me for acupuncture at 25 weeks suffering from vulval varicose veins and varicose veins in both legs. This was Sasha's third pregnancy – she had two boys aged 12 months and 2 years – and she had suffered badly with varicose veins in each pregnancy. She presented with extreme pain which made standing and walking for any length of time unbearable. The pain was also present during the night and she was now totally exhausted.

At her first appointment, I needled GV-20 and LR-5 for only 20 minutes with even technique; as she was so exhausted I added BL-23. This seemed to help with the pain immediately as standing up after the treatment, Sasha commented that her legs felt lighter.

At her second treatment, 1 week later, the improvement in the pain had continued, even though there was no change in the size of the varicose veins.

Treatment continued with fortnightly appointments and I added in SP-8, the empirical point of vessels, and BL-20 to her treatments, which now lasted 45 minutes. The vulval veins began to reduce and the leg veins, although prominent throughout her pregnancy, caused much less pain. Sasha gave birth to a healthy girl at 38 weeks.

The lower back includes the lumbar spine, the sacrum, the sacroiliac joints, the coccyx and associated tissues and muscles. It covers the base of the spine and bears most of the weight of the trunk, head and arms, transferring this weight to the hips.

Causes

Back strain in a pregnant woman can be caused by various factors: the weight of the pregnant uterus; altered posture to compensate for altered shape; tiredness leading to poor posture; instability of the joints caused by lax ligaments, the result of progesterone and relaxin softening and relaxing the ligaments of the pelvis; or increased lumbar curve.

This condition is often dismissed as 'par for the course' in pregnancy because there is very little that Western medicine can do to relieve it. Women may be offered physiotherapy, given back exercises and advice on posture, or supplied with a Fem Brace, which gives support to the lower back.

Chinese viewpoint

The most common cause of acute back ache in pregnancy is stagnation of the Blood and Qi. This is the most frequent problem that I encounter and the one with which I have the highest success rate.

Excessive lifting and physical work weaken the back by putting a strain on the Kidney Qi, which in turn will weaken the back muscles. The lower back is dominated by the Bladder, Kidney and Du channels. In pregnancy and childbirth, a strain is put on the back not only by the extra weight but also by weakened Kidney Qi. This is especially apparent in a woman whose constitution is weaker or who has had a number of children in quick succession.

External factors, such as Cold and Damp, affect the Gate of Vitality and cause the invasion of pathogenic factors in the back channels. The back area should be protected from the weather (for example, women should avoid jogging or playing sports in poor weather wearing insufficient clothing).

Working long hours without adequate rest over a long period of time depletes the Kidney Yin.

Diagnosis

Caution: in pregnancy it is very important to establish that the pain is due to back ache rather than a kidney infection (see Urinary tract infections, p. 128).

Questions to ask include the following.

- Is the pain aggravated by rest or improved by movement and light exercise?
- Is the area tender to the touch?
- Does it improve with the application of heat, damp or cold?
- Is there marked stiffness?
- Is there restricted movement such as inability to extend and turn?
- Is the pain radiating down the leg?
- Is the pain worse in the morning or evening?
- Is the pain worse when the patient is overtired (this is often the case in women who have had IVF treatment)?

The first consultation

Women are often very wary about acupuncture and seek reassurance about the success rate of treatment. Their pain is such that they do not want to risk doing anything that may make their condition worse. Often their pain can be so severe that they can walk only with difficulty, their gait is very stiff and often they have to be transported to clinic because they are unable to drive themselves.

The first thing to try to establish is whether the pain is acute or chronic (Box 6.1). Pain that is severe and stabbing, worse with rest, better with light exercise and tender to the touch is connected to stagnation of Qi and Blood.

If the back ache improves with light exercise it is due to local stagnation but if it improves with rest it is due to Kidney deficiency.

Treatment for acute back ache

At a first consultation I ask the patient to lie on her side on the bed, with the affected side uppermost. For acute back ache, I have found great success with Ah Shi points. These are selected according to tenderness. Ascertain where the greatest pain is felt by using the thumbs to press hard over the area while the patient indicates where the pain is. The commonest Ah Shi points are generally BL-54, 28 and 36 and GB-30. I use 34-gauge needles, 3.8–5 cm long, on Ah Shi points in the buttock and insert them all the way in. (Obviously, back points do not go in as far.) Leave the needles in using even technique for 20–30 minutes.

Box 6.1 Acute and chronic back ache

Acute	Chronic
Stagnation of Qi and Blood	Kidney deficiency
Severe pain	Dull ache
Improves with exercise	Improves with rest
Worse at the start of the day	Better upon waking
Improves as the day goes on	Gets worse as the day goes on
Worse for cold and damp, better for heat	Worse for heat, better for application of cold

A large area of pain can indicate an invasion of Cold and Dampness or a Kidney deficiency. An area of cold on the backs of the legs may indicate a Kidney Yang deficiency.

Note: Care should be taken with the points on the lower back, depending on where a woman is in her pregnancy. Also, prior to 37 weeks, avoid BL-31 and 32. (These points are not likely to be treated by mistake as they are hard to find at the best of times.)

POINTS TO TREAT

- **If the pain is radiating down the back of the leg and knee, I will use BL-40 bilaterally or unilaterally, leaving the needles in.**
- **If the pain is going down the side of the leg, I will use GB-34 and LR-3, again leaving the needles in.**
- **Moxa is good for back ache in pregnancy to warm a cold area or for Kidney Yang deficiency.**

This would constitute a first treatment and it is generally highly effective.

Treatment for chronic back ache

Chronic back pain is more difficult to treat and is usually caused by Kidney deficiency. The pain comes sporadically and is a dull ache which improves with rest. If the cause is a Kidney Yang deficiency, there will be an area of cold around the area of pain. The application of heat will improve the back ache.

CASE STUDY 6.2

Tina was 37 weeks' pregnant and suffering from severe pain that radiated down her leg. The pain was worse when she woke in the morning but improved as the day went on and was better for the application of heat. Her job was stacking shelves in a supermarket but she was having difficulty in walking and had a pronounced limp. She was using an umbrella as a walking stick and had to be driven to her treatment. The Western diagnosis was sciatica and weakness of the sacroiliac joints; the Chinese diagnosis was acute back ache caused by stagnation of Qi and Blood.

She lay on her side and I placed a pillow between her legs to make her as comfortable as possible. I palpated the area, which was not cold, and then used Ah Shi points on the lower back, BL-54 and out towards GB-30. I also needled GB-34 as the pain was spreading down her leg. I left the needles in for 20 minutes using even technique (although the texts recommend reducing techniques in acute cases, I find that even techniques are generally very effective). Although the area felt warm, I used a moxa stick over the lower back to help relax the muscles.

Improvement after the treatment was marked and although the pain did not disappear completely, Tina was able to walk with far more ease.

POINTS TO TREAT

It is useful to concentrate on the underlying weakness.

- **For Kidney deficiency, tonify BL-23 and Ki-3, do not leave the needles in.**
- **For Spleen weakness, tonify BL-20 and SP-3.**
- **BL-23 tonified is good in any case of chronic back ache.**

Symphysis pubis pain

This is pain around the area of the pubic bone, caused by separation of the symphysis pubis joint or swelling within the joint. The hormones of pregnancy are thought to cause an increase in the width of the symphysis pubis.

Symptoms

These usually occur in the second or third trimesters of pregnancy and the onset may be experienced gradually or suddenly. Pain will be felt in the pubic area and the groin, sometimes radiating to the inner thighs or lower back. It could initially be mistaken for an infection of the urinary tract. Movement may be limited, difficulty experienced with walking and sitting, getting in and out of bed or climbing the stairs, and sleep may be affected.

Management of the pain

Help offered includes physiotherapy and the use of a Fem Brace, a support belt that may give relief by supporting the pubic bone. Analgesia or painkillers may be prescribed. For some women the pain is so severe that they are admitted to hospital for bedrest and administered strong injections of painkiller.

Acupuncture treatment

When I first started treating these conditions, I used points such as LR-3, which I felt would traverse the pubic area and help the pain. As I gained experience and grew braver in my treatments, I began to use points actually on the pubic bone itself. (Although I advocate never using abdominal points, this is one of the few occasions when I break the rules.) Use 3.8 cm needles, inserted to a depth of half a cun, left in with even technique.

I use Ah Shi points on the pubic bone, palpating to find the centre of the bone, which is usually tender. I then insert the needle on a parallel to CV-2 but down slightly, and I also use CV-2 itself. I then come out about an inch on either side to feel whether the point is tender again and insert two more needles. I find this to be excellent as a first treatment on its own and the patient usually notices an immediate difference. The longer the needles can be left in place, the greater is the effectiveness of the treatment.

Treatment is given according to where the pain is situated. Most women experience pain centrally on the pubic bone but for some it is under the pubic arch. Once again, I feel the area of pain to locate the exact spot, placing needles with caution wherever the pain is.

I appreciate that I am at an advantage by virtue of being a midwife and female when giving these treatments. But once women have felt a benefit, they are very willing to try anything to help with their pain.

Recent research

There are two published articles from studies carried out in Sweden on pelvic pain relief for pregnant women. Both articles concluded that acupuncture relieves low-back and pelvic pain without any serious side-effects. However, the studies are noted to have used acupuncture points which are forbidden in TCM texts. The 2001 study by Kvorning Ternov et al used local painful points and mainly LR-3 and LI-4; the acupuncture was performed by midwives in a maternity unit. The more recent study by Elden et al, published in the British Medical Journal in 2005, concluded that acupuncture was more efficacious than stabilising exercises in the management of pelvic girdle pain in pregnancy. In this randomised single-blind controlled trial, the acupuncture was given by medical acupuncturists, using mainly GV-20, LI-4, BL-60 and ST-36 and a selection of local painful points.

Nutrition during the second trimester

Vitamins and minerals are in great demand for both the growing fetus and the mother. The role of specific vitamins and minerals, together with food sources, was discussed in Chapter 3. In addition, the following is recommended daily as the basis of a healthy diet:

- four servings of vegetables, in particular the green leafy ones such as broccoli, spinach and watercress
- four servings of fruit
- two servings of wholegrains, legumes, nuts and seeds (sesame, sunflower and pumpkin), lean meat or fish (in particular the oily ones)
- three servings of calcium-rich foods (soft and blue-veined cheeses should be avoided)
- one litre of fluid (water, diluted fruit juice and herbal teas). Drinks containing alcohol, caffeine and excess sugar should be avoided.

CASE STUDY 6.3

Imogen came to me for acupuncture at 34 weeks in her third pregnancy. She had severe pubic pain, could hardly walk and was not getting any sleep. She had tried physiotherapy and a Fem Brace to no avail. Because she could not drive, she was housebound. She couldn't do the shopping, carry a basket, push a trolley or even a pushchair. Needless to say, she was very miserable and fed up.

At the first treatment, I needled LR-3 to see whether this would have any effect. I suspected that it wouldn't make a huge difference but my first priority was to put Imogen at ease. When women first come along they are often very nervous and unsure about the treatment and the needles.

At the second treatment, there had been no improvement at all, so I explained to Imogen what I wanted to do. I placed 1-inch needles along the pubic bone and inserted them half a centimetre apart. Then I left them in place for 40 minutes. The difference was marked and she felt relief almost immediately.

At the third treatment, the pain had improved by 50%. Over the next week her sleep also improved and though she was still in pain, by comparison it was much, much better.

At the fourth treatment, I again put the needles along the pubic bone but I also added one to the perineum. I got her to sit up on the bed and point to where the pain was. Then I inserted another 1-inch (2.54 cm) needle, just under the pubic arch. Once again, the improvement was significant.

Prior to treatment, she had been making a weekly appointment to see her GP, demanding that she be induced because she could not go on. Acupuncture really helped her to get through the last weeks of her pregnancy.

Summary

- Common problems in the second trimester include: heartburn, varicose veins, bowel problems, haemorrhoids, acute or chronic back ache and sciatica, and symphysis pubis pain.

- Acupuncture points during the second trimester include:
  - *heartburn*: CV-12 to 14, ST-44 and 45, LI-11
  - *varicose veins*: LR-5 and 8, SP-5, GV-20 and LR-3 (vulval veins)
  - *bowel problems*: BL-17, ST-36 and LR-8 (Blood deficiency); GB-34, LR-2, 3 and 11 (Liver Qi stagnation); BL-23, KI-3 and 6 (Kidney Yin deficiency)
  - *haemorrhoids*: LR-11 with SP-10, LR-2, BL-17; plus GV-1 and 20, BL-57 and 58, GV-20 (Blood stasis)
  - *acute back ache and sciatica*: BL-28, 36 and 54, GB-30; plus BL-40 (pain radiating down back of leg), GB-34 and LR-3 (pain radiating down side of leg)
  - *chronic back ache*: BL-23 and KI-4 (Kidney deficiency), BL-20 and SP-3 (Spleen weakness)
  - *symphysis pubis pain*: LR-3, Ah Shi points on the pubic bone, CV-2.

References

Elden H, Ladfors I, Fagevik Olsen M, Ostaard H, Hagberg H 2005 Effects of acupuncture and stabilizing exercise as an adjunct to standard treatment in pregnant women with pelvic girdle pain: a randomized single blind controlled trial. British Medical Journal 330(7494): 761

Fitzpatrick TB, Elsen AZ, Wolff K 1979 Dermatology in general medicine. McGraw-Hill, New York

Kvorning Ternov N, Grennert L, Aberg A, Algotsson L, Akeson J 2001 Acupuncture for lower back and pelvic pain in late pregancy: a retrospective report on 167 consecutive cases. Pain Medicine 2(3): 204–207

Further reading

Hytton F 1990 The alimentary system in pregnancy. Midwifery 6: 201–204

7 Third trimester: 28 to 40 weeks

Chapter outline

During the final 3 months of pregnancy, most women start to feel much larger and heavier. There is often a spurt of weight gain, which is probably due to the weight of the growing baby and the increase in amniotic fluid.

Although some women may still be enjoying the traditional 'bloom' of pregnancy, many will be feeling very tired and uncomfortable. They may also be suffering from such minor problems and discomforts as breathlessness, insomnia, back ache, constipation, piles and heartburn.

Common terms used in the third trimester

CPD. Cephalopelvic disproportion is failure of the fetal head to descend through the pelvis despite strong uterine contractions.

Doppler. Doppler ultrasound is a way of imaging blood flow in vessels using the Doppler effect; the frequency shift in the echo from flowing blood indicates the nature of the flow.

IUGR. Intrauterine growth retardation is when the baby fails to gain weight or its weight falls suddenly below the norm, perhaps because of congenital malformation but more usually because the amount and quality of nourishment received from the placenta have declined.

Oblique (or transverse) lie. Here the fetus lies horizontally across the womb rather than with its head down. A shoulder presentation would make vaginal delivery impossible and, if suspected in late pregnancy, should be confirmed by ultrasound diagram to show oblique lie.

OP position. Occipito-posterior (OP) position is a malposition of the vertex presentation (Fig. 7.1).

Placental insufficiency. This is an inability of the placenta to perform its functions properly, putting the fetus in jeopardy.

Small for dates. This indicates babies who are growing but consistently fall below the accepted norm for size.

Unstable lie. Here the fetus keeps changing position in the womb after 36 weeks.

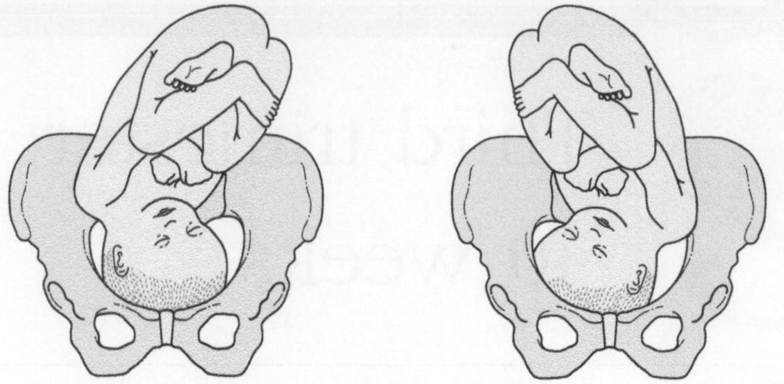

Figure 7.1 Right and left OP positions. (Reproduced with permission from Sweet 1997, p. 632.)

Anatomy and physiology

By week 28, breast tissue will be developing and the breasts will be starting to produce colostrum, the fluid that precedes milk.

By week 32, the blood volume circulating round the body will have increased by around 40% to accommodate the needs of the fetus, the placenta, the uterus and the breasts.

By week 36, pressure from the uterus may be pressing against the lungs and causing slight breathlessness.

The pelvic joints will be starting to soften and expand in preparation for birth.

Importance of the placenta in the third trimester

In most women the placenta reaches its maximum efficiency at around 37–38 weeks. As detailed in Chapter 2, the placenta acts as a substitute lung, liver and kidney for the fetus; it also stores energy as glycogen to feed the baby as required, and it provides an immune barrier.

In addition, the placenta produces a number of hormones, including:

- Human chorionic gonadotrophin (HCG), which increases absorption of calcium and stimulates milk production
- oestrogen, which stimulates the breasts and uterus and regulates fetal growth
- progesterone, which helps to maintain the pregnancy, stimulates the breasts and relaxes the muscles
- relaxin, which softens the cervix and loosens the ligaments in preparation for birth.

If the placenta stops working efficiently before 38 weeks, the baby's development is affected, leading to low birthweight.

By the end of the third trimester the placenta is usually around 17.5–20 cm wide and 2.5 cm thick, and weighs about one-sixth of the baby's birthweight. It is delivered during the third stage of labour.

Mental and emotional aspects

Bringing a new life into the world requires all sorts of emotional adjustments and can throw up many difficult feelings, which need to be worked through. This goes far beyond a superficial 'loss of body image' or 'resentment of loss of freedom'. Mothers need time to prepare, emotionally as well as practically and physically, for the transformations involved in becoming a parent. First-time mothers in particular, many of whom work much longer and later in their pregnancies, leave themselves little time for mental preparation before their baby arrives. It is possible this may have a detrimental affect on the fetus, whose growth rate can slow down if the mother does not take time to rest and prepare herself.

It is too easy to dismiss negative feelings as the result of hormonal changes, and women need to be able to express such feelings in a supportive environment in order to accept and come to terms with them.

Every woman responds in her own unique and individual way, depending on:

- her personal circumstances
- her self-image – the way she sees herself as a woman and as a mother
- her relationship with her own mother and her maternal role models
- her relationship with the baby's father
- the way she views her own place in society
- ambivalence about the pregnancy – whether or not the baby was wanted and planned for
- ill health experienced as a result of the pregnancy.

As full term approaches, some women also experience increasing anxiety about the labour and delivery. This can range from mild worry to a full-blown panic attack. It may be based on ignorance, on misinformation (too much listening to old wives' tales and the gossip of other mothers), or it may be the result of a bad experience in a previous pregnancy. Whatever the reason, talking such fears through with a sympathetic midwife or practitioner can go a long way to reassure and encourage.

Common ailments of the third trimester

To ensure the well-being of mother and baby, the frequency of antenatal visits increases from every 4 weeks to every 2 weeks in the third trimester. Abdominal examinations after the 28th week will determine the lie, presentation and position of the fetus, as well as the height of the uterine fundus, and from 36 weeks it may also be possible to determine engagement of the head.

Anaemia

Oxygen is needed by every single cell in the body. It is transported by a pigment in the red blood cells called haemoglobin. These cells are formed in the bone marrow and released into the blood, where they circulate for approximately 120 days. When they die, they are destroyed by the spleen. Under normal circumstances, a woman's haemoglobin level is between 11 and 15 g (Sweet 1997). A stable level is maintained in the blood by the body strictly balancing the number of red cells produced in the bone marrow and the number destroyed by the spleen. If this balance is upset and the number of red blood cells reduced, anaemia results and it can take quite a while to bring the haemoglobin back up to normal limits.

Total blood volume increases during pregnancy but the number of red blood cells does not increase at the same rate, so that the level of haemoglobin in the blood is reduced. Opinion about safe levels of haemoglobin varies, but usually ranges between 10 and 13 g/dl.

It is important that blood is taken at between 28 and 32 weeks to check haemoglobin levels, as anaemia could pose a threat to the health of both mother and baby if left untreated.

The *effects* of anaemia in pregnancy include: undermining of general health, lowered resistance to infection, exacerbation of minor pregnancy disorders such as digestive problems, intrauterine hypoxia (in severe cases), risk of premature labour, increase in perinatal mortality, risk of antepartum and postpartum haemorrhage, higher risk of thromboembolic disorders and increase in maternal mortality.

There are five different *types* of anaemia:

- iron deficiency anaemia – the most common form in pregnancy
- folic acid deficiency anaemia
- haemoglobinopathies, which include sickle cell disease and thalassaemia
- anaemia as a result of blood loss or secondary to infection
- aplastic varieties, rare in pregnancy.

The *symptoms* of iron deficiency anaemia include: shortness of breath, tiredness, dizziness and fainting, pallor, palpitations, loss of appetite and headaches.

Those most at risk of iron deficiency anaemia are women who:

- are poorly nourished
- generally lose excessive amounts of blood during menstruation (women who have had heavy periods before conception may enter pregnancy already marginally anaemic)
- have repeated pregnancies, especially ones that are close together
- have a multiple pregnancy
- use alkaline preparations to relieve heartburn
- have a diet low in vitamin C
- suffer from repeated vomiting or diarrhoea
- suffer bleeding from haemorrhoids or antepartum haemorrhage
- suffer from internal parasites such as hookworm
- have malabsorption problems such as coeliac disease.

Western medicine generally treats anaemia with iron preparations, sometimes in combination with folic acid.

Diet advice for anaemia

Iron, protein, copper, folic acid and vitamins B6, B12 and C are all necessary for the formation of red blood cells, so a deficiency in any of these nutrients can cause anaemia. (For good food sources of these, see Ch. 3.) But iron deficiency anaemia can occur even if the diet is rich in iron, because a lack of B vitamins can result in poor absorption of iron. Factors which interfere with iron absorption include: high zinc intake, tea and coffee, antacids given for heartburn, and dairy products; try to eat dairy-rich and iron-rich foods separately.

To absorb iron more efficiently, take your supplement with vitamin C – a glass of fresh orange juice or a portion of blackberries.

Treatment with acupuncture

In Chinese medicine, the Blood is seen as more than just a collection of cells. Blood is Yin and is regarded as receptive and sensitive, the seat of our emotions. So the relationship between the Blood and our emotional state is very important. If the Blood is low, a woman is likely to feel weak, anxious and depressed.

The function of the Blood is also to cool and moisturise. If the Blood is weak, there will be symptoms of Heat: flushes, dry skin, constipation, joint tingling and numbness.

Blood is created from the nutrients in the food we eat by the action of the Spleen, combined with the Kidney Essence known as the Jing. Most of our Jing is stored in the Bone Marrow.

The organs responsible for the blood in Chinese terms are the Heart, the Liver (because it stores the Blood), the Spleen (because it makes the Blood) and the kidneys (because of the Essence and Bone Marrow). Any disturbance in these organs can lead to problems with Blood imbalance. Anaemia is usually linked to Blood deficiency. The actual manifestation depends on which organ is involved. For example, Heart symptoms would include palpitations, poor memory, insomnia, dreams and disturbed sleep, and pale complexion and colourless lips.

If a woman enters pregnancy having had a lot of emotional problems, she will generally be Qi and Blood deficient. A Spleen Qi deficiency is usually at the root of this, as the Spleen generates the Blood.

POINTS TO TREAT

All the points mentioned below (see Fig. 7.2) are tonified.

- **BL-17 is an influential point for the Blood and I use it in all cases of anaemia (moxa cones can be applied).**
- **If a woman is very deficient, then combine BL-17 with BL-15, the Back Shu point of the Heart, which tonifies the Heart Qi.**

When treating the Heart, the Kidney may also need to be treated. When the Heart is settled, the balance between the Yin and Yang of the Kidneys can be maintained.

Liver Blood symptoms would include: tiredness, weakness, cramps, blurred vision, tingling or numbness of the limbs, brittle nails, dry skin and dull hair.

POINTS TO TREAT

Once again, all the points require tonification.

- **BL-17 is an influential Blood point combined with BL-18, the Back Shu point of the Liver; heat with moxa.**
- **LR-8 nourishes the Liver Blood.**

If the Spleen is deficient, it cannot make Blood and this will in turn affect the Liver, causing Liver Blood deficiency. If you are treating Liver Blood deficiency, add Spleen points and also tonify BL-20.

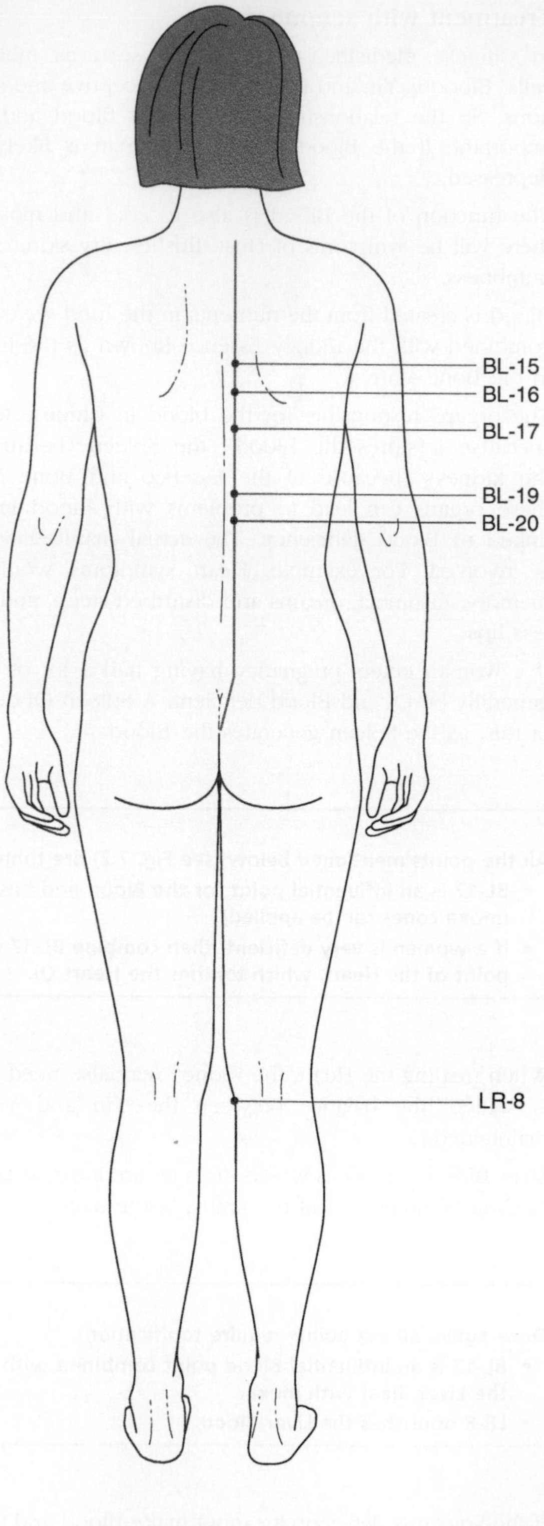

Figure 7.2 Points useful for the treatment of anaemia.

CASE STUDY 7.1

Elizabeth was now 28 weeks' pregnant. She had had a difficult early pregnancy when she was nauseated and vomited small amounts till 14 weeks' gestation.

Elizabeth worked for a busy fashion PR company and it had been difficult to take any time off work as she didn't want to let the team down. She had missed several antenatal appointments but had been told by a friend that acupuncture had really helped her in pregnancy.

She presented in my clinic, with palpitations, insomnia and, when she did sleep, very vivid dreams; she looked pale and agitated. My first advice was to see her midwife as soon as possible. At her first treatment I needled only two points, HT-7 even technique and ST-36, as she was so deficient.

The next week she had taken my advice and had been thoroughly checked out by her midwife and doctor who informed her she was anaemic. She was now on iron supplement medication.

I continued to treat her weekly, focusing on blood building points, and she realised she needed to take care of herself and her baby. Elizabeth shortened her working day and took early maternity leave at 33 weeks.

Cramps

Muscular cramps, usually in the legs, can be very painful and are often reported by pregnant women. The cause is unknown, although it may be linked to a deficiency of magnesium, calcium or vitamin B.

Regular gentle exercise (walking, swimming or yoga) may help to improve the circulation and prevent cramps. In an attack, stretching and extending the limb and firmly massaging the calf muscle may help to relieve the pain. Night cramps can also be helped by massaging the legs before going to bed and by raising the foot of the bed by 20–25 cm.

There is always the slight possibility that cramps could be associated with deep vein thrombosis, so if they keep recurring this should be checked out medically.

Treatment with acupuncture

Use tonification of LR-8.

Insomnia

These days women very often work much later into their pregnancy. Often it is difficult for them to unwind and their minds are too active at night to let them get the rest they badly need. They start to get tired and complain about lack of sleep, especially from around 34 weeks. The discomfort of a growing abdomen adds to the problem. Many women find it increasingly difficult to get comfortable in bed. Sleeping on the back can cause feelings of faintness, because the pressure of the baby weighs on the main internal blood vessels. Sleeping on the tummy becomes impossible, for obvious reasons. But sleeping on the side is not comfortable for some women. Nights can also be broken by the need to get up to pass urine.

Heartburn, the reflux of acidic stomach contents causing a burning sensation in the oesophagus, can be exacerbated by lying down, so can add to sleep disturbance. This is commonly worse towards the end of pregnancy, when the growing baby pushes upwards, compressing the space between the oesophagus and the stomach. Sleeping in a more upright position can be helpful.

There is little that Western medicine can offer the pregnant insomniac, other than general advice about allowing time to relax and unwind in the evening, taking a warm bath, a hot soothing drink or a relaxing massage.

Chinese viewpoints

Mental as well as physical overwork, long hours spent working without adequate rest over many weeks and months, plus the strain of a pregnancy – all this weakens the Kidney Yin. This fails to nourish the Heart Yin, so the Kidneys and Heart are not harmonised.

Worry also affects the Spleen and if it is already deficient, it cannot produce Blood and the deficiency affects both the Heart and the Mind. This usually falls into two patterns: either Full and Excess conditions or Deficient conditions. Deficient conditions affect the Heart, Spleen and Liver.

Heart and Spleen Blood deficiency is very common in women who are anaemic. Women suffering from this will experience: difficulty in falling asleep, palpitations, tiredness, poor memory and mild anxiety.

POINTS TO TREAT

Treatment would be to tonify the Spleen and the Heart:

- **tonify ST-36 and BL-20 to help produce the Blood**
- **tonify BL-15 to nourish the Heart Blood**
- **tonify BL-17 to calm the mind for sleep; moxa can also be added.**

I find sometimes in women who have had IVF (in vitro fertilisation) treatment or fertility drugs, both of which can be very taxing on the Kidneys, that the Heart and Kidneys are not harmonised. Symptoms include: waking frequently at night, night sweats, a poor memory, mental restlessness and back ache.

POINTS TO TREAT

- **BL-15 and 23 to harmonise the Heart and Kidneys.**
- **HT-7 to calm the Mind.**

Recent research

A small pilot study from Brazil (Guerreiro da Silva et al 2005) studied a group of 30 pregnant women suffering from insomnia. Seventeen women had acupuncture and 13 were in the control group. The study decided to use predefined points with an option of up to four additional points. The most commonly used points were: HT-7, PC-6, GB-21, Anmian, Yintang, GV-20 and CV-17. The acupuncture treatment was mainly once per week although occasionally twice over an 8-week period. The outcome was that acupuncture was both efficacious and showed no side-effects. It was recommended that larger cohort studies should be carried out in the future. However, it must be noted that GB-21 is listed in TCM (traditional Chinese medicine) texts as a forbidden point in pregnancy, and care must be taken.

Abdominal pain

There will always be some degree of abdominal pain in pregnancy but if it is severe I would insist that the woman contact her doctor as well as offering treatment myself.

Abdominal pain may be due to ectopic pregnancy (a pregnancy that occurs outside the uterus in the fallopian tubes). This is usually accompanied by vaginal bleeding as well as abdominal pain and is potentially fatal.

Another possibility is fibroids; these may have been present before the pregnancy but, due to the increased blood supply in pregnancy, a fibroid may enlarge, often causing abdominal pain. (This equates in Chinese medicine to Blood stasis.) Do not treat fibroids in pregnancy.

Treatment with acupuncture

In Chinese terms, the main reason for abdominal pain would be Blood stasis, poor circulation of Qi and Blood, and Blood deficiency. A pre-existing Blood deficiency is also likely to cause abdominal pain, as the blood is diverted to nourish the fetus. Emotional problems, especially anger and resentment, will cause Liver Qi stagnation.

POINTS TO TREAT

I have tried a variety of points (Fig. 7.3), always avoiding the abdomen directly, and have found BL-17 and BL-20 to be effective. Tonify with moxa cones. The Spleen is considered the foundation of postnatal life and the source of Blood and these points strengthen the Spleen and the Blood, especially where the pain is due to Blood deficiency.

If the cause is stagnation of Qi, the symptoms will be a distending pain in the lower abdomen. Such women are usually very irritable and depressed, and probably suffered a lot of Liver Qi stagnation prior to getting pregnant. Use even technique on PC-6 and LR-3 together, to calm the mind and move the Qi.

One woman I treated was admitted to hospital with severe abdominal pain. She was very irritable and depressed. Although given every test possible, no medical explanation could be found for her pain. I treated her with acupuncture and there was a definite improvement using the above points.

If the pain is due to Cold and the woman finds that the pain improves when she uses heat, moxa can be used on CV-12 and ST-36 (depending on how many weeks pregnant she is).

Oedema

Mild swelling of the ankles, feet and hands is considered normal in the later stages of pregnancy. It usually occurs during the third trimester and is experienced by over half of normotensive women. For a few women, however, the swelling becomes severe and so painful that they are unable to walk. Swelling of the hands is known as carpal tunnel syndrome (see below, p. 114).

Water accounts for three-fifths of the body's weight and is constantly being exchanged between blood and tissues. Various disorders can interfere with this process. During pregnancy, the blood becomes more dilute and greater in volume, and because of the force of gravity the excess tissue fluid tends to gravitate towards the extremities. Provided the blood pressure and urine are tested frequently and remain normal, nothing needs to be done medically. This type of swelling tends to subside with rest. Gentle exercise to keep the circulation moving, flexing the calf muscles and rotating the ankles, and sitting or lying with the feet raised can all help.

Oedema can be accompanied by high blood pressure and protein in the urine (a possible sign of pre-eclampsia). I see this most frequently in women who are

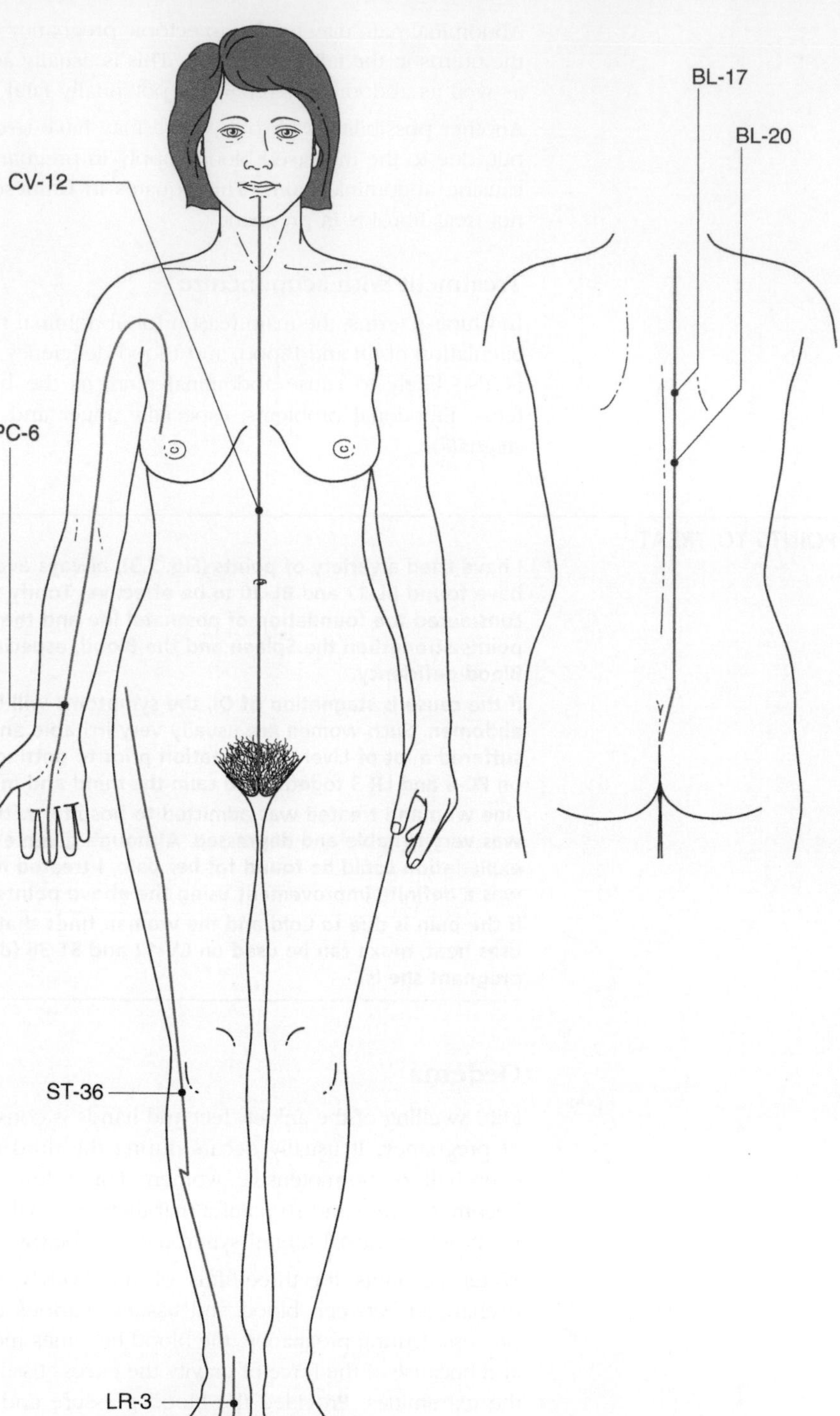

Figure 7.3 Points useful for the treatment of abdominal pain.

overweight prior to getting pregnant and in women who have had problems conceiving. If there is severe swelling of the hands and feet and any headache, the patient must contact her doctor or midwife as this also could be a sign of pre-eclampsia.

Causes

These include: increased blood volume, hot weather, standing for long periods of time, and carrying twins.

General advice

Patients should be advised to:

1. elevate the feet for 20 minutes, 3–4 times a day, especially during the peak time for the Water element, 3 p.m. to 7 p.m.
2. drink between meals rather than with meals
3. lie on the side when sleeping to improve circulation and reduce swelling
4. wear flat shoes and avoid tight shoes or socks
5. remove rings if the fingers are swelling
6. avoid crossing the legs.

Dietary advice

Parsley, onion and garlic are all good circulation tonics, so meals rich in these should be eaten. Choose foods or juices that act as natural diuretics, such as carrots, cucumber, grapes, lentils, legumes, peas, pineapple, seaweed, spinach, watercress and watermelon. Vitamin C also has a mild diuretic action, so increase the intake of C-rich fruits. Avoid ordinary table salt and instead buy a natural form of salt from a healthfood shop.

Treatment with acupuncture

Oedema in pregnancy is difficult to treat because it tends to get worse as the pregnancy progresses owing to the increasing volume of fluids. As it tends to occur in the last trimester, no abdominal points can be treated.

In the Chinese view, oedema is connected to poor diet. Too much raw or cold food in pregnancy can cause oedema by affecting the Spleen Yang, causing a failure of transportation.

Overwork is also thought to affect the Kidney Yang. Emotional factors such as worry, fear and anxiety can all lead to Stagnation of the Qi.

The most common pattern to find is Kidney Yang deficiency and the main treatment is to tonify the Yang. The Kidneys tend to become weaker as pregnancy progresses.

POINTS TO TREAT

- **BL-23 to tonify Kidney Yang.**
- **KI-3 to tonify the Kidneys.**
- **GV-4 could be used with moxa but only as a last resort.**

Other points to use for oedema include:

- **BL-20: tonify with moxa if the oedema is caused by Spleen Yang deficiency**
- **SP-3 tonification**
- **ST-36 tonification is effective in all cases of oedema.**

Carpal tunnel syndrome

Carpal tunnel syndrome is very common in pregnancy. It is caused by compression of the median nerve in the wrist. The symptoms are more common at night and include numbness, tingling and pain in the fingers.

Western medicine usually treats the condition with splints or bandages. Acupuncture works very well but a daily treatment is required. I use PC-5 with the needle angled towards the carpal tunnel, and ST-36, the empirical point of the wrist. Obtain Deqi and leave the needles in with even technique.

Relief is usually given for the first night but the pain returns again next morning. The condition improves spontaneously after the baby is delivered.

Anxiety

Although pregnancy is a normal, physiological life event, impending motherhood can also give rise to a great deal of anxiety, stress and fear. This may be caused by:

- fear of the unknown (in a first pregnancy)
- fear of pain, of having an abnormal baby or of losing control
- fear of repetition of a bad experience (such as a previous induced abortion, a still birth, a neonatal death or a bad obstetric experience)
- ambivalence about the pregnancy (which could be caused by a whole range of factors, such as the attitude to the conception, unhappy family circumstances, problems with finances or inadequate housing)
- personal problems (such as breakdown of the relationship with the partner or the death of a family member)
- feelings of ill health
- guilt about failure to give up smoking
- chronic stress (due to a stressful occupation, too much time spent travelling, or not enough time for mental preparation as the end of pregnancy approaches).

Probably the best way to help alleviate fears and anxieties is to provide a woman with a safe environment to talk them through, offering counselling where appropriate.

It is probable that maternal anxiety may increase the perception of pain, increasing the need for pain relief in labour. It may also interfere with normal uterine activity in labour, slowing down contractions. Therefore the more realistic reassurance that can be given to a woman to help her to handle her fears, the better.

Chinese viewpoint of anxiety in pregnancy

Emotional problems such as worry, fear and anger may lead to Qi stagnation (see Ch. 5), which in turn leads to Fire, which in turn will affect the mind. Pregnant women suffer a lot from Heat and anxiety in pregnancy is often Heat related.

Empty-Heat is generally caused by Yin deficiency. Symptoms include mental restlessness, fidgeting, dry mouth, hot flushes and night sweats.

POINTS TO TREAT

- **CV-15 relaxes the Mind and the chest; use even technique and leave the needles in for 20 minutes.**
- **KI-2 clears Empty-Heat; use even technique.**
- **KI-6 nourishes Kidney Yin, reinforcing tonification.**
- **Point Zero and Shenmen (auricular points).**

If the Liver is affected there will be more irritability and dream-disturbed sleep.

POINTS TO TREAT

- **LR-2 drains Liver Fire.**

Phobias may be caused by Phlegm.

- **ST-40 relieves Phlegm.**
- **ST-8 even technique.**

Baby not growing

To assess fetal growth, the age of the fetus must be established prior to 24 weeks of pregnancy. Regular abdominal examinations at antenatal visits will assess the height of the uterine fundus. If the baby appears small for its gestational age, an ultrasound scan will give further guidance, and babies that appear to be at risk will be closely monitored. The head circumference and the abdomen will be measured every 4 weeks.

Intrauterine growth retardation is caused by chronic, slowly progressive hypoxia (lack of oxygen), and the fetus will generally show asymmetrical growth patterns. If the hypoxia continues, the fetal organs can begin to fail, the placenta will age rapidly and the renal blood flow will fall, causing decreased amniotic fluid. Lack of oxygen to the central nervous system will lead to decreased fetal and respiratory movements and tone, and a drop in the variability of the fetal heart rate, which will be picked up on a CTG (cardiotocograph) (see Ch. 10).

Another test carried out is Doppler ultrasound, a non-invasive test using a device similar to the one used by midwives to listen to the baby.

Biophysical profiling may also be used, another non-invasive test to check fetal well-being in a fetus that does not appear to be growing. This measures the fetal heart rate, fetal tone, breathing movements and the volume of amniotic fluid. It also measures blood flowing through the umbilical artery.

Fetal distress and retardation of fetal growth are often related to social factors in the mother's profile:

- low socioeconomic status (this is not just a question of income but of education, nutrition, physical health and physique)
- maternal age (young teenagers and mothers over the age of 35 seem to be at higher risk)
- smoking (nicotine leads to decreased uterine blood flow and carbon monoxide reduces the transport of oxygen)
- maternal drug misuse in pregnancy (linked to intrauterine growth retardation, hypoxia, preterm labour and perinatal death)
- overwork: high-powered professional women who continue to work right through their pregnancy without giving themselves any time to rest
- poor obstetric history (previous abortions, preterm labours or still births).

Treatment with acupuncture

In Chinese terms, the reason for the fetus failing to grow would be deficient Blood in the mother or failure of the Kidneys to nourish properly; I always find some form of Kidney deficiency in such cases. This is also common in women who have previously had infertility problems, women with weak constitutions and women who work long hours.

I generally recommend to women that they try and put their feet up for an hour or two during the afternoon, to give themselves a chance to rest.

POINTS TO TREAT

The main points to use are ones that build up the Kidneys, Blood and Spleen.

- **BL-17, 20 and 23 to strengthen the Spleen and Kidney and to build up the Blood; use tonification with moxa if there are a lot of Yang signs of the Spleen and Kidney.**

On one occasion I used the Directing and Penetrating Vessels with a woman whose baby was very small at 32 weeks. A CTG tracing showed the heartbeat to be slow and the medical staff were anxiously trying to postpone doing a caesarean section. I used PC-6 (left) and SP-4 (right), inserting the needle to get the Deqi and leaving the needles in with even technique for 20 minutes. I also used LU-7 (right) and KI-6 (left). My intention was to try and improve the flow of blood to the placenta. Although this is purely anecdotal evidence, I am pleased to say that the tracing did start to improve while the needles were in.

Premature labour

Premature or preterm labour is defined as that occurring before the end of the 37th week of pregnancy (full term is between 38 and 42 weeks). It is found in between 6% and 10% of births in developed countries, with less than a quarter of preterm deliveries occurring before 32 weeks (Griffin 1993). Preterm birth is responsible for 75–90% of neonatal deaths.

Preterm birth may occur as a result of: elective preterm delivery (because of severe pre-eclampsia, maternal renal disease or severe intrauterine growth retardation), premature rupture of the membranes (see below), complicated emergency delivery (placental abruption, eclampsia, Rhesus isoimmunisation, maternal infection, prolapsed cord) or uncomplicated spontaneous preterm labour of unknown cause (the largest group, accounting for up to 40% of preterm births).

There are many risk factors associated with preterm labour (these are not the causes but can help to indicate those women most at risk):

- maternal age (less than 15, more than 35)
- low maternal bodyweight (less than 50 kg at conception)
- poverty or social deprivation
- marital status (preterm labour is more common in unmarried women)
- maternal employment that involves hard physical work
- psychological distress (emotional disturbance can affect nutritional status)
- cigarette, alcohol or drug abuse
- short gaps between pregnancies

- late antenatal booking and poor attendance for antenatal care
- maternal history of hypertension, renal disease or diabetes mellitus
- maternal viral or generalised infections or genital tract infection
- maternal history of preterm birth
- bleeding in the current or in a previous pregnancy
- uterine abnormality
- failure to gain weight adequately in the current pregnancy
- abdominal surgery
- multiple pregnancy (46% deliver preterm)
- polyhydramnios
- fetal malformation
- rhesus disease
- fetal death.

Prevention of preterm birth depends on preventing uterine activity or cervical dilation, or both. Bedrest is usually recommended. Antibiotic therapy may sometimes help and skin patches of glyceryl nitrate can be effective at suppressing contractions. Cervical cerclage, carried out under anaesthetic, may be helpful in cases in which there is a recognised cervical weakness.

Taking the minerals magnesium and calcium may help to prevent preterm labour.

Treatment with acupuncture

Before treating a patient with an irritable uterus (the term given to a uterus that keeps on contracting and is usually better with rest), with early contractions or preterm labour, it is vital to make sure that Western care is also being given. Anything that acupuncture can do will be in addition to this. Bear in mind also that you may have to see some women at their own homes, as exerting energy to go out for treatment could make the contractions much worse.

From the Chinese viewpoint, preterm labour is caused by a deficiency of Qi and Blood (the same as anaemia). If the cause is Blood deficiency, the solution is to tonify Blood points.

POINTS TO TREAT

- **BL-17, 20 and 23 to build up the blood; these points are good for deficiency conditions; heat with moxa and use tonification.**
- **BL-23 and 17: where there is a background of Kidney deficiency then tonification and moxa may be used.**
- **KI-6 and BL-23. use tonification but do not use moxa in cases of Kidney Yin deficiency.**
- **Other points I have found to be useful (here again my evidence is anecdotal) are on the Girdle Vessel; if the Girdle Vessel is deficient, the Spleen, Liver and Kidney also become deficient. Use GB-41 on the right side and TE-5 on the left side; obtain Deqi and leave the needles in with even technique for 20 minutes.**

CASE STUDY 7.2

Vicki has been pregnant seven times (including two miscarriages and twins in her fourth pregnancy). On each occasion she suffered from preterm labour and/or an irritable uterus that kept on contracting, and had to be repeatedly admitted to hospital from 20 weeks on for complete bedrest. Throughout the last three pregnancies, I have given her a weekly treatment from about 8 weeks of pregnancy.

Vicki's main problem is Kidney Yang deficiency, and Blood deficiency.

When the uterus is contracting, I needle the Penetrating Vessel PC-6 on the right side and SP-4 on the left side, as well as LU-7 and KI-6 to ease the abdominal pain and calm any anxiety in the patient. This treatment was really helpful in Vicki's case and I was able to treat her again 3 days later, when I added further points, BL-17 and 23, to tonify and build up her Blood and Kidney energy. On this occasion I used moxa on the points.

In her most recent pregnancy, Vicki was not admitted to hospital until 32 weeks (as opposed to 20 weeks in her previous pregnancies), and she delivered normally at 38 weeks.

CASE STUDY 7.3

Annabel was an IVF pregnancy with a history of infertility. She came to me at 24 weeks suffering frequent contractions and an irritable uterus. Problems with contractions are often linked to Kidney deficiency and an excess of heat. However, in Annabel's case, she was also very angry and frustrated by the contractions. She was suffering greatly from back ache and a feeling of heaviness in the abdomen: she felt like the baby was going to drop out. She also had a number of Yin symptoms, such as a dry mouth, thirst and heat at night. Movement made the contractions worse so I treated her at home.

I treated the Girdle Vessel points GB-41 on right side and TE-5 on the left side, PC-6 on the right side and LR-3 on the left side. After obtaining Deqi, I left the needles in for 45 minutes. The aim of the treatment was to calm her anxiety and move her Qi. I finished treatment by tonifying BL-23 and KI-6 to nourish her Yin.

I feel there is nothing to be lost by treating a woman with acupuncture in preterm labour, and possibly much to be gained (see Case studies 7.1 and 7.2).

Preterm rupture of the membranes

Preterm rupture of the membranes occurs when the fetal membranes (or the amniotic sac) spontaneously rupture before 37 weeks' gestation and before labour commences. The cause is unclear but may be associated with cervical incompetence or genital tract infection. Labour often starts soon after but if several days elapse without this happening, then the uterine cavity and the fetus may be colonised by bacteria, which increases the risk to the fetus. There is also the danger of prolapse of the umbilical cord.

If rupture occurs at home, the woman should be admitted to a hospital with a neonatal unit. Temperature and pulse should be recorded at least twice a day if labour does not start at once, and antibiotics prescribed if there is evidence of infection. It is also important to check for signs of bleeding, in case of placental abruption due to the reduction in liquor volume. Steroids may also be prescribed if the woman is between 24 and 32 weeks, to help promote lung maturity in the fetus and reduce the risk of respiratory disease syndrome at birth.

Different hospitals have different policies about when a women should go into hospital or not. I have never treated preterm rupture of the membranes with acupuncture because I do not believe it is appropriate to do so.

Nutrition in the third trimester

Although, as detailed in Chapter 3, the baby is growing rapidly during this period, the mother only needs to consume approximately 200 extra calories a day. Any more could lead to excess weight gain that she will find hard to shed later. A balanced diet is recommended, containing plenty of fruit, vegetables, nuts, cereals, seeds, lentils and wholegrains, high in fibre, low in fats and sugar. The body's need for protein also increases slightly.

All the main vitamins and minerals are needed. These and their food sources are dealt with in detail in Chapter 3.

So far as the baby is concerned, the mature brain is made up of 60% lipids or fats, particularly 'long chain polyunsaturated fatty acids' or LCPs. The two most important for the development and functioning of the brain are arachidonic acid (AA) and docosahexaenoic acid (DHA) (see Ch. 3).

Summary

- Common problems in the third trimester include: anaemia, cramps, insomnia, abdominal pain, oedema and carpal tunnel syndrome, the baby not growing, anxiety, premature labour and preterm rupture of membranes.
- Acupuncture points to use during the third trimester include:
  - *anaemia*: BL-17 and 15 (Spleen Qi deficiency); BL-17 and 18, LR-8 (Liver Blood deficiency)
  - *cramps*: LR-8
  - *insomnia*: ST-36, BL-20, 15 and 17 (Heart and Spleen Blood deficiency); BL-15 and 23, HT-7 (Heart and Kidney not harmonised)
  - *abdominal pain*: BL-17 and 20; plus PC-6 and LR-3 (Liver Qi stagnation), CV-12 and ST-36 (moxa, for Cold)
  - *oedema and carpal tunnel syndrome*: BL-23, KI-3, GV-4 (with moxa, as a last resort); plus BL-20 (moxa, for Spleen Yang deficiency), SP-3 and ST-36; PC-5 and ST-36 (carpal tunnel)
  - *anxiety*: CV-15, KI-2 and 6, Point Zero and Shenmen; plus LR-2 (Liver Fire), ST-40 and 8 (Phlegm)
  - *baby not growing (IUGR)*: BL-17, 20 and 23
  - *premature labour*: BL-17, 20 and 23 (for deficiency), BL-23 and KI-6 (Kidney Yin deficiency); plus GB-41 (right) and TE-5 (left).

References

Griffin J 1993 Born too soon. Office of Health Economics, London

Guerreiro da Silva JB, Nakamura MU, Cordeiro JA, Kulay L 2005 Acupuncture for insomnia in pregnancy – a prospective, quasi-randomised, controlled study. Acupuncture in Medicine 23(2): 47–51

Sweet BR (ed.) 1997 Mayes' midwifery, 12th edn. Baillière Tindall, New York, p 584

Further reading

Barker DJP 1992 Diet for a lifetime. Mothers' and babies' health in later life. Churchill Livingstone, New York

Crawford M, Doyle A 1989 Fatty acids during early human development. Journal of Internal Medicine 225: 159–169

Department of Health 1991 Dietary reference values for food energy and nutrients for the United Kingdom. HMSO, London

8 High-risk pregnancies

Chapter outline

This chapter is intended as a reference guide for the acupuncturist. When giving acupuncture to women who are considered a high risk medically, it is as well to have a background knowledge of the possible complications. It is my strong opinion that any woman with complications should always be treated in conjunction with her midwife and doctor.

A high-risk pregnancy means simply that the fetus is at risk (OPCS 1994).

Twins and other multiple pregnancies

The incidence of multiple pregnancies (Fig. 8.1) is currently rising in many countries. In 1994 there were approximately 13 twins per every thousand live births (rising from 10 per thousand in 1982) and 14 triplets (plus) per thousand (rising from 9 per thousand in 1982) (Sweet 1997). This rise is in the main related to the increased use of fertility treatments.

Complications

Multiple pregnancy should not be regarded as abnormal. However, with more than one baby the minor disturbances in pregnancy such as morning sickness, heartburn, back ache, sleeplessness and exhaustion are all more likely to be exaggerated.

The mother should be encouraged to rest as much as possible to minimise the risk of such problems. Good nutrition from a well-balanced diet is especially important.

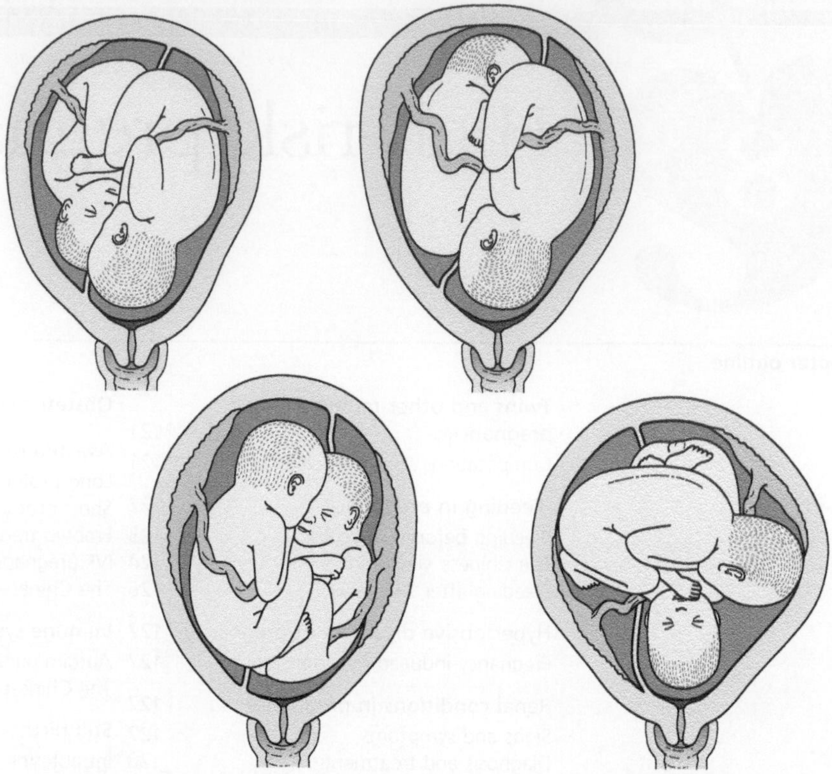

Figure 8.1 Positions of twins in the uterus.

During labour there are greater risks to both mother and babies. Policy on managing the risk varies, and it will depend on the individual hospital whether the mother will be offered a caesarean section or allowed to deliver the twins vaginally. Medical complications that can arise are:

- *pregnancy-induced hypertension (PIH)*: more common in twin pregnancies
- *anaemia*: not surprisingly, greater demands are made on the mother's stores of iron and folic acid when there is more than one baby, which can result in anaemia
- *preterm labour*: a common risk, and babies are typically also light in weight for their dates
- *antepartum haemorrhage*: significantly increased in multiple pregnancy
- *placenta praevia*: more common because of the large placental site.

Bleeding in pregnancy

An irregular and unbalanced diet over a long period of time may lead to Blood and Qi deficiency. Blood deficiency means that the fetus is not adequately nourished. Emotional problems, worry, anger, fear and grief may lead to Liver Qi stagnation. Over a long period of time, this may turn to Heat, which causes bleeding. Overwork and working long hours without adequate rest over time can cause Kidney Yin deficiency.

The significance of the bleeding depends on whether it occurs in early or in late pregnancy. The 24th week is regarded as the watershed.

Bleeding before 24 weeks

Prior to week 24, bleeding may be caused by: implantation, abortion, hydatidiform mole, ectopic pregnancy, cervical lesions or vaginitis. Any bleeding vaginally is considered abnormal and should be reported to a doctor.

Implantation bleeding

There may be a little bleeding when the ovum embeds into the uterus. It is usually bright red and of short duration. Implantation takes place 8–10 days after fertilisation.

Abortion

Spontaneous abortion

In at least 15% of confirmed pregnancies, spontaneous abortion occurs before the 12th week of pregnancy (Lewis & Chamberlain 1990). It is more common in a first pregnancy. Spontaneous abortion is caused by the following.

- *Maldevelopment of the fetus*: chromosomal abnormalities account for 70% of defective conceptions (Lewis & Chamberlain 1990).
- *Maternal disease*: an acute illness such as influenza, rubella, appendicitis or pneumonia, particularly when accompanied by a high temperature, can result in spontaneous abortion. Infections such as toxoplasmosis and listeria are also a danger, as are urinary tract infections (pyelonephritis) caused by pregnancy. Other medical diseases, including diabetes and thyroid disease, are also associated with a high risk of abortion.
- *Maternal immune response*: see separate section below.
- *Uterine abnormalities*: there may be structural abnormalities in the uterus, which prevent it from sustaining a healthy pregnancy.
- *Environmental factors*: lead pollution, radiation, drugs, alcohol and smoking can all cause abortion.
- *Stress*: severe emotional upset can lead to abortion.
- *IVF (in vitro fertilisation) pregnancy*: about 21% of IVF pregnancies abort spontaneously.

Threatened abortion/miscarriage

Slight bleeding may occur during the first 3 months of pregnancy. It may be painless or it may be associated with abdominal pain or back ache even though there is no dilation of the cervix. Conventional Western treatment is to recommend bedrest (often in hospital) until the bleeding stops.

Increased bleeding is an ominous sign that abortion may occur, but 'bedrest and let's see what happens' is all that Western medicine can advise. This is a good example of where acupuncture can, by comparison, make a very positive contribution.

Inevitable abortion

The conditions described above are all treatable with acupuncture but if the cervix is dilating, abortion is the unavoidable outcome. The bleeding is more severe than in a threatened abortion.

Missed abortion

You may hear the term 'missed abortion' to describe the retention (rather than abortion) of a dead fetus. This may not be identified until several weeks after the fetus has died.

Recurrent abortion

This is a term used when three or more consecutive abortions have occurred. It is also known as habitual abortion. Following three or more miscarriages, the patient is usually investigated and tests may indicate one of the following: abnormality of the uterus, incompetent cervix, maternal disease, genetic causes, hormonal deficiency or maternal immune response.

The Chinese viewpoint

I am often asked if intervention with acupuncture is somehow 'going against nature'. The Chinese view of threatened abortion is that it is an imbalance of the natural state that it is quite appropriate to redress. The Chinese differentiate between uterine bleeding (where the bleeding is scanty and the only symptom) and what they describe as 'restlessness of the fetus' (where there is lower abdominal pain and lumbar soreness). Each denotes a different stage of the same problem.

Causes

The main cause of spontaneous abortion is disharmony of the Qi and Blood in the Directing and Penetrating Channels. The Penetrating Vessel is the Sea of Blood and is needed to nourish the fetus. If the fetus cannot grow, it becomes weakened and a miscarriage is the potential result.

POINTS TO TREAT THE PENETRATING VESSEL

- **ST-30**
- **SP-4 and PC-6**

Other factors can also play a part. Stomach or Spleen deficiency can cause sinking of Qi and consequent failure to hold the fetus. There may also be a Kidney deficiency, a constitutional weakness or a Heat pattern. Emotional factors, such as worry, fear, anger or grief, can all contribute. The eventual result will be to affect the Liver Qi, which will turn to Liver Fire and Blood Heat.

If a woman has had any previous miscarriages, it is vital to mitigate the risks with good preconceptual care. Optimum nutrition is an important part of this care, to ensure an adequate intake of vitamins and nutrients such as zinc, magnesium and essential fatty acids (see Ch. 3).

A woman suffering from a deficiency of Qi and Blood usually looks pale, weak and tired. This overall impression will be matched by a pale tongue and weak pulse.

POINTS TO TREAT

Typically I treat by tonifying the following points.

- **BL-17 and 20: this is a good combination to treat with moxa for the Blood and production of the Blood.**
- **BL-17 and 18: treat with moxa for Liver Blood.**
- **ST-36: to tonify Qi.**

I always treat the empirical point SP-1, using up to 10 moxa cones on the point. Depending on the severity of the bleeding, I may needle the point and leave the needles in place. I also instruct the patient in applying moxa to herself, so that she can continue regular treatment at home. My experience has shown this sustained treatment to be very effective in stopping bleeding.

Kidney deficiency

When symptoms of threatened miscarriage include back ache, period-type pains, slight dizziness and the frequent passing of urine, Kidney deficiency is indicated. This is more likely to occur in patients who have had a previous miscarriage.

POINTS TO TREAT

Treatment in this case would concentrate on the Kidneys.

- **Tonify points BL-17 and 23, and the Source point of the Kidney, KI-3.**
- **Use moxa on SP-1, and encourage the patient to continue use at home.**

CASE STUDY 8.1

Celia had had three pregnancies, all the result of IVF, but all had ended in miscarriage. In one pregnancy she sadly lost the baby at 24 weeks. She came to me for acupuncture in desperate hope, prior to her fourth IVF attempt.

Her main weakness was a Kidney deficiency, which was exacerbated by all the IVF drugs. She became pregnant but at 5 weeks she started to bleed. The treatment I gave her concentrated on SP-1, which I heated with moxa cones. I also gave her sufficient cones to take away, so that her partner could treat her once a day. I tonifed BL-17 (for the Blood) and BL-23 (for the Kidneys). The bleeding stopped.

The same thing happened again every 2–3 weeks. She was understandably very fearful and refused a scan, as she was worried about the effect of the ultrasound and did not feel the benefits were worth the risk. She kept up the acupuncture treatments and the bleeding continued at intervals with no known cause until she was 20 weeks. She went on to deliver a healthy boy at 39 weeks.

Heat

I have found Heat to be quite a common cause of miscarriage. Typically patients suffer abdominal pain and constipation, with bright red bleeding. The tongue will be red with a yellow coating.

Acupuncture should be aimed at clearing the heat and will depend on the severity of the bleeding.

POINTS TO TREAT

- **At a first treatment I would use SP-10 and LI-11, leaving the needles in place for 30–40 minutes; these points are known to cool the Blood.**
- **To conclude treatment I would tonify BL-23 and always tonify BL-17.**

Figure 8.2 Placenta praevia, types I–IV. (Reproduced with permission from Sweet 1997, p. 253.)

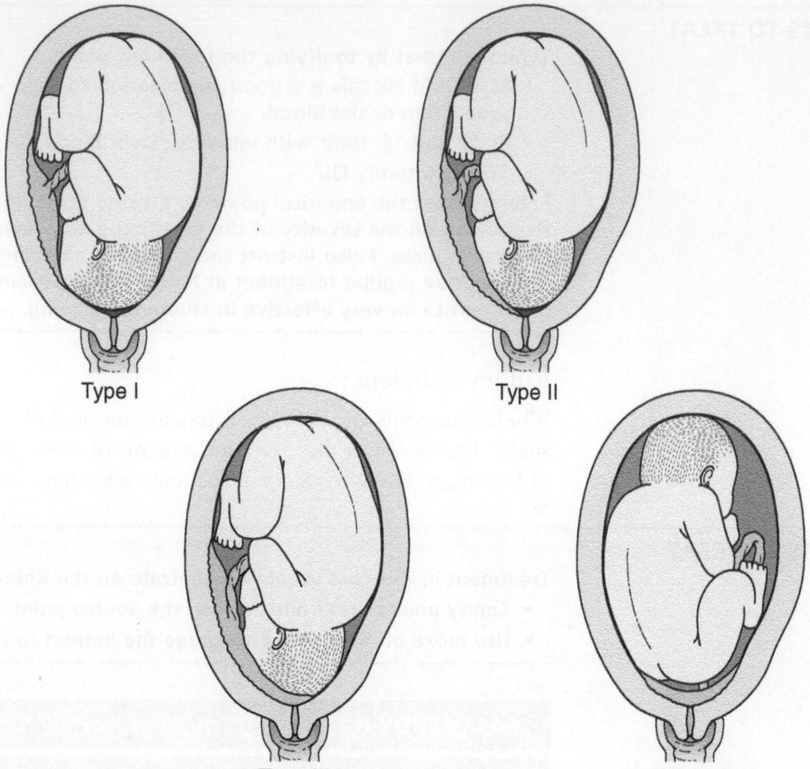

Recurrent abortion

I use points on the Chong and Ren channels, since conception can only occur when the Ren channel is normal and the Sea of Blood Chong channel is sufficient. In cases of recurrent abortion there is always some degree of Kidney deficiency. The same principles apply as for threatened miscarriage and the aim should be to work on the Kidney channel and strengthen the Kidneys prior to a pregnancy.

POINTS TO TREAT

As a preventive measure before the woman is pregnant, these are:

- **CV-6, which tonifies the Kidney**
- **CV-7, which nourishes Kidney Yin.**

Bleeding after 24 weeks

Antepartum haemorrhage

Bleeding after 24 weeks of pregnancy is known as an antepartum haemorrhage. This is a serious complication, which can result in death of the mother and the baby. There are two varieties:

- *placenta praevia*: bleeding as a result of separation or abnormality of the placenta which can lie over the cervix (Fig. 8.2)
- *abruptio placentae*: bleeding from separation of the placenta (Fig. 8.3).

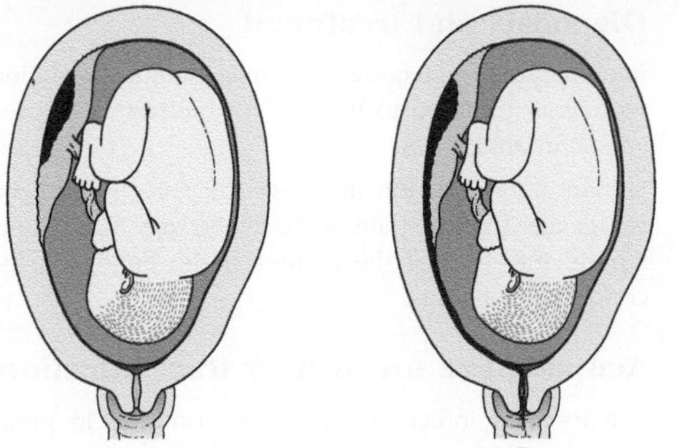

Figure 8.3 Abruptio placentae: A concealed; B revealed. (Reproduced with permission from Sweet 1997, p. 527.)

I would not recommend using acupuncture for bleeding in later pregnancy. A woman who has any bleeding in later pregnancy must be under medical supervision, as heavy blood loss may result in loss of the baby.

Hypertensive disorders of pregnancy

Pregnancy-induced hypertension (PIH)

Hypertension, or high blood pressure, is defined as a level of 140/90 or more. It is considered potentially serious when measured at this level after the 20th week of pregnancy and on at least two separate occasions after that. It is usually accompanied by protein in the urine and by oedema.

Although much research has been done on PIH, the causes remain uncertain. Certain women have more predisposing factors:

- primigravidae or first-time mothers
- young teenagers
- women over 35 years of age
- women with an obesity problem.

I rarely treat pregnant women for PIH but if necessary will help with acupuncture points for stress.

Renal conditions in pregnancy

Pyelonephritis is an inflammatory state of the urinary tract, due to bacterial infection. It is more likely to occur in pregnancy because of the physiological changes that take place and it is found in 1–2% of all pregnancies (Sweet 1997). The organism responsible is *Escherichia coli*.

Signs and symptoms

Onset commonly occurs around the 20th week of pregnancy. The woman may complain of pain in the loin (often on the right side), she may have a headache and nausea, raised temperature and increased pulse rate, and suffer pain and a frequent need to pass urine.

Diagnosis and treatment

Pyelonephritis is diagnosed by microscopical examination of a urine specimen. The woman is admitted to hospital for bedrest and observation and prescribed broad-spectrum antibiotics.

Urinary tract infection increases the risk of abortion or preterm labour and there is a danger that the pain of the illness may mask the uterine contractions of preterm labour. Infection of the mother at the time of delivery puts the infant at risk of congenital infection.

Acupuncture for urinary tract infections

Urinary tract infections are quite common in pregnancy but should always be treated as they can result in a miscarriage or premature labour if the pregnancy is advanced. Western medicine is required for this, but simple acupuncture points may also help.

POINTS TO USE

- **BL-63 Accumulation point clears Heat and stops pain.**
- **KI-2 and HT-6 helps clear Empty-Heat.**

Diabetes

Diabetes is a medical condition in which the pancreas fails to produce sufficient insulin. Although the effect is mainly seen in relation to glucose metabolism, most of the metabolic pathways are disturbed and the disease affects all the systems of the body. Perinatal complications and mortality are increased.

Types of diabetes

Insulin dependent

The patient will have an abnormal glucose tolerance test and an almost complete lack of insulin. The symptoms are significant (including excessive urination and dehydration) and treatment is required. It is most common in juveniles.

Non-insulin dependent

The patient will have abnormal glucose tolerance test but no symptoms. It is more frequent in later life and among those who are obese.

Gestational diabetes

A woman can develop glucose intolerance during pregnancy due to impaired insulin secretion and action. It is generally treated by diet and insulin therapy. Recent studies have shown that gestational diabetes has increased alongside the rise of general obesity around the Western world. Although investigations are ongoing, some studies have shown that untreated gestational diabetes has been linked to an increased risk of obesity and diabetes of those children as young adults. Lifestyle changes and the use of oral medication are now being looked at as less costly treatment (Catalano et al 2003, Metzger 2006, Svare et al 2001).

Obstetric cholestasis

This is a condition caused by an overflow of bile passing through to the placenta. It is toxic to the baby and if left untreated can result in still birth.

The symptoms are severe itching in the third trimester, from 28 weeks – itching so severe that the woman will have to scratch herself constantly.

Diagnosis is by a blood test and a liver function test and the woman is usually delivered at 37–38 weeks.

Always be wary if asked to treat a woman with very bad itching. It is important that she consults her doctor or midwife, and I only treat in conjunction with the doctor. Acupuncture can help with the skin itching but it does not get rid of the underlying condition.

POINTS TO TREAT

Use points to cool the Blood:

- **SP-10**
- **LI-11**
- **tonify BL-17 and BL-19 to build up the Liver Blood.**

Assisted reproductive techniques

Over the last 20 years assisted reproductive techniques (ART) have increased and may offer couples their only chance of having a child. Those who decide to go down this route will have undergone numerous tests to find out if there is a reason for their inability to conceive.

- *Female tests*: hormone assessment, tubal assessment, infection and immunological sceening, endometriosis, fibroids, polycystic ovary syndrome.
- Male tests: semen analysis, hormone assessment and infection screening.

Since 1978 and the birth of the first 'test tube baby', in vitro fertilisation (IVF) and/or intracytoplasmic sperm injection (ICSI) have become the most common ART procedures in the Western world. IVF is the fertilisation of an egg by a sperm in a laboratory Petri dish. ICSI will follow the same procedures as IVF but the sperm is injected directly into the egg. The fertilised egg is transferred into the womb. ICSI is the preferred treatment if there is male factor infertility, such as poor sperm count, high proportion of abnormal forms, the sperm have to be obtained surgically or there was a low fertilisation rate in previous IVF cycles.

There are two main types of IVF protocols – long and short. However, all IVF clinic programmes will differ slightly; some clinics like to put the woman on the oral contraceptive pill to rest the ovaries prior to commencement.

Long protocol

This is generally used on women who have regular menstrual cycles and whose hormone profiles are within the normal limits. Following natural ovulation, the woman will take gonadotrophin-releasing hormone (GnRH) agonists, in the form of either a nasal spray or injection. The GnRH will prevent the pituitary gland from producing follicle-stimulating hormone (FSH) and luteinising hormone (LH), thus putting the body into a temporary state of menopause. This is known as 'down-regulation' and may take around 2 weeks but can be longer. The clinic will monitor the process via blood tests and ultrasound scan.

If all tests are within the normal range the next stage of the treatment will begin. This is stimulation of the follicles by injection of FSH or FSH and LH. This stage is very carefully monitored once again by scan and blood tests, as too little of the drugs could result in an unsuccessful cycle and too much can lead to overstimulation and the serious side-effect of ovarian hyperstimulation syndrome (OHSS; see below). Some clinics will check blood levels of oestrogen daily. After approximately 10–14 days of stimulation, the follicles should be mature enough for egg collection. A trigger injection of human chorionic gonadotrophin (HCG) is given 36 hours prior to egg collection, which prepares the follicles for egg release.

Short protocol

This can be called a 'flare' or 'boost' cycle and takes advantage of the natural levels of FSH which will be tested on day 2 or 3 of a cycle. The woman will take both the GnRH agonist and the FSH drugs at the same time. The follicle development is monitored as before in the long protocol.

Egg collection is normally via the vagina using ultrasound scan to guide a needle into each follicle in the ovaries. Most clinics will use light sedation, some will give a general anaesthetic. The number of eggs will vary depending on age and other unknown factors, but it is quality rather than quantity which matters.

The sperm donated during the egg retrieval stage are washed and sorted into the best motile sperm, in the laboratory. The eggs then meet the sperm in a culture medium in a dish or tube and are incubated overnight at 37°, identical to a woman's body temperature. If ICSI is the option then an embryologist will choose a single sperm and inject it into the egg under a microscope.

Embryo transfer

This will take place between 2 and 5 days following fertilisation. A 5-day embryo is called a blastocyst; in natural conception this is the stage at which the embryo will implant in the uterus. However, in IVF embryos may stop developing at any stage and although longer culture can allow the embryologist to choose the best-quality one, it could also leave the couple with no embryos to transfer back.

The transfer is a simple procedure: the embryos are put into a thin catheter, which is inserted via the vagina into the uterus. The embryos are released and the catheter slowly and carefully removed and checked to ensure that no embryos have remained within it. The current ruling by the Human Fertilisation and Embryology Authority (HFEA) is that a maximum of two embryos may be transferred in women under 40 and three in women over the age of 40.

Following transfer, I would recommend, if possible, that the woman puts her feet up for a minimum of 3 days. There is no research to show that this will increase the chances of getting pregnant but my belief is that you should give those embryos every possible chance to implant. One of the factors important for successful implantation is good blood flow through the womb lining. Physical activity diverts blood to the extremities and vital centres, whereas lying down allows for a good flow of blood to the womb.

Then there is a 2-week wait until a pregnancy test can be taken. During this time the woman will be on various medications.

- Progesterone: in the form of injection, vaginal pessary or suppository. This can help to sustain the pregnancy and prepare the womb lining for implantation.

- HCG: injection; maintains the womb lining.
- Heparin: injection; thins the blood and is used if there is any history of recurrent miscarriage and/or immune problems (see below).
- Aspirin: tablet; also used to thin the blood and if there is any history of recurrent miscarriage and/or immune problems (see below).
- Steroids: this can be in the form of injection – intravenous immunoglobulin (IVIG) – or tablet. Common brand names are prednisolone or dexametasone (see below).

IVF pregnancy complications

The use of ART in industrialised countries has become a routine infertility treatment. In the last 10 years there have been many research articles comparing pregnancy complications and obstetric risk in twin and singleton IVF/ICSI pregnancies, with those of a natural conception (Lambers et al 2007, Ochsenkuhn et al 2003, Tallo et al 1995).

A recent study from Canada (Allen et al 2006) which reviewed articles from 1995 to 2005 on the effect of ART on perinatal outcomes and obstetric risk showed that there is a definite link to a higher risk of perinatal complications, due mainly to the higher incidence of multiple pregnancies. These include pregnancy-induced hypertension, preterm birth, low birthweight, abruptio placentae and placenta praevia. The outcomes of that study and others have lead to a push from the medical world for single embryo transfer in ART, especially at blastocyst stage (Jansen & Sullivan 2006, Pinborg et al 2004). However, the study stated: 'it remains unclear if these increased risks are attributable to the underlying infertility, characteristics of the infertile couple, or use of the assisted reproductive techniques' (Allen et al 2006).

Ovarian hyperstimulation syndrome

During an IVF cycle some women may be more sensitive to the drugs used to stimulate follicle production, and produce a large amount of follicles. This can cause the ovaries to increase in size and raise blood oestrogen levels. As a result it can lead to leakage of fluid into the abdominal cavity and lungs causing breathlessness, reduced urine production and blood clotting problems. This is known as ovarian hyperstimulation syndrome (OHSS).

The most common time for this to occur would be near to egg collection or after embryo transfer. The IVF cycle may be abandoned completely or slowed down by 'coasting' – FSH drugs are withdrawn until oestrogen levels drop to a safe level. The higher risk patients for OHSS are younger women and those diagnosed with polycystic ovary syndrome (PCOS).

Women who go through an IVF cycle are carefully monitored via blood samples and ultrasound scans and therefore OHSS is a rare occurrence. As an acupuncturist treating through an IVF cycle it is important to be aware of the signs and symptoms:

- severe lower abdominal pain
- difficulty breathing
- nausea and vomiting
- very swollen abdomen
- dizziness, feeling faint
- passing small amounts of urine.

If a patient presents with these symptoms it is vital to refer them back to their IVF consultant as soon as possible.

The Chinese viewpoint on infertility

In Chinese medicine the menstrual cycle is divided into four phases – period, post-menstrual, mid-menstrual and premenstrual. The Kidney energy is the most vital aspect: 'The treatment of infertility according to the four phases is always based principally on treating the Kidneys, because the phases are a result of the waxing and waning of Kidney-Yin and Kidney-Yang and because the Kidneys are the source of the Heavenly *Gui* which is the basis for reproduction' (Maciocia 1998, p. 695).

Acupuncture treatment through an IVF cycle can help in many ways.

- Increase implantation rates.
- Increase blood flow to the ovaries to boost follicular development.
- Increase blood flow to the endometrium.
- Relieve side-effects of the drug.
- Relax and reduce anxiety levels.

There are now a number of research articles pertaining to acupuncture treatment and an increased success rate of IVF. The treatments below are only a basic starting point as each patient will present with varying patterns of disharmony, at different stages of their treatment.

Downregulation phase

At this time the woman's hormone system is being shut down, putting her into a menopausal state. She may present with headache and irritability and other signs of Liver Qi stagnation.

POINTS TO TREAT

- **Yintang, LI-4, LR-3, LR-14, GB-34, Shenmen**

Follicular stimulation phase

The ovaries are being stimulated via injections of FSH. The woman may now become bloated and irritable and experience the most commonly seen side-effect, exhaustion. Her stress levels may be increasing as she has to visit the clinic for blood tests and scans on a daily basis.

POINTS TO TREAT

- **Yintang, Chong and Ren Mai**

Transfer phase

Recent studies from Germany and Denmark have shown a remarkable, almost 50% increase in success rates in women who had acupuncture 25 minutes before and after embryo transfer. The studies used the same acupuncture points which, according to TCM (traditional Chinese medicine) principles, would increase blood circulation and energy to the uterus as well as relax the patient (Paulus et al 2002, Westergaard et al 2006).

Three of the extraordinary channels are important in fertility treatment. The follicles, ovum and corpus luteum are Yin in nature and relate to the Ren and Chong Mai. For fertilisation to take place, there has to be a change from Yin to Yang, for which the Du Mai is responsible, thus maturing the follicle to release the egg and the thickening of the corpus luteum. Therefore in acupuncture treatment during an IVF cycle, it would be appropriate to use these channels.

Immune system

In recent years there has been much research into the role of the immune system and the body's inflammatory response during pregnancy. However, many of the new theories remain controversial. For a pregnancy to survive to term, the woman's immune system must recognise what is going on and not reject the fetus. It is thought that recurrent miscarriage may be due to a failure in the immune mechanisms, from either an autoimmune reaction or the inability of the mother's immune system to respond protectively (Balen & Jacobs 2003).

Autoimmunity

Obstetrical antiphospholipid syndrome

Since the 1950s it has been known that the presence of a high concentration of antiphospholipid antibodies (APAs) can cause numerous obsteteric complications such as miscarriage, intrauterine growth retardation and pre-eclampsia (Sarig et al 2002).

APAs are a type of antibody – 'proteins that are made by the immune system as a primary defense against infection or injury by foreign proteins. (The immune system is able to distinguish between proteins that are "self" and those which are foreign, or "nonself".)' (Sher et al 2005).

The APAs are said to attack the placental cells and blood supply. Treatment with low-dose aspirin and heparin has been shown to significantly reduce the risk of miscarriage. In fact, studies have shown that with no treatment, the live-birth rate can be as low as 10%, with heparin only 40% and with the combined aspirin and heparin a remarkable 70% (Rai et al 1997). More recent studies have looked at the management guide of antiphospholipid syndrome as combining aspirin, heparin and intravenous immunoglobulin (Asherton et al 2006, Erkan & Lockshin 2006).

Antinuclear antibodies (ANAs)

These are thought to be related to women who suffer from systemic lupus erythematosus (SLE) or rheumatoid arthritis. The ANAs attack the cells of the placenta and uterus, leading to an inflammatory response which can impede implantation and cause early miscarriage. These can be treated with an oral corticosteroid such as prednisolone.

Natural killer (NK) cells

These cells are part of the immune system's first line of defence against life-threatening diseases such as cancer. In pregnancy there is an abundance of NK cells in the uterine lining, which work with the fetal trophoblast to help develop the placenta (Hanna et al 2006). However, recent research from around the world has shown that an overabundance of NK cells can be toxic to the trophoblast cells and lead to cell death and early abortion (Quenby & Farquharson 2006).

Further studies on the immunology of pregnancy have noted that abnormal function of NK cells during pregnancy may lead to pre-eclampsia (Le Bouteiller & Tabiasco 2006, Sargent et al 2006). The present treatment of choice for women who are tested via a blood sample and show raised levels of NK cells is oral steroid – prednisolone and or administration of intravenous immunoglobulin (IVIG) (Clark et al 2006). A recent study in Italy looked at the use of progesterone gel administered via the vagina that showed a reduction of NK cells in women with recurrent spontaneous abortions (De Carolis et al 2006).

The Chinese viewpoint

In Chinese medicine there is no discourse on the immune system as such. However, according to Professor Yu Jin of Shanghai Medical University, 'The Kidneys are said to be the essence of life, while the Liver has a common source with the Kidneys. Both relate to growth and reproduction, and can thus be associated with the functions of the hypothalamus, pituitary, ovaries, adrenals, and thyroid, which also comprise the body's immuno-neuroendocrine framework' (Yu Jin 1998).

There may also a link between the Kidney Essence, *jing*, the bone marrow and the immune system, as in Western medicine the immune response is thought to come from a stem cell in the bone marrow (Maciocia 1994).

POINTS TO TREAT

To tonify Kidney and Liver Qi:

- **KI-3: tonifies both Kidney Yin and Yang**
- **KI-7: nourishes Kidney Yang**
- **LR-14: nourishes the Liver**
- **BL-23: Kidney Qi**
- **BL-52: Kidneys**
- **GV-4: general Yang tonic.**

In TCM the acupuncture point ST-36 is said to strengthen the immune system and boost the body's resistance to disease (Ross 1995). The Spleen's function of constantly transforming what is consumed into new Qi and Blood also plays a part in the body's defence system (Liang 2003). Recent studies from Korea and Taiwan have shown an impact on autoimmune diseases such as SLE and arthritis with electro-acupuncture and moxibustion on ST-36 and SP-6, by 'suppressing autoimmunity and modulating immune abnormality' (Kung et al 2006, Yun-Kyong et al 2007).

CASE STUDY 8.2

Anna was 33. She had suffered three spontaneous abortions between 5 and 8 weeks of pregnancy in the past 2 years. Recently she decided to try IVF and had bloods taken to check her immune system, which showed raised NK cells. Anna was told by her specialist that she would require treatment with oral steroids and intravenous immunoglobulin for a successful outcome. Anna felt she would like to try a more natural approach for 4–6 months. She came for acupuncture and on initial consultation showed weakness in the Stomach and Kidney energy.

Anna had weekly acupuncture for 6 weeks, specifically focusing on points to regulate the immune system and tonify Kidney Qi – ST-36, SP-6, Ren-12, Ren-4, BL-23, BL-20, BL-17. She also made lifestyle changes to her diet and exercise regimes.

In the third month of treatment Anna called to say she had conceived naturally. She had no problems during her pregnancy and continued with acupuncture every 6–8 weeks, with ST-36 and BL-23 used in each session. Anna gave birth to a healthy boy at 40 weeks.

Still birth

The definition of still birth is a baby who has been born after 24 weeks of pregnancy but did not breathe or show any signs of life.

It is usually the result of some congenital abnormality or fetal anoxia. Fetal anoxia is starvation of oxygen, which can occur because of: cord prolapse, the placenta not functioning properly, the placenta coming away from the uterine wall, medical conditions such as diabetes, intrauterine infection or a traumatic delivery. Acupuncture after a still birth can be of benefit to the mother and can do a great deal to restore the spirit.

Intrauterine death

This may be due to fetal distress and may be indicated by reduced fetal movements. At least 75% of women will start labour spontaneously but if this does not happen, they will be brought in to hospital for an induction once it has been diagnosed. Acupuncture can be used to get a woman started but if a uterine death occurs before the due date then only an induction will get a woman into labour.

Summary

- A high risk is associated with: twins and other multiple pregnancies, bleeding in pregnancy, hypertensive disorders of pregnancy (PIH), renal conditions, diabetes and obstetric cholestasis.
- Acupuncture points for high-risk pregnancies include:
  - *recurrent abortion*: CV-6 and 7
  - *threatened abortion*: BL-17, 18 and 20, ST-36 (Qi and Blood deficiency); BL-17 and 23, KI-3 (Kidney deficiency); SP-10, LI-11, BL-23 and 17 (Heat)
  - *renal conditions*: BL-63, KI-2 and HT-6
  - *obstetric cholestasis*: SP-10, LI-11, BL-17 and 19.

References

Allen VM, Wilson RD, Cheung A 2006 Pregnancy outcomes after assisted reproductive technology. Journal of Obstetrics and Gynaecology Canada 28(3): 220–250

Asherton RA, Frances C, Iaccarino L et al 2006 The antiphospholipid antibody syndrome: diagnosis, skin manifestations and current therapy. Clinical and Experimental Rheumatology 24(1 suppl 40): S46–51

Balen AH, Jacobs HS 2003 Infertility in practice, 2nd edn. Churchill Livingstone, Edinburgh

Catalano PM, Thomas A, Huston-Preslegh L et al 2003 Increased fetal adiposity, a very sensitive marker of abnormal inutero development. American Journal of Obstetrics and Gynecology 189(6): 1698–1670

Clark DA, Coulam CB, Stricker RB 2006 Is intravenous immunoglobulin (IVIG) efficacious in early pregnancy failure? A critical review and meta-analysis for patients who fail in vitro fertilization and embryo transfer (IVF). Journal of Assisted Reproduction and Genetics 23(1): 1–13

De Carolis C, Ruggiero G, Dal Lago A et al 2006 Progesterone gel reduces NK cells in recurrent abortion. Human Reproduction 21(suppl 1): i168

Erkan D, Lockshin MD 2006 Antiphospholipid syndrome. Current Opinion in Rheumatology 18(3): 242–248

Hanna J, Goldman-Wohl D, Hamani Y 2006 Decidual NK cells regulate key developmental process at the human fetal–maternal interface. Nature Medicine 12(9): 1065–1074

Jansen RPS, Sullivan E 2006 Monozygotic twinning with blastocyst culture and single blastocyst transfer: increasing incidence predates zona manipulation and blastocyst culture. Human Reproduction 21(1): 79

Kung YY, Chen FP, Hwang SJ 2006 The different immunomodulation of indirect moxibustion on normal subjects and patients with systemic lupus erythematosus. American Journal of Chinese Medicine 34(1): 47–56

Lambers MJ, Mager E, Goutbeek J et al 2007 Factors determining early pregnancy loss in singleton and multiple implantations. Human Reproduction 22(1): 275–279

Le Bouteiller P, Tabiasco J 2006 Immunology of pregnancy: renewed interest. Medecine Sciences (Paris) 22(8–9): 745–750

Lewis T, Chamberlain GVP 1990 Obstetrics by 10 teachers. Hodder and Stoughton, London

Liang L 2003 Acupuncture and IVF. Blue Poppy Press, Boulder, Colorado

Maciocia G 1994 The practice of Chinese Medicine. Churchill Livingstone, Edinburgh

Maciocia G 1998 Obstetrics and gynaecology in Chinese medicine. Churchill Livingstone, Edinburgh

Metzger BE 2006 Diet and medical therapy in the optimal management of gestational diabetes. Nestle Nutritional Workshop Series Clinical Performance Programme 11: 155–169

Ochsenkuhn R, Strowitzki T, Gurtner M et al 2003 Pregnancy complications, obstetric risks, and neonatal outcome in singleton and twin pregnancies after GIFT and IVF. Archives of Gynecology and Obstetrics 268(4): 256–261

OPCS 1994 GRO Scotland and GRO Northern Ireland, Table 1. OPCS, London

Paulus WE, Zhang M, Strehler E, El-Danasouri I, Sterzik K 2002 Influence of acupuncture on the pregnancy rate in patients who undergo assisted reproduction therapy. Fertility and Sterility 77(4): 721–724

Pinborg A, Loft A, Nyboe Andersen A 2004 Neonatal outcomes in a Danish national cohort of 8602 children born after in vitro fertilization or intracytoplasmic sperm injection: the role of twin pregnancy. Acta Obstetrica et Gynecologica Scandinavica 83(11): 1071–1078

Quenby S, Farquharson R 2006 Uterine natural killer cells, implantation failure and recurrent miscarriage. Reproductive Biomedicine Online 13(1): 24–28

Rai R, Cohen H, Dave M, Reagan L 1997 Randomised controlled trial of aspirin plus heparin in pregnant women with recurrent miscarriage associated with phospholipid antibodies (or anti-phospholipid antibodies). British Medical Journal 314: 253–257

Ross J 1995 Acupuncture point combinations. Churchill Livingstone, Edinburgh

Sargent IL, Borzychowski AM, Redman CW 2006 NK cells and human pregnancy – an inflammatory view. Trends in Immunology 27(9): 399–404

Sarig G, Youris JS, Hoffman R, Lanir N, Blumenfield Z, Brenner B 2002 Thrombophilia is common in women with idiopathic pregnancy loss and is associated with late pregnancy loss. Fertility and Sterility 77: 342–347

Sher G, Marriage Davis V, Stoess J 2005 In vitro fertilization: the A.R.T. of making babies, 3rd edn. Checkmark Books, New York

Svare JA, Hansen BB, Molsted-Pedersen L 2001 Perinatal complications in women with gestational diabetes mellitus. Acta Obstetrica et Gynecologica Scandinavica 80(10): 899–904

Sweet BR (ed.) 1997 Mayes' midwifery, 12th edn. Baillière Tindall, New York, p 556

Tallo CP, Vohr B, Oh W et al 1995 Maternal and neonatal morbidity associated with in vitro fertilization. Journal of Pediatrics 127(5): 794–800

Westergaard LG, Mao Q, Krogslund M, Sandrini S, Lenz S, Grinsted J 2006 Acupuncture on the day of embryo transfer significantly improves the reproductive outcome in infertile women: a prospective, randomized trial. Fertility and Sterility 85(5): 1341–1346

Yu Jin 1998 Handbook of obstetrics and gynecology in Chinese medicine. Eastland Press, Seattle

Yun-Kyong Y, Hyun L, Kwon-eui H et al 2007 Electroacupuncture at acupoint ST36 reduces inflammation and regulates immune activity in collagen-induced arthritic mice. eCam 4(1): 51–57; doi10.1093/ecam/ne1054

Further reading

Goel N, Tuli A, Choudry R 2006 The role of aspirin versus aspirin and heparin in cases of recurrent abortions with raised anticardiolipin antibodies. Medical Science Monitor 12(3): CR132–136

Kupferminc MJ 2003 Thrombophilia and pregnancy. Reproductive Biology and Endocrinology 1:111.

Wu O, Robertson L, Twaddle S et al 2006 Screening for thrombophilia in high-risk situations: systematic review and cost-effectiveness analysis. The Thrombosis: Risk and Economic Assessment of Thrombophilia Screening (TREATS) study. Health Technology Assessment 10(11): 1–110

Wu S, Stephenson MD 2006 Obstetrical antiphospholipid syndrome. Seminars in Reproductive Medicine 24 (1): 40–53

9 Abnormal positions of the fetus

Chapter outline

The previous chapter deals with normal positions of the baby. This chapter will explain abnormal positions and the consequences for labour.

With the important exception of breech presentation, there is little that the acupuncturist can do by way of treatment in these circumstances, but the following notes will provide greater understanding and awareness of the potential problems caused by abnormal fetal positions.

Abnormal positions of the fetus are:

- breech presentation (Fig. 9.1)
- transverse and unstable lie
- face presentation (Fig. 9.2)
- brow presentation (Fig. 9.3)
- shoulder presentation (Fig. 9.4).

Breech presentation

Between weeks 29 and 32 of pregnancy, approximately 15% of babies are in the breech position (Kauppila 1975). Only 3–4% of these continue in the breech position until labour. However, the longer this position is maintained into the

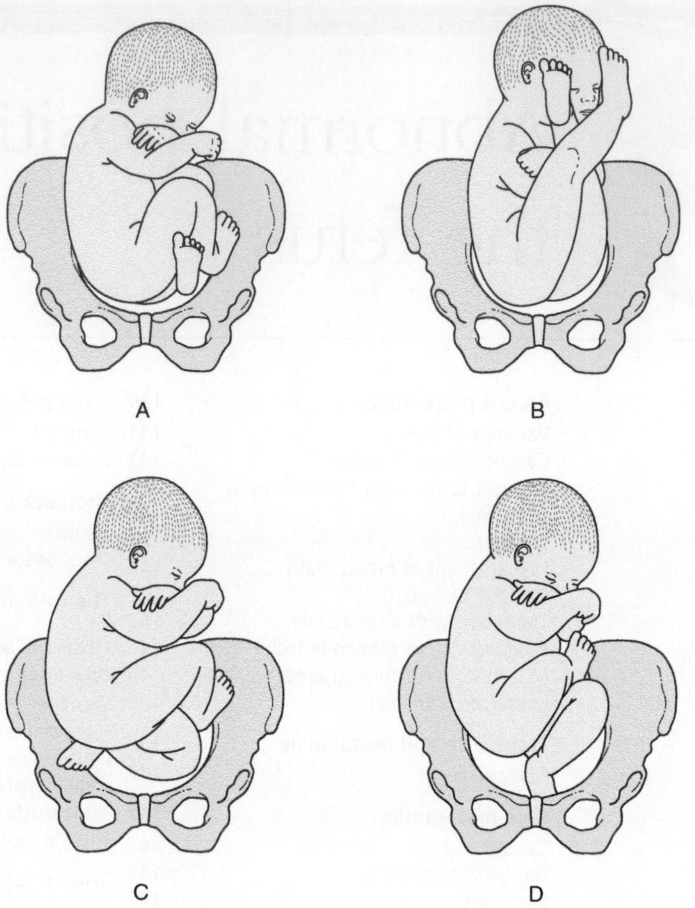

Figure 9.1 Types of breech presentation: **A** flexed; **B** extended; **C** knee; **D** footling. (Reproduced with permission from Sweet 1997, p. 640.)

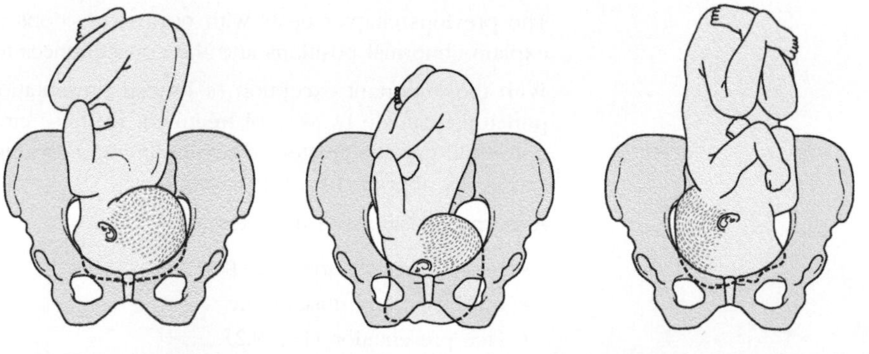

Figure 9.2 Face presentations. (Reproduced with permission from Sweet 1997, p. 652.)

pregnancy, the less chance there is of the baby turning. Nowadays, the usual management of delivery if the baby is still in the breech position at 38 weeks is to do a caesarean section. The result is that many midwives have sadly lost the skills of delivering breech babies.

Note: It is worth explaining to mothers the risks involved in delivering a breech baby vaginally, but the final decision is always that of the mother.

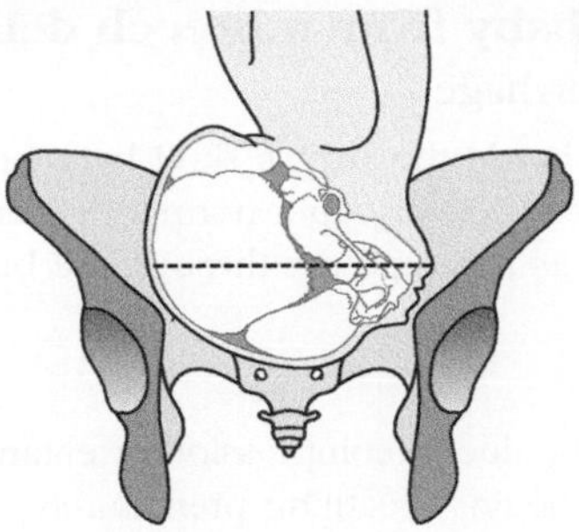

Figure 9.3 Brow presentation. (Reproduced with permission from Sweet 1997, p. 654.)

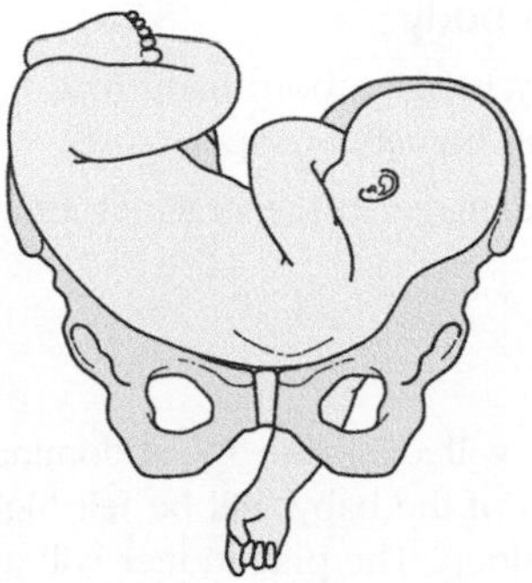

Figure 9.4 Shoulder presentation with prolapse of one arm. (Reproduced with permission from Sweet 1997, p. 652.)

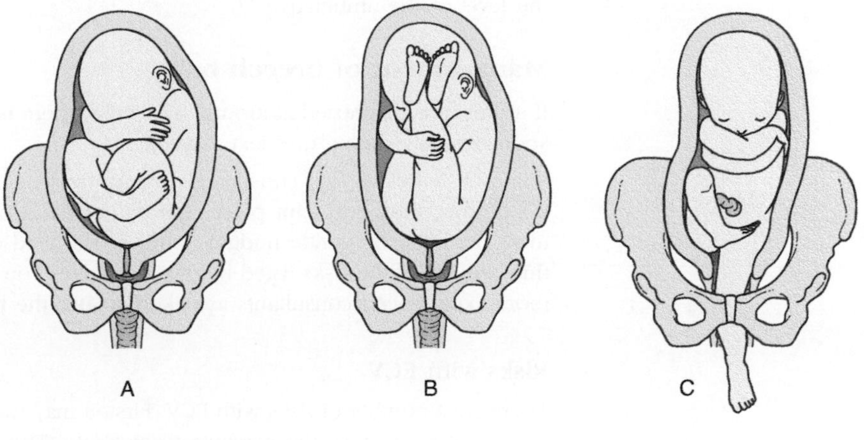

Figure 9.5 Varieties of breech: **A** full; **B** frank; **C** footling.

Varieties of breech

These include:

- complete breech: flexed thighs and flexed legs (Fig. 9.5A)
- frank breech: legs extended upwards (Fig. 9.5B)
- footling breech: the feet are above the cervix (Fig. 9.5C).

Causes of breech position

One in four babies will present by breech at some stage of pregnancy, but by 34 weeks most of these will have changed. In the majority of cases there are no obvious reasons for a breech position but the cause may be: a low-lying placenta, premature birth, multiple pregnancy, polyhydramnios, hydrocephalus, fibroids or an unusually shaped uterus.

Dangers to the baby from a breech delivery

Intracranial haemorrhage

Bleeding may occur inside the baby's skull because of the rapid compression of the aftercoming head at delivery. In a normal delivery the head comes first so that it has time to mould as it progresses through the birth canal.

Hypoxia

Lack of oxygen may be due to compression or entanglement of the umbilical cord, or because the baby begins breathing prematurely.

Injuries to the baby's body

For example, if the baby is being born hand first, efforts to get the head out may result in a fracture of the humerus (upper arm).

Other dangers include damage to the brachial artery, and crushing of the spinal cord.

Diagnosis

The midwife or doctor will diagnose by abdominal palpation during a routine antenatal visit. The head of the baby will be felt high up in the uterus rather than in the normal lower position. The practitioner will also listen for the baby's heartbeat; usually it would be heard low down, but in a breech baby it would be nearer the level of the umbilicus.

Management of breech baby

If a breech is diagnosed at around 32 weeks, there is still a chance that it may turn spontaneously during the next 2 weeks.

Some obstetricians will consider doing *external cephalic version (ECV)* (Fig. 9.6). To do this, the consultant places his or her hand on the mother's abdomen and turns the baby by gentle nudging until it lies head down. Not all doctors will do this because of the risks listed below; nowadays you generally find that only older, more experienced consultants are likely to use the technique.

Risks with ECV

There are a number of risks with ECV. First, it may cause the membranes to rupture. Second, it may cause the placenta to separate. Third, it would not be carried out if the mother's blood group is Rhesus negative, because of the risk of her blood mixing with the baby's and the possibility of the baby's blood group being positive (see Ch. 4). Fourth, there may be problems if the mother has high blood pressure. Finally, if the mother has had a previous caesarean section, the weakness of the scar may cause complications.

Chinese viewpoint

The Dai Mai channel links the Kidneys with the uterus. To the Chinese, if there is a constitutional deficiency of the Kidneys because of excessive sexual activity or excess childbirth, this may injure the Kidneys and lead to deficiency of Jing and Blood. After pregnancy, Jing and Blood accumulate to nourish the fetus via the Bao Mai channel. If the Kidneys are lacking, the fetus cannot maintain its position.

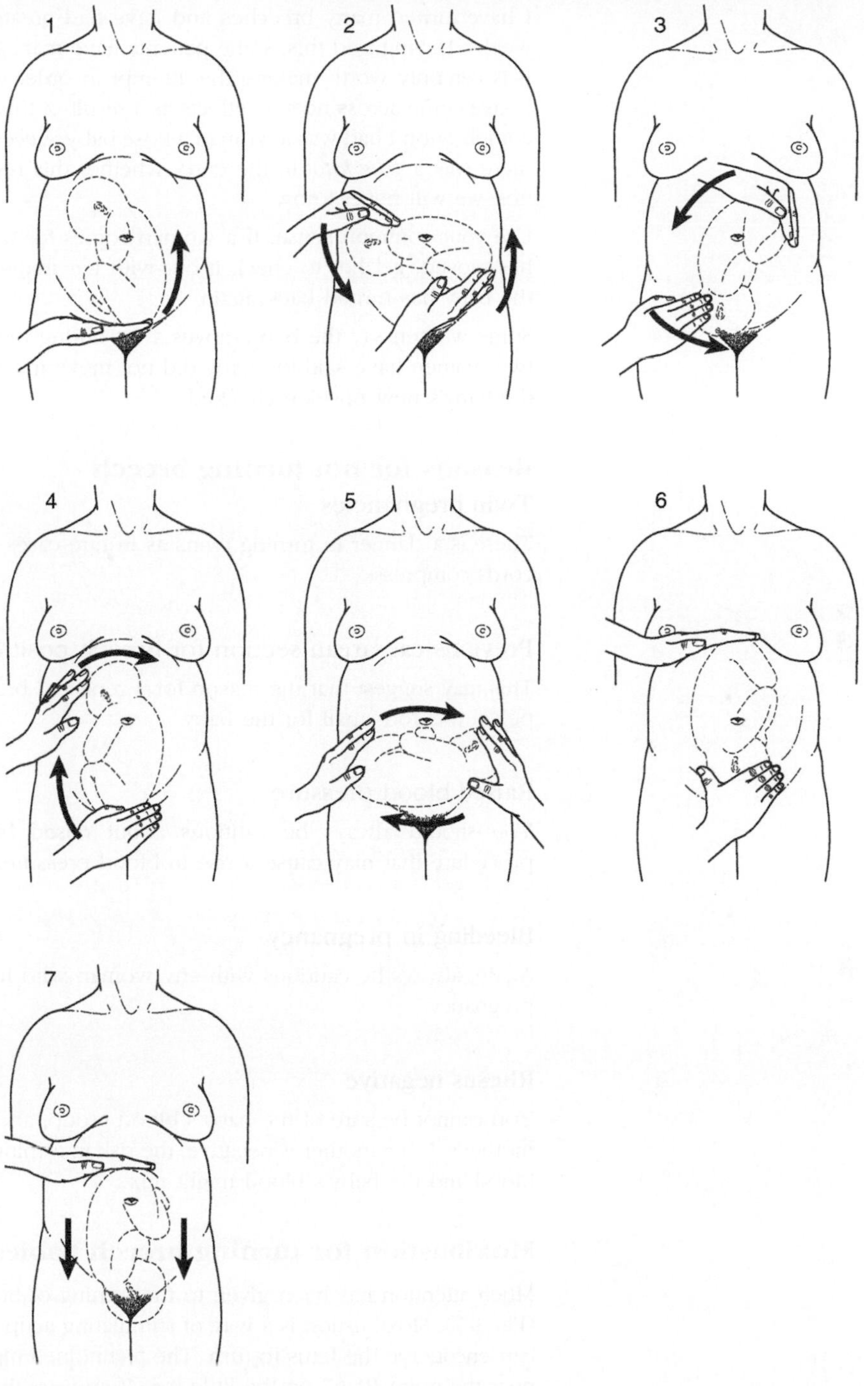

Figure 9.6 Steps in external cephalic version. (Reproduced with permission from Sweet 1997, p. 697.)

Treatment with acupuncture

Considering all the potential outcomes and dangers of having a breech baby, it is not surprising that women will turn to acupuncture for help rather than have a caesarean section. However, a strict code should always be followed to ascertain the safety of the process, and a number of points to watch are listed below.

I have turned many breeches and have had greatest success between 32 and 35 weeks. Having said this, some patients have managed to turn as late as 38 weeks. It is certainly worth making the attempt in order to avoid caesarean section, and I have come across no side-effects as a result of this treatment. The most significant complication I had was a woman whose baby successfully turned but at the delivery there was a *true knot* in the cord; whether this resulted from the acupuncture or not, we will never know.

Use your common sense. If a woman comes for treatment and says that the baby has moved, get her to check it out with her midwife; you do not want to treat if the baby has turned back again.

Some women say the baby moves a lot during the moxa treatment, while one or two women have said the baby did not move much. The important thing is to get the baby's new position checked.

Reasons for not turning breech

Twin pregnancies

There is a danger in turning twins as in rare cases the heads may interlock or the cords compress.

Previous caesarean section for breech position

This may suggest that the reason for a repeated breech could be that the mother's pelvis was too small for the baby.

Raised blood pressure

You should always be cautious about raised blood pressure and avoid any procedure that may cause a rise in blood pressure.

Bleeding in pregnancy

Again, always be cautious with any woman who has a history of bleeding during pregnancy.

Rhesus negative

You cannot be sure of the baby's blood group, and it may not be the same as the mother's. If the mother is negative, the risk in turning the breech is that the mother's blood and the baby's blood might mix.

Moxibustion for turning breech babies

Much attention has been given to the turning of breech babies using moxibustion (Fig. 9.7). Moxibustion is a way of stimulating acupuncture points with heat, which can encourage the fetus to turn. The technique employs a lighted moxa stick held near the point BL-67 on the little toe. It appears that by stimulating production of maternal hormones (placental oestrogens and prostaglandin) (Budd 1992) (Fig. 9.8), it encourages the lining of the uterus to contract, which in turn stimulates fetal activity. Certainly mothers on whom I have used moxibustion invariably report that they feel the baby moving almost immediately I light the stick, even if ultimately the baby does not actually turn, although no formal survey has yet been made.

The reasons for not turning a breech, listed above, also apply to moxibustion.

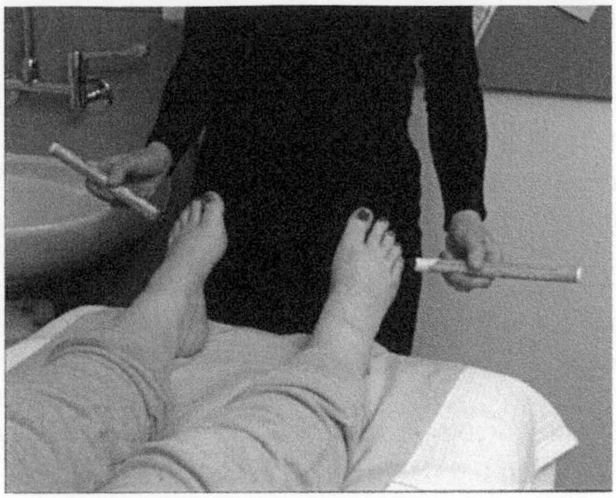

Figure 9.7 Moxibustion for turning breech babies.

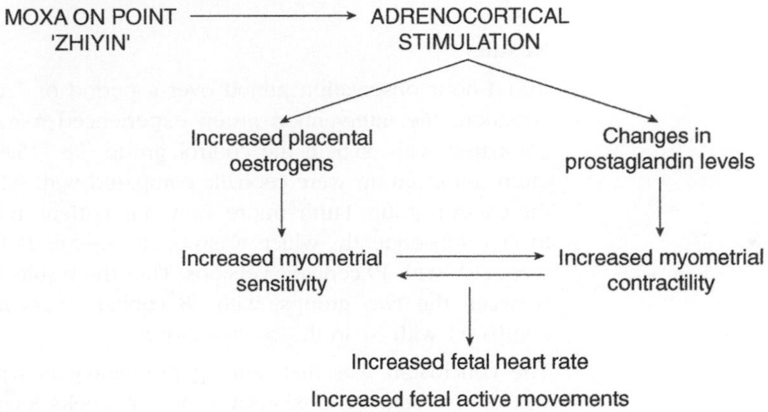

Figure 9.8 Hypothetical hormonal effects of moxa on Zhiyin point. (Reproduced with permission from Tiran & Mack 1995, p. 232.)

Technique

The patient can also use this technique at home, with help from her partner.

1. Get the woman to sit comfortably, with her legs raised. She should be wearing loose clothes, especially over her abdomen.
2. Her therapist, or partner, should light the moxa sticks and hold them just over BL-67, on both feet at the same time.
3. The sticks should be held still and bilaterally over the points until the woman feels they are too hot. The therapist will remove the sticks briefly and then reapply them to the point. This will be continued throughout the treatment.
4. Treat for 15 minutes, once or preferably twice a day, for 10–14 treatments.
5. The patient may feel the baby start to move noticeably once the moxa sticks are applied.
6. If the patient feels the baby move significantly, treatment should be stopped for the midwife to check whether the baby's position has changed.
7. Moxa ignites very easily so make absolutely sure that you put it out after use. Do not allow the sticks to get wet.

If the baby does not turn, it is best to accept the inevitable. Babies who persist in this position have made a choice to be born this way. Take it as an early lesson to mothers that not all children do what we want them to!

Research on breech

Studies in China have shown varying success rates, ranging from 80% to 90% (Cardini & Weixin 1998). Research has also shown that the optimal time to carry out moxibustion is at 34 weeks.

Cardini & Weixin (1998) carried out a randomised controlled trial in Italy. Their patients were 260 primigravidas in the 33rd week of pregnancy, all with normal pregnancies and diagnosed as breech position by ultrasound; 130 of the women were randomised to the intervention group and received stimulation to the acupuncture point BL-67 with moxa for 7 days. They were given treatment for a further 7 days if the fetus was still in the breech position. The other 130 were randomised to the control group and received routine care but no intervention. Subjects with persistent breech (after 32 weeks) could undergo external cephalic version any time between 35 weeks and delivery.

Results

In a 1-hour observation period over a period of 7 days during the 35th week of gestation, the intervention group experienced a mean of 48.5 fetal movements compared with 35.5 in the control group; 98 (75.4%) of the 130 fetuses in the intervention group were cephalic compared with 62 (47.7%) of the 130 fetuses in the control group. Furthermore, only one patient in the intervention group agreed to ECV subsequently, which was not successful; 24 from the control group underwent ECV with 19 cephalic versions. Thus the results were still significantly different between the two groups, with 98 cephalic versions in the intervention group compared with 81 in the control group.

The conclusion was that, among primigravidas with breech presentation at 33 weeks of gestation, moxibustion for 1–2 weeks increased fetal activity during the treatment and the incidence of cephalic presentation after the treatment. As a secondary observation, it was noted that 82 of the 98 cephalic versions were obtained during the first week and 16 during the second week of treatment. After the 35th week all remaining breech presentations remained unchanged, except for the 19 successfully treated with ECV.

More recent studies from Italy and Japan have also shown that stimulation of acupuncture point BL-67, with both acupuncture and moxibustion, is a safe and effective treatment in revolving the fetus in a breech presentation (Kanakura et al 2001, Neri et al 2004). In Italy, Neri et al (2004) studied a total of 240 pregnant women at 33–35 weeks gestational age, carrying a breech presentation baby. The primary outcome of the study was fetal presentation at birth. One hundred and fourteen women were randomised to observation only, and 112 to acupuncture and moxibustion at the acupuncture point BL-67. At delivery, there was a significantly higher cephalic presentation in the acupuncture group (53.6%) than in the observation group (36.7%). However, so far in my own practice I have only ever used the moxibustion treatment.

Transverse and unstable lie

An unstable lie is the term used from 36 weeks to describe the baby's position when it is not established head down, and is found to vary from one weekly examination to the next.

Management

The mother is admitted to hospital usually around 37 weeks and remains there until she delivers. The reason is the risk that, if she went into labour, the cord might prolapse because the lower part of the uterus is empty.

The mode of delivery is usually by caesarean section. Please note that I have never used moxa to turn an unstable lie and feel that it is better to leave well alone.

Face presentation

In a normal delivery, the baby's head is flexed. In about one case in every 500 (Sweet 1997) the head is extended, giving a face presentation as shown in Figure 9.2.

Causes

These include: women who have had multiple pregnancies and whose abdominal muscles are consequently lax, women with a small pelvis, polyhydramnios or anencephaly.

Dangers to the baby

First, the cord could prolapse because there is not a well-fitting part. Second, the head could become stuck; this is an obstetric emergency (see next section).

Diagnosis

A face presentation is difficult to diagnose in the antenatal period. It should be picked up in a vaginal examination when instead of the smooth hard surface of the head, the soft and irregular features of the face are felt.

Labour management and outcome

When the face comes first, it does not have the same good fit that the head does, and it therefore does not stimulate good contractions or good dilation of the cervix. Seventy-five percent of babies are born spontaneously (Sweet 1997).

Brow presentation

The causes for brow presentation are the same as for face presentation, but the brow is the leading part of the head (see Fig. 9.3).

Diagnosis

A brow presentation may be suspected from the unusually large width of the head that can be felt during vaginal examination.

Labour management and outcome

If the mother has a large pelvis and a small baby, it may be possible for the baby to be delivered by forceps. However, the majority of cases give rise to obstructed labour and a caesarean section will probably be necessary.

Shoulder presentation

In about one case in every 250, the shoulder presents first (Sweet 1997) (see Fig. 9.4). This is the result of the baby lying transversely in the uterus. The occurrence is five times greater in women who have had many children.

Causes

These include: premature baby, multiple pregnancy or polyhydramnios.

Diagnosis and management

A shoulder presentation ought to be diagnosed antenatally because of the obvious transverse lie. Failure to diagnose before labour would be serious mismanagement, and the consequences could be dire. Shoulder presentation can result in obstructed labour, rupture of the uterus, and maternal and fetal death. A caesarean section *must* be carried out.

The role of the acupuncturist

Face, brow and shoulder presentation are all self-explanatory terms that you may hear used to describe abnormal head-first deliveries, and they are described briefly here for information. They all carry complications and are sometimes hard to diagnose when the midwife or doctor palpates. You may see these diagnoses written in the notes, or your patient may be admitted to hospital because of them.

As an acupuncturist, there is little you can do to treat these conditions directly, but you can of course help to relieve any anxiety and stress they might cause to the mother. It is also important that you are familiar with the terminology so that you have a greater understanding of what is happening in a complicated labour. In all cases, even if complications are not previously diagnosed, labour would begin normally. You would therefore use the same acupuncture treatments as for a normal delivery.

You are most likely to become aware that there is a problem following the midwife's vaginal examination of the mother. If the midwife is unsure of the position of the baby or observes that the fetal heart rate is dipping, she may call a doctor. Understandably, the mother's anxiety is going to be heightened in such circumstances. The acupuncturist can support the mother emotionally, in order to relax her and keep her as calm as possible.

POINTS TO TREAT

- **A useful point is HT-7, which is good for shock and anxiety. Insert, tonify and remove.**

Obstetric emergencies and operative procedures explained

Other complications can occur that may result in emergencies. All obstetric emergencies have potentially catastrophic outcomes, resulting in the death or retardation of the baby, or the death of the mother. It is important for acupuncturists to be aware of the seriousness of these events, even though there is little direct action that they can take. There is overriding urgency for immediate action by the patient's doctors and midwives.

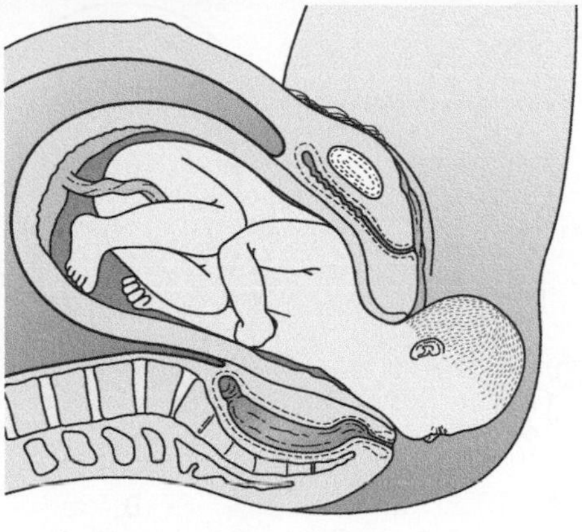

Figure 9.9 Shoulder dystocia. (Reproduced with permission from Sweet 1997, p. 661.)

The following complications are explained:

- shoulder dystocia
- presentation and prolapse of the umbilical cord
- obstructed labour
- cephalopelvic disproportion
- uterine rupture.

Shoulder dystocia

Shoulder dystocia refers to a delivery in which the baby's shoulders get stuck (Fig. 9.9). It occurs in about two deliveries per 1000 (Sweet 1997). It is unexpected and alarming for the whole team, who have to manoeuvre the baby with its head out, possibly trying to breathe and going blue.

Diagnosis

Although careful observations during labour should alert the midwife to a potential problem, the first sign that something is actually wrong will be at delivery, when the chin remains tight against the perineum as the head emerges.

Labour management and outcome

Midwives are taught special techniques to deliver the baby. Specific manoeuvres aim to deliver the baby as quickly as possible, in order to minimise the risk to it, but more force is involved than in the gentle downward motion of a normal delivery. Doctors are immediately called to assist.

Possible maternal outcomes include: haemorrhage, possibly fatal, and vaginal lacerations.

Possible fetal outcomes include: asphyxia and meconium aspiration.

Presentation and prolapse of the cord

Emergencies involving presentation and prolapse of the cord occur in approximately one birth in 300 (Lewis & Chamberlain 1990). In presentation of the cord, a loop of the cord lies below the baby's head in the birth canal (Fig. 9.10A). The membranes hold the cord in position until they rupture, when the cord will fall down before the head and is then described as prolapsed (Fig. 9.10B).

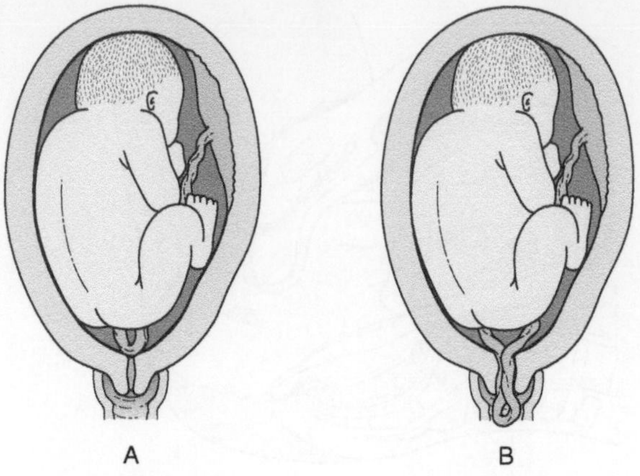

Figure 9.10 A Cord presentation; B Cord prolapse. (Reproduced with permission from Sweet 1997, p. 669.)

In these circumstances, the cord will become compressed by the head during birth, cutting off the blood supply in the vessels of the cord to the baby. This can result in brain damage.

Causes

These include: long umbilical cord, breech presentation, preterm baby or abnormal position of the fetus.

Dangers to the baby

First, death may occur owing to interruption of oxygen supply. Second, there may be brain damage.

Diagnosis

The problem can usually be seen on an ultrasound scan. Vaginal examination in labour may reveal the soft distinctive form of the cord to the midwife's touch. If the membranes are ruptured, vaginal examination will show that the cord is prolapsed, and the fetal heart will be slow.

Management

The mother will be put into the 'knee–chest' position, which keeps pressure from the head off the cord.

The midwife will also manipulate the head with her fingers to relieve pressure coming from the mother's contractions.

Doctors will be called.

Obstructed labour

Obstructed labour occurs whenever there is a barrier to the passage of the fetus through the birth canal.

Causes

These include: cephalopelvic disproportion (CPD), large fetus or malposition.

Signs and symptoms

These include: no progress in labour, the baby's head remaining high in labour, and failure of the cervix to dilate.

If the condition is allowed to continue, the contractions will become stronger and more frequent. The mother will be in continuous pain and very distressed. She may be vomiting and showing signs of dehydration. Her pulse will be very rapid.

Prevention

Good antenatal care and close observation in early labour should avert an obstructed labour. If this occurred at a home delivery, the midwife would immediately call the emergency obstetric team and arrange for an ambulance to transfer the patient to hospital. In hospital, treatment is always an immediate caesarean section to deliver the baby.

Cephalopelvic disproportion (CPD) and obstructed labour

CPD is the failure of the head to descend into the pelvis during uterine contractions. It is not in itself an obstetric emergency, but is frequently the cause of obstructed labour. If there are good contractions, the head should descend easily, suggesting that failure to do so is caused by a misfit between the head and the mother's pelvis, or a malpresentation, as discussed above. The head is the largest part of the fetus so if it is able to pass through, then the rest of the body will also be able to.

Diagnosis

There may be a previous history in the mother of spinal injury or congenital abnormality of the pelvis, or a previous labour that was prolonged or difficult and resulted in a caesarean section. In the last few weeks of pregnancy it will usually be found that the head is not engaged, and in some cases cannot be made to engage.

Uterine rupture

Uterine rupture is a serious obstetric emergency that frequently results in fetal death, and can sometimes result in maternal death. The incidence of uterine rupture is higher in parts of the world where antenatal and labour care are rarely available.

Causes

In modern obstetrics, uterine rupture is almost always due to the misuse of oxytocic drugs. These are used to initiate and maintain the mother's contractions (see Ch. 12, Augmentation of labour).

Uterine rupture

Scar rupture. Previous surgery from a caesarean section may leave a physical weakness in the uterine wall. This can occur in late pregnancy or in early labour.

The unscarred uterus. Sixty to seventy percent of uterine ruptures are reported to occur where the uterus is unscarred.

Traumatic rupture. Where external factors are the cause, the condition is described as traumatic rupture. Typically it results from the use of instruments or misuse of oxytocic drugs.

Spontaneous rupture. When external factors cannot be identified, the condition is described as spontaneous rupture. This may occur because of very strong uterine contractions. The cause is not always clear, but may often be due to unidentified trauma or scarring from previous pregnancies.

Signs and symptoms

Uterine rupture is usually associated with the acute and dramatic collapse of the mother's condition. She will go into shock, manifested by pallor, rapid pulse, shallow breathing and a fall in blood pressure. She will suffer severe pain and bleeding.

Incomplete rupture

An incomplete rupture is far less dramatic but harder to diagnose, as the signs and symptoms become apparent more gradually. The mother may complain of constant abdominal pain. Management of an incomplete rupture will depend on the particular condition of the mother, but an immediate caesarean section is always undertaken.

Trial of labour

In cases of shoulder dystocia, a previous history of obstructed or difficult labour, or suspected CPD, mothers may be offered a 'trial of labour' to see whether they can progress naturally. This is conducted as an ordinary labour in hospital, but a particularly close watch is kept on the mother. Its purpose is to give the mother maximum opportunity to have a normal delivery but at the first signs of distress, it is normal to deliver the baby by caesarean section.

Conclusion

This chapter is not intended to alarm the acupuncturist, but to give information about what is happening during the management of labour if complications or emergencies should occur. In these circumstances, action has to be taken very quickly, and there is little time to explain to others what is happening. As the medical staff respond, very often both the mother and her partner become confused and frightened. A great deal of support can be given by the acupuncturist, easing the way for midwives and doctors to get on with urgent technical procedures. Seconds can make the difference between life and death, and every action that the acupuncturist can take to settle and reassure the patient is vital.

Summary

- Abnormal positions of the fetus include: breech presentation, transverse and unstable lie, face presentation, brow presentation and shoulder presentation.
- Obstetric emergencies include: shoulder dystocia, presentation and prolapse of the umbilical cord, obstructed labour, cephalopelvic disproportion and uterine rupture.
- Acupuncture points for abnormal positions of the fetus include:
  - *turning a breech:* moxa on BL-67
  - *shock and anxiety:* HT-7.

References

Budd S 1992 Traditional Chinese medicine in obstetrics. Midwives Chronicle 105 (1253): 140–143

Cardini F, Weixin H 1998 Moxibustion for the correction of breech babies: a clinical study with retrospective controls. Journal of the American Medical Association 280(18): 1580–1584

Kanakura Y, Kometani K, Nagata T et al 2001 Moxibustion treatment of breech presentation. American Journal of Chinese Medicine 29(1): 37–45

Kauppila O 1975 The perinatal mortality in breech deliveries and observations on affecting factors: a retrospective study of 2227 cases. Acta Obstetrica et Gynecologica Scandinavica 44(suppl): 13–19

Lewis T, Chamberlain GVP 1990 Obstetrics by 10 teachers. Hodder and Stoughton, London

Neri I, Airola G, Contu G, Allais G, Faccinetti F, Benedetto C 2004 Acupuncture plus moxibustion to resolve breech presentation: a randomized controlled study. Journal of Maternal, Fetal and Neonatal Medicine 15(4): 247–252

Sweet BR (ed.) 1997 Mayes' midwifery, 12th edn. Baillière Tindall, New York, pp 640, 652, 654, 661, 669, 697

Tiran D, Mack S (eds) 1995 Complementary therapies in pregnancy and childbirth. Baillière Tindall, London, p 232

10

Preparation for labour

Chapter outline

Every labour is a voyage into unknown waters for the mother to be, especially if this is her first experience of giving birth. Support from the professionals around her, from her birthing companion and from you – her acupuncturist – will go a long way to reassure her, support her and allay her fears. It is therefore important for you to be familiar with hospital procedures and medical interventions, as well as with the physiological and emotional processes of your patient. This chapter and the next will introduce you to the various aspects of labour that you are likely to encounter.

Topics in this chapter include:

- how to recognise the onset of labour
- admission to hospital
- induction
- optimum nutrition in the final week before labour.

Recognising the onset of labour

A number of physiological changes in late pregnancy indicate that labour is imminent. Most women will follow a similar pattern but there will be individual variations, as women have different pain perceptions, different responses and different expectations of labour.

The show

The show is often the first sign that labour is imminent or has begun. This show is a plug of mucus, often bloodstained, which has passed from the vagina, where it plugged the canal around the cervix. Its appearance is an indication that there is a degree of cervical activity.

Uterine contractions

In the later stages of pregnancy, women will generally be aware of painless, irregular contractions known as Braxton-Hicks. At the onset of labour, these will become regular and painful uterine contractions, which may coincide with sacral or lower abdominal pain, or both. As labour progresses, the contractions get longer and stronger, more frequent and more painful, resulting in progressive effacement of the cervix.

False labour

A false (or spurious) labour occurs when there are regular (and painful) uterine contractions but they are not accompanied by effacement of the cervix. This is more common in women who have had more than one child. It can be very distressing for the woman, who feels she has started her labour, begins to contract – and then stops without making any real progress. Giving her reassurance and moral support is very important.

Rupture of membranes

As the cervix starts to efface, membranes form a small bag of amniotic fluid that protrudes into the cervix. As the baby's head descends, it separates the small bag in front, the *forewaters*, from the rest, the *hindwaters*. The forewaters help early dilation, whereas the hindwaters help to equalise the pressure in the uterus during uterine contractions, so helping to protect the uterus and placenta.

Rupture of the membranes can occur before labour begins or at any time during labour. Although significant, it is not a true sign of labour unless there is also dilation of the cervix. The amount of fluid lost depends on the position of the baby. If the head is not well engaged in the pelvis, fluid loss may be significant. But if the head is well engaged, loss may be minimal and further seepage may be mistaken for urinary incontinence. If the waters are intact and there is minimal leaking of amniotic fluid, this suggests that it is the hindwaters that have ruptured.

Once a woman's membranes have ruptured and if contractions do not start of their own accord, she is generally admitted to hospital because of the risk of uterine infection and prolapse of the umbilical cord.

Management

Home birth

Home births are being given more encouragement now than in recent years. Women who choose to give birth at home have more personal control and more privacy, and are more comfortable in their own familiar surroundings, in an unhurried, relaxed environment. They feel safe and secure and have greater intimacy with their children and partners. A home birth allows for more emotional and physical spontaneity. Also, many women choose a home birth because they may have had bad previous experiences in hospital, or because they are more likely to know their midwife and so feel safer. Midwives have observed that women are less likely to need pharmacological analgesia at home.

Preparation for a home birth

The midwife will have organised with the mother for the following to be available: running water, heating, lighting, plastic sheet, binliners, towels, blankets and a prepared bag in case of transfer to hospital. The midwife attending a home birth will also have all the medical equipment necessary.

For the acupuncturist it is therefore a case of bringing:

- an electroacupuncture machine
- a supply of needles for use in the ear: 1 inch and $1^1/_2$ inches (2.5 cm and 3.8 cm)
- labour massage oil
- Rescue remedy
- a drink to sustain energy.

Preparation for a water birth at home

Pools for water birth are purpose made and are supplied with thermometers. The temperature is usually around 36.5–37.5°C (i.e. just below blood heat). Women who choose to have a water birth at home will usually hire their pools independently.

There are certain criteria that a woman has to meet before she would be allowed a water birth at home. These are:

- the technique must be used at her request
- she must have a normal healthy pregnancy
- the baby must not be preterm; that is, before 36 weeks of pregnancy
- the baby's head must be cephalic, head down
- the woman and her partner must agree to leave the pool if the midwives request it
- the mother's and baby's observations must be normal.

Having a water birth does not necessarily mean actually having the baby in the water. Some women like to labour in the pool and then get out to deliver the baby.

When to go to hospital

Whether or not the mother intends to have a hospital or home delivery, she will be most at ease during the first part of labour at home, in a familiar environment where she can make herself most comfortable.

Her midwife will usually be the first person to be informed of the onset of labour. The acupuncturist will have made arrangements with the mother as to when to attend. If the mother is going into hospital, the best guide as to when to go there will be the intensity, strength and duration of the contractions. Once these are lasting 60 seconds or more, the cervix will be dilating. Acupuncture treatment can be started at once.

On admission to hospital

A swift initial assessment of the stage of labour needs to be made upon arrival at hospital, so as to determine the most appropriate course of action. A fuller examination can then be carried out.

Building a good relationship between the care givers and the woman and her partner is vitally important, to foster confidence and trust and to minimise the woman's feelings of anxiety and loss of control.

The role of the midwife

The midwife must carefully read the mother's antenatal and other relevant records, including her birth plan. (She may, of course, already be well acquainted with the woman and her history.)

General observations will be made and recorded, including taking the blood pressure and temperature, and testing the urine for glucose, protein and ketone bodies.

The midwife will feel the mother's abdomen to determine which position the baby is in, which way it is lying and whether the head is engaged.

She will listen to the baby's heart, which should be strong and regular with a rate of between 110 and 150 beats per minute.

An internal vaginal examination will be made, to assess the progress of dilation of the cervix. The rate of cervical dilation is the most exact measurement of how labour is progressing. It is reckoned in centimetres, from 0 to 10 cm so, as a rough guide, if the mother is 4–5 cm dilated on admission then she is approximately halfway through her labour.

The midwife may also do a CTG (cardiotocograph), which is an electronic trace of the baby's heartbeat (see Fig. 11.5, p. 176). Two electrodes are placed on the mother's abdomen, one measuring the strength of contractions and the other recording the fetal heart activity. It is usually left in place for 20–30 minutes to check that the baby is responding normally.

All the findings from the examination will be plotted on a partogram, the chart form on which the midwife will record all her information to show how the woman is progressing through her labour.

Unless contraindicated, the woman may enjoy a warm bath or shower. A loose cotton nightdress is probably the most comfortable garment to wear, which can be changed as often as necessary.

Routine shaving and the giving of enemas are no longer regarded as of any value in contributing to the safe outcome of labour.

Induction of labour

Induction is the deliberate attempt by artificial means to pre-empt the spontaneous and natural start of labour. Rates of induction vary greatly between different maternity units and different consultants, but in general there are far fewer now than in previous decades, as the adverse affects of unjustified induction have begun to be felt.

There are a number of situations where the risk of continuing the pregnancy would be considered greater than the potential risk of intervention:

- women over 41 weeks' gestation
- hypertension
- medical conditions such as diabetes
- pre-labour spontaneous rupture of the membranes
- placental abruption
- poor obstetric history
- evidence of diminished fetal well-being
- fetal death
- Rhesus isoimmunisation
- severe congenital abnormality.

There are a number of methods that can be used to induce labour:

- cervical ripening by administering small doses of prostaglandins, usually by vaginal pessary
- sweeping the membranes from the lower uterine segment
- rupturing the membranes (amniotomy)
- intravenous infusion of oxytocin.

Alternative remedies to induce a baby

Sex. Sperm contains prostaglandins and can work in the same way as prostaglandin gel. Although the prostaglandin is less concentrated in the semen, frequent sex is reputed to help.

Castor oil. This is a traditional treatment; although too revolting to the palate to recommend seriously, it does sometimes get women into labour.

Curry. This is a purgative that works on the same principles as castor oil.

Homeopathy. Caulophyllum 30 can be taken every half an hour until contractions start.

Cranial osteopathy. This is very good to get working on the pituitary glands, which are the source of certain hormones important in labour.

Copper. This is another old treatment to bring on labour; a copper penny was placed under the tongue. It is known that copper levels rise at the end of pregnancy, although the reason is not understood.

Induction of labour is a deliberate attempt to make a woman go into labour by artificial means. Policies on induction vary greatly from hospital to hospital but there is an overall trend away from the practice when possible. There are, nevertheless, circumstances where the continuation of the pregnancy beyond 40 weeks, or even before 40 weeks, would be dangerous or even life threatening to the mother and the baby and when induction is therefore advisable.

Indications for induction of labour

Postmaturity

The term 'postmaturity' is used when the baby is 7 or more days beyond term. Hospital policy is particularly variable in this regard, and certain hospitals allow some pregnancies to continue for as long as 14 days beyond term. The hospital staff may ask the mother to be aware of and report changes in the baby's movements, and often the mother will be brought into hospital for scans and monitoring.

Hypertensive disorders

Hypertensive disorders relate to raised blood pressure, and a decision to induce the birth would depend on the severity of the condition. Considerations typically include the level of protein in the urine and how mature the baby is. In some cases induction as early as 34 weeks can be desirable if the lungs are adequately matured. A caesarean section may be necessary for pre-eclampsia or pregnancy-induced hypertension (PIH).

Diabetes

Diabetes of the mother is known to cause fetal death in late pregnancy, so a caesarean section is usually performed at about 37 weeks if there is evidence of diminished fetal well-being. Indications that the baby is not well may include lack of growth, sluggish movements or a poor fetal heart rate.

Early rupture of membranes

Induction of labour is the usual response to early rupture of membranes.

Other considerations

Other conditions that are taken into consideration include: older mothers and a poor obstetric history; that is, women who have previously had still births, babies with abnormalities, etc.

Induction for non-medical reasons

Sadly there are increasing numbers of women who want to know exactly when their baby is going to be born and who actually press for induction. All inductions carry a risk, and this must be stressed most emphatically. There are possible complications with inductions, and I have so often seen one problem lead to another in a downward spiral. If you kick against nature it has a nasty habit of kicking back at you!

The downward spiral of induction (Fig. 10.1)

Most labours start spontaneously, so that women are able to get used to the pain; the natural endorphins that are released enable them to cope with the pain as it comes along. With induction this natural process is short circuited, so that the pain comes quickly and acutely. It is inevitable that many women will lose control much earlier. They then want pain relief earlier and they may end up with an epidural when they are dilated as little as 2 cm. Following an epidural there is a higher incidence of forceps and caesarean delivery, with all the attendant risks.

The success of induction

The success of induction in labour can depend on several factors.

The state of the cervix. If it is soft or dilating, the process can be successful. If it is hard and unyielding, it is likely that it is going to be much more difficult for the woman to go into labour.

The period of gestation. The nearer the pregnancy is to term, the better is the chance of the mother going into labour.

The level of the fetal head. If the head is well down on the pelvis, success is more likely.

The sensitivity of the uterus to respond. A responsive uterus will go into labour more easily.

How an induction is started and performed

Induction protocols will vary from hospital to hospital. Some women will be admitted the night before, others on the morning of the induction.

The midwife will assess the state of the cervix for its dilation, length and position. Each factor is scored according to a system known as the Bishop's score, and the overall assessment is made on the total score.

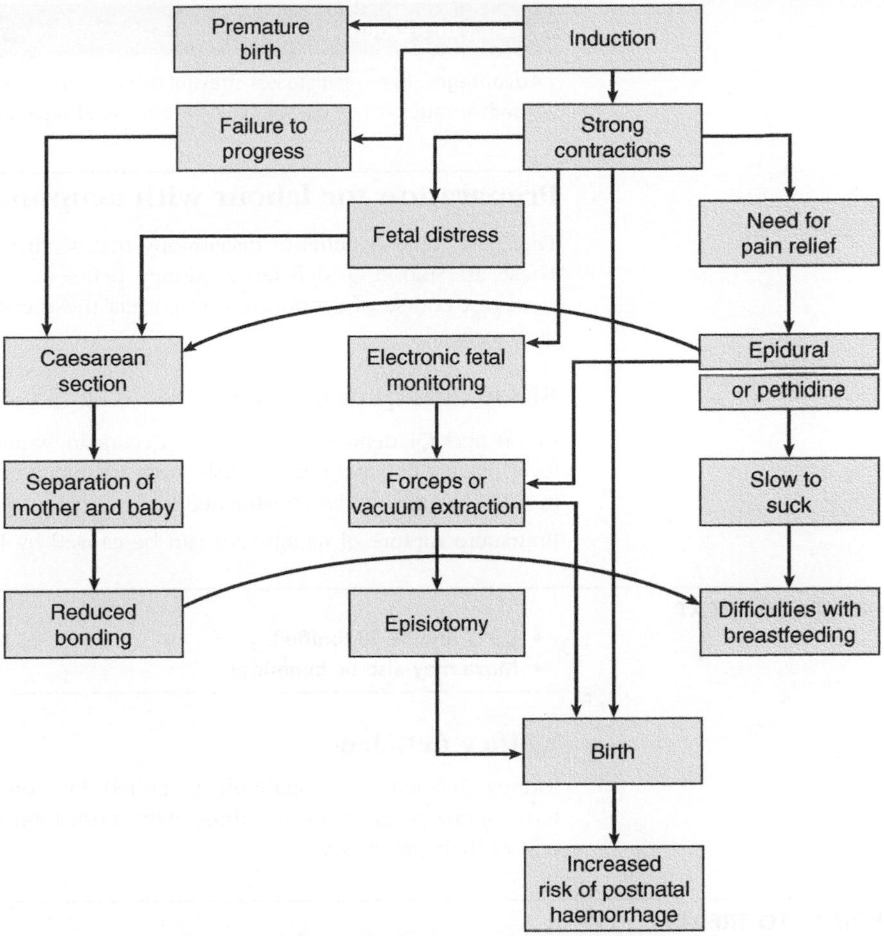

Figure 10.1 The 'cascade of intervention' in birth.

If induction is indicated, prostaglandin gel is then inserted into the vagina and the woman remains in bed for an hour to allow her body to absorb it. The midwife will monitor the fetal heart and contractions.

Prostaglandin

Prostaglandins are hormones that stimulate contractions. Prostaglandin gel is used before term to help soften the cervix prior to induction, and to induce labour. At term, it helps to initiate the labour without using a drip or rupturing the membranes.

The prostaglandin gel is applied to the area around the cervix. A repeat dose may be given after 6 hours if contractions have not begun. It would not be used for women whose membranes have already ruptured.

Effects of prostaglandin on the mother

Advantages. It may initiate a more physiological labour than an induction by other means.

Disadvantages. First, it may cause severe spontaneous labour if the cervix is already ripe. Second, there may be an increased risk of infection. Third, nausea, vomiting and diarrhoea may occur. Finally, there may be an increased risk of postpartum haemorrhage.

Effects of induction on the baby

Advantages. It may initiate less stressful labour than induction by other means.
Disadvantages. There may be an increased risk of fetal distress.

Preparation for labour with acupuncture

There are three patterns of disharmony that seem related to problems in labour. These are: Blood/Qi deficiency, Kidney deficiency and Stomach/Spleen Qi deficiency. A course of acupuncture to correct these conditions prior to delivery will be beneficial.

Blood and Qi deficiency

Blood and Qi deficiency frequently occurs in women with a low haemoglobin level. They will benefit enormously from acupuncture prior to labour (see Anaemia in Ch. 7 for appropriate treatments).

Premature rupture of membranes can be caused by Blood and Qi deficiency.

POINTS TO TREAT

- **BL-17 and ST-36 tonified.**
- **Moxa may also be beneficial.**

Kidney deficiency

Kidney deficiency is commonly identified in women who have IVF (in vitro fertilisation) pregnancies and those who work long hours and/or right up to the end of their pregnancy.

POINTS TO TREAT

- **BL-23 to tonify the Kidneys.**

Stomach and Spleen Qi deficiency

Typically Stomach and Spleen Qi deficiency are related to lack of sleep and lack of appetite in the final weeks.

POINTS TO TREAT

- **BL-17 and 20 to tonify the spleen.**

Acupuncture and induction

I find that acupuncture works very well for women who are being induced (Figs 10.2, 10.3). Its main benefit is in reducing the acute pain that is often associated with induced labours (see above). Ear points such as Uterus and Shenmen are particularly effective if the needles are attached to a V-TENS machine.

I have induced many women using acupuncture but I will use it only in normal, healthy, pregnant women who have had no complications in their pregnancy. I would not use it where a mother had suffered from conditions such as severe pre-eclampsia, kidney disease, a heart condition, diabetes, any bleeding, or if they had previously delivered by caesarean section.

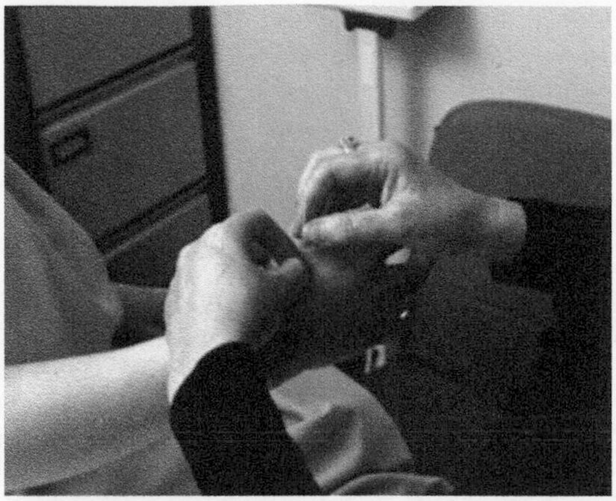

Figure 10.2 A mother with needles inserted for induction.

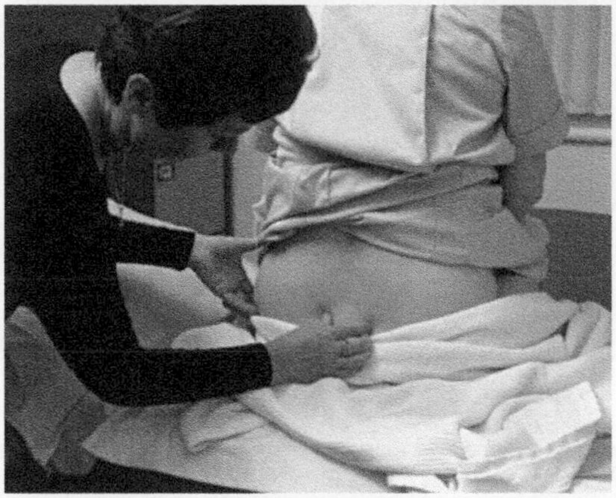

Figure 10.3 Induction.

As a word of caution, there are many medical reasons why a woman may be induced. You should only treat a client if you are confident about treating pregnant women and have some background knowledge around pregnancy, and always make sure the midwife or GP is happy that you are doing this.

Initially I get the patient to sit up on the bed, with her legs on a chair at the side, so that I have access to her back. I then insert four needles, $1^1/_2$ inches (3.8 cm) long, 34 gauge, into BL-31 and 32 bilaterally. Because these are straight into the sacral plexus, I consider that this is what initiates the contractions.

I also put needles into LI-4 bilaterally and SP-6 or LR-3, which tends to be my preferred point. I then go to the back and I stimulate the four needles in BL-31 and 32 as strongly as I can, for as long as 10 minutes at a time, breaking briefly every minute.

Finally I return to the other points, LI-4 and LR-3. I have found this sequence to be the most effective.

Frequency of treatment

Ideally the patient's first treatment would last for 45 minutes. This is quite sufficient, as most women do not find it very pleasant. Success depends on how far beyond term the pregnancy is, with the best results at 10–14 days over.

Treatment will usually start the uterus hardening, and contractions may get going. However, the contractions are often not sustained and repeat sessions are necessary. In practice, it is often not possible to provide treatments more than once a day, but twice or more would ensure greater success (Kubista et al 1975). The research that has been done shows that acupuncture takes from 3 to 60 hours to initiate contractions.

CASE STUDY 10.1

Sharon was 10 days over her dates and due to come into hospital to be induced on day 14. She came along to me to try acupuncture. She had been feeling niggles of pain and thought she would go into labour at any time. I sat her on the bed with her feet placed on a chair, inserted the needle into BL-31 and 32 and began to manipulate them very strongly for 2–4 minutes. I then came from around the back of the bed and placed the needles in LI-4 and LR-3, and again manipulated the needles very strongly.

I carried on working my way around the points for 35 minutes, every now and then stopping to see whether there was a contraction. The uterus started to contract after about 20 minutes. Sharon then began to feel back ache and a slight niggling, period-type pain in her groin.

The contractions continued after I took the needles out and while she was up and about, carrying on well into the evening and then stopping at around 11 p.m. I gave the same treatment again the next day, and again it worked throughout the day and into the evening. It then stopped for a couple of hours and started again, and she went into labour at 7 a.m. the next morning, with regular contractions.

CASE STUDY 10.2

A friend and neighbour of mine was 7 days past her dates and came to my home every evening for five nights. Nothing happened and she had to be admitted to hospital to be induced.

However, when the gel was inserted, she went into labour very quickly and delivered 3 hours later, at 2 a.m. Sadly, I was at home asleep and missed the birth!

What the points do

- BL-31 and 32 are into the sacral plexus, affecting the uterus and so getting the contractions going.
- LI-4 increases contractions.
- SP-6 helps to dilate the cervix angle, with the needle perpendicular and aiming it at the uterus.
- LR-3 is a very strong point, and I have found it very effective in getting contractions going.
- I have also used Uterus and Bladder ear points with a quarter-inch (0.6 cm) needle to get things going.

I prefer to stimulate the needles strongly using my hands as I find this works better for me.

CASE STUDY 10.3

This case shows how acupuncture may help to get a patient over the first hurdle of pain, without resorting to an epidural. Caron's induction was started at 7 a.m. She was overdue and was 2–3 cm dilated. When a woman is induced she does not have time for the natural build-up of endorphins (see Ch. 11), so that the pain comes on very quickly. It can quite literally take her breath away, leaving her unable to deal with the pain, and she will often request pain relief at an early stage. The induction process can enter a downward spiral of interventions (see Fig. 10.1) at this point. Women in this state need a lot of reassurance and support, as they are rarely prepared for the severity of the pain. They are very likely to lose confidence in themselves and fail to cope. Caron was in a lot of pain and very distressed.

Initially I got Caron to sit straddling a chair, and I got her comfortable with pillows to support her bump, while maintaining full access to her back to be able to stimulate the necessary points. I used my V-TENS machine setting on 2.5 and 200 Hz with the pads on BL-31 and 32 on both sides. I kept them there for 20 minutes. I used V-TENS because she was already in a lot of pain and she did not want needles. After about 20 minutes she was becoming less tense and seemed to be in more control, so I then took the pads off and placed quarter-inch (0.6 cm) needles in her ears on the Uterus and Shenmen points. I attached the needles to the V-TENS machine on the previous setting. Caron was still, and felt a warm throbbing sensation in her ear. After 20 minutes the treatment started to take effect, so that she was able to get up and walk, and to breathe through her contractions. She was able to remain more in control and to deal with the pain. The needles were kept in for 2 hours, by which time she was 4–5 cm dilated and ready to get into the birthing pool for labour.

Not only does acupuncture help women who have had inductions to get through the most painful part, the support that the acupuncturist provides through the treatment is vital in building the patient's confidence and reducing the anxiety and tension that contribute physiologically to the pain.

Research on acupuncture for the induction of labour

Acupuncture for induction has been used in a number of clinical trials, including the effect on prolonged rupture of membranes and after the membranes have been ruptured (Kubista et al 1975). The relation between the force of contractions and degree of dilation of the cervix has been studied. The results of the hundreds of studies have shown that virtually any hormone neurotransmitter may affect the appropriate acupuncture stimulation.

A study in Germany has shown a reduction in the *length of labour* of women who had received prenatal acupuncture. Tsuei & Leuizi have looked at the use of electroacupuncture for induction of labour. In the first study (Tsuei & Leuizi 1977), 12 women were enlisted at various stages of pregnancy between 19 and 43 weeks. *These would have included induced abortions.* The main points chosen were SP-6 (taken from the ancient text) and LI-4. Three of the women delivered vaginally with electroacupuncture. The time from the start of contractions to delivery varies from 3 to 60 hours.

Other studies have been undertaken using TENS on SP-6 and LR-3 (Dunn et al 1989).

More recent studies from the USA, Germany and Austria have once again shown that acupuncture can influence cervical ripening and induction of labour. Zeisler et al, in 1998, treated women from 36 weeks gestation using the following acupuncture points: GV-20, HT-7 and PC-6. The result was a shortening of the first stage of labour.

Rabl et al, in 2001, carried out a randomised controlled trial on 45 women who were either given acupuncture or were allocated to a control group on their due date. The acupuncture points selected were SP-6 and LI-4. The outcome was that acupuncture again shortened the first stage of labour.

The above points, SP-6 and LI-4 plus BL-31 and 32, were used in the 2006 study by Harper et al on term nulliparous women. The outcome showed an increase in spontaneous labour and reduction of caesarean sections in these women, compared to the control group.

Nutrition in preparation for labour

The final weeks of pregnancy are very important in the countdown to labour and there is a great deal that the mother can do to prepare herself. Great changes are happening in the body and the baby's growth is faster than at any other time in pregnancy. The mother should try to get the extra calories she needs from foods rich in nutrients: fresh fruit and vegetables, wholegrains, seeds, pulses and nuts, fish and poultry, milk and eggs.

Complex carbohydrates are the body's main energy source and stocking up at this stage will ensure that glycogen reserves stored in the muscles and liver tissues are filled to capacity, ready to provide sustained energy for labour. Lack of energy in labour can trigger a downward spiral of tiredness, dehydration, weakness and demoralisation, very often leading to the need for medical intervention.

Eating the above foods should ensure that the mother gets a sufficiency of the main vitamins A, B, C and E, to prepare the body for making milk. These were discussed in Chapter 3; however, the following are particularly significant in the period immediately before birth.

Vitamin K

Vitamin K is particularly important in the last weeks of pregnancy to prevent haemorrhagic disease in the newborn. A baby cannot manufacture vitamin K itself until several days old, so depends on the mother for what it needs. (This vitamin is discussed in detail in Ch. 14.)

Vitamin F (EFAs)

Essential fatty acids form a large part of the membranes of all cells and give rise to prostaglandins. EFAs affect all systems of the body, activate many enzymes, are involved in the production of hormones (Crawford 1992, Crawford & Doyle 1989) and are essential for the baby's brain and eye development (see Ch. 3 for further details).

From 36 weeks, drinking raspberry leaf tea is said to have a toning effect on the uterus. It can also be drunk during labour to assist with contractions.

Other advice

Antenatal care of the perineum

The perineum is the diamond-shaped area between the thighs and the buttocks, which includes the area around the vagina and anus.

Perineal massage involves massaging the perineum for 5–10 minutes a day. From 34 weeks, women may be encouraged to massage the perineum with oil to increase flexibility and elasticity. Research suggests that this can help to prevent tearing during delivery, so may help to avoid the need for an episiotomy and is worth suggesting to patients. They should begin by emptying the bladder and having a bath to soften the tissues. It may help them initially to use a mirror so that they become familiar with the area. The patient should place her thumbs inside the vagina and, in a U-shaped motion, move them upwards along the sides. Either olive oil or wheatgerm oil is suitable. With regular daily massage, women should notice the tissues start to relax and stretch.

Pelvic floor exercises

Toning the pelvic floor antenatally will also help with delivery of the baby, as exercised muscles stretch and recoil more easily. Women should be encouraged to do these exercises regularly. They can be practised in any comfortable position, with the legs slightly apart.

Instructions are to begin by closing the back passage as though preventing a bowel action, then close the front passages as though preventing the flow of urine. Hold this action for up to 10 seconds, breathing normally throughout, then relax and rest. Repeat up to 10 times, as often as possible.

Summary

- Problems when preparing for labour are related to: Blood and Qi deficiency, Kidney deficiency, and Stomach and Spleen deficiency.
- Acupuncture points to use in preparation for labour include:
  - *Blood and Qi deficiency:* BL-17 and ST-36
  - *Kidney deficiency:* BL-23
  - *Stomach and Spleen Qi deficiency:* BL-17 and 20
  - *induction of labour:* BL-31 and 32, LI-4 and SP-6 or LR-3; plus Uterus and Bladder ear points.

References

Crawford M 1992 The role of dietary fatty acids in biology: their place in evolution of the human brain. Nutritional Reviews 50: 3–11

Crawford M, Doyle A 1989 Fatty acids during early human development. Journal of Internal Medicine 225: 159–169

Dunn PA, Rogers D, Halford K 1989 Transcutaneous electrical stimulation at acupuncture points in the induction of uterine contractions. Obstetrics and Gynecology 73: 286–290

Harper TC, Coeytaux RR, Chen W et al 2006 A randomized controlled trial of acupuncture for the initiation of labour in nulliparous women. Journal of Maternal, Fetal and Neonatal Medicine 19(8): 465–470

Kubista E, Kucera H, Riss P 1975 Initiating contractions of the gravid uterus through electro acupuncture. American Journal of Chinese Medicine 3: 343

Rabl M, Ahner R, Bitschnau M, Zeisler H, Husslein P 2001 Acupuncture for cervical ripening and induction of labour at term – a randomized controlled trial. Weiner Klinische Wochenschrift 113(23–24): 942–946

Tsuei J, Leuizi YF 1977 The influence of acupuncture stimulation during pregnancy. Obstetrics and Gynecology 50: 479–488

Zeisler H, Tempfer C, Mayerhofer K, Barrada M, Husslein P 1998 Influence of acupuncture on the duration of labour. Gynecologic and Obstetric Investigation 46: 22–25

11 Labour

Chapter outline

One of the most important considerations in labour should always be to reduce the mother's fear and to reassure her. If you are guided by her natural behaviour patterns, everything should in most cases progress well. A basic understanding of how hormones affect pain in labour and the role of the pelvis will also help your acupuncture treatments.

This chapter covers:

- the role of the pelvis in labour
- positions of the baby's head prior to labour
- different types and lengths of labour
- emotional aspects of labour
- the hormonal system in labour
- monitoring
- pain relief options for labour
- an explanation of the different obstetric interventions
- general uses of acupuncture in labour.

Anatomy and physiology

The pelvis in labour

The pelvis is a bony cradle that supports the growing baby during pregnancy and forms a tunnel for the baby to pass through at birth. The pelvic ligaments are affected by hormones during pregnancy (see below). Progesterone and relaxin increase elasticity in the joints to allow movement between the pelvic bones during labour.

Posture and gravity

When the head is engaged and pressing tightly on the cervix, dilation of the cervix is encouraged. The more upright the mother is, the more effective this will be, allowing gravity to exert its natural pull and bring the weight of the baby to bear. Remaining upright has been shown to decrease the length of labour and to make contractions less painful.

Engagement

Engagement of the fetal head is measured in fifths, which is the amount of fetal head palpated above the brim of the pelvis.

5/5 The fetal head is five-fifths palpable; that is, the whole head can be palpated above the brim of the pelvis.

4/5 Four-fifths of the fetal head is palpable above the brim of the pelvis; one-fifth is therefore below the pelvic brim.

3/5 Three-fifths is palpable above the brim of the pelvis and two-fifths below.

2/5 Two-fifths palpable above the brim of the pelvis and three-fifths below.

1/5 One-fifth of the fetal head is palpable above the pelvic brim and four-fifths are below; the head is described as 'deeply engaged'.

These details are usually recorded on the woman's notes.

Positions of the baby prior to labour

The range of positions is shown in Figure 11.1.

Occipito-anterior (OA) position (Fig. 11.2)

This is the ideal position to go into labour. The baby's head and spine are flexed and the arms are crossed over the chest. In this position the fetus forms a complete ovoid, fitting nicely into the uterus head down. Records will note it as left occipito-anterior or right occipito-anterior depending on the position in which the baby is lying in the mother's pelvis.

In this position the baby's spine is against the soft abdomen of the mother. When the head is flexed it presents the smallest diameter to pass through the pelvis, and normal labour is usual. With the head flexed and engaged in this position, it presses evenly on the cervix and good contractions are likely to ensue.

Occipito-posterior (OP) position (Fig. 11.3)

In contrast, in the occipito-posterior position, the baby's spine is aligned *against* the mother's spine. Flexion of the head is more difficult and if the head is not flexed, it has a more difficult job ahead entering the pelvic brim. The analogy is with an egg lying sideways in an eggcup. There is a risk in an OP position that the head will be *deflexed* (i.e. bent backwards at the neck) rather than forwards in the normal *flexed* position. This means that the smallest diameter of the head is not presented to the cervix. Contractions will not be as effective and dilation of the cervix is likely to be uneven because the head is not pressing tightly on the cervix.

The cause of an OP position is not known, but it is often associated with women who have an android-shaped pelvis (see Ch. 8).

Diagnosis of an OP position

Diagnosis of an OP position is made by the midwife by abdominal examination. Often the abdomen is slightly flatter and may have a dip below the umbilicus. If

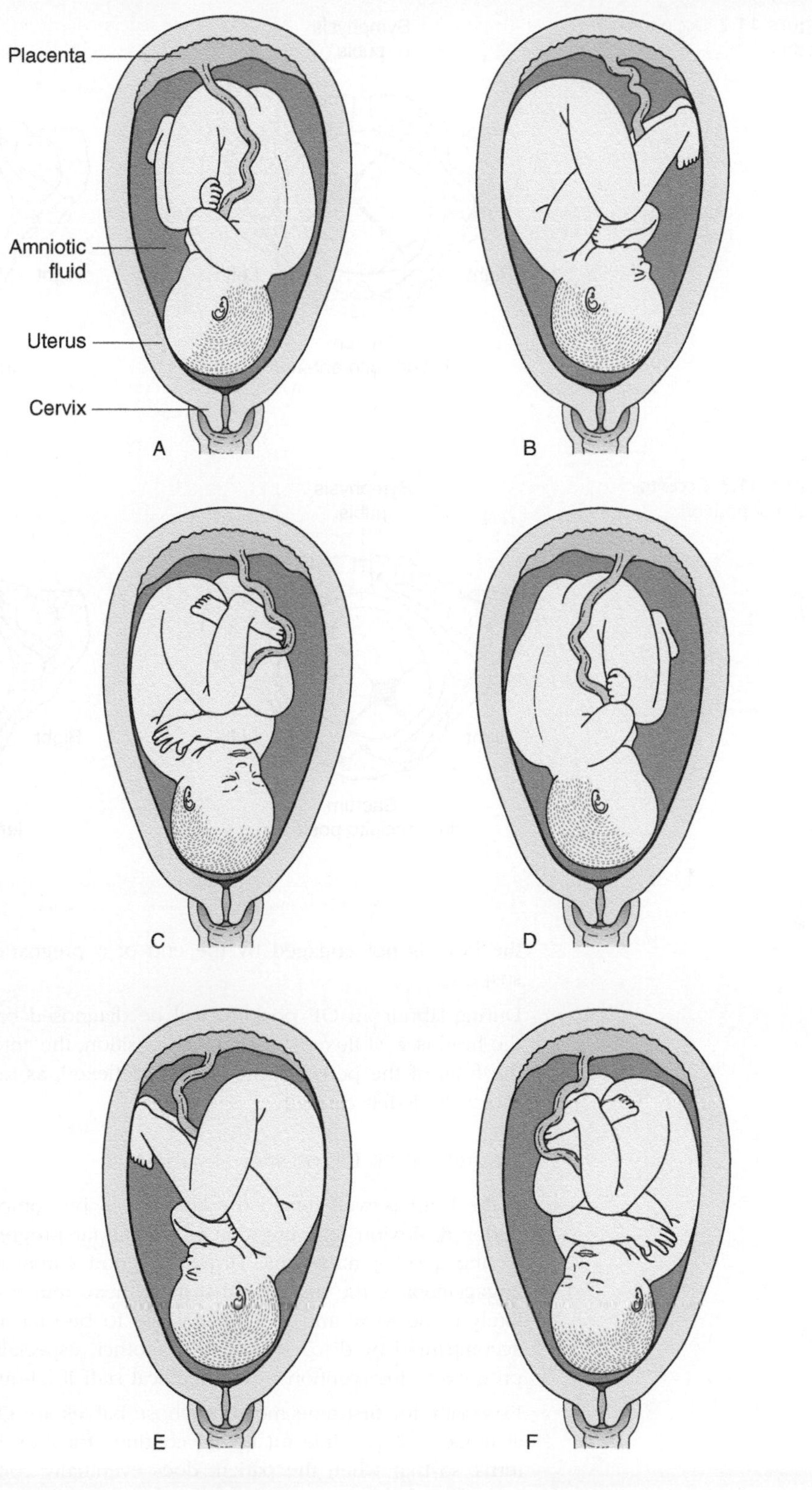

Figure 11.1 Positions of the baby prior to labour: **A** left occipito-anterior; **B** right occipito-lateral; **C** right occipito-posterior; **D** right occipito-anterior; **E** left occipito-lateral; **F** left occipito-posterior.

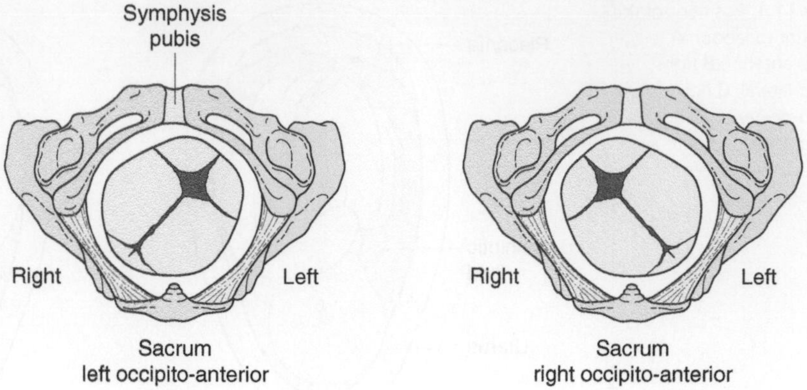

Figure 11.2 Occipito-anterior position.

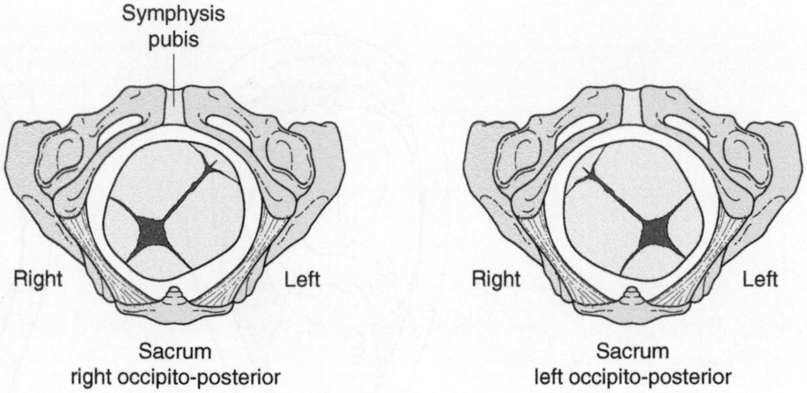

Figure 11.3 Occipito-posterior position.

the head is not engaged by the end of a pregnancy, an OP position is always suspected.

During labour an OP position will be diagnosed on vaginal examination. When the head is well flexed, as in an OA position, the anterior fontanelle is felt towards the front of the pelvis. If the head is deflexed, as in an OP position, the anterior fontanelle is felt centrally.

Progress of an OP position in labour

If the head is well flexed the labour will be completely normal. If the head is deflexed, flexion may improve as the labour progresses providing the woman is having good contractions. However, good contractions are also dependent on engagement of the head, so that if the head remains high in the pelvis, labour is likely to be slow and to take a while to become established. OP positions are accompanied by discomfort for the mother, especially back ache. Often they will progress to intervention by the medical staff if labour fails to develop.

Especially for first-time mothers whose babies are OP, labour may start and stop at home. It is possible for this to continue for 2 or 3 days, interrupting sleep patterns, so that when the patient does eventually come into hospital, she may be very tired and exhausted.

How long is a labour?

It is impossible to anticipate how long a labour will take as there are so many variables and each woman has her own individual way of giving birth. In general, the birth of a first baby takes longer than those of subsequent children. The average length of labour is between 12 and 14 hours. The second stage can last from hour up to 2 hours. As long as mother and baby are doing well, there is no cause for concern.

Different types of labour

Slow, weak labour, back ache labour

These kinds of labour usually mean that the baby is in the posterior position, facing the mother's front with its back facing the mother's spine. Such a labour may be very protracted, as it can take the baby a long time to turn into the anterior position facing the mother's back.

Precipitate labour

This is very fast and can be quite unpleasant, because there is no gradual build-up of the rhythm of contractions, and no time for the woman to appreciate what is happening. It can all be over in a few hours, before contractions have been felt or the membranes ruptured. Often the mother may be in shock afterwards as a result.

Emotional aspects of labour

Every woman enters labour with a different agenda and a different history. I find today that many women work right through their pregnancies, up to around 36 weeks, often going into labour about 2 weeks later, without giving themselves time for the mental preparation that will help them to cope with the baby after the birth.

Emotional stress has a huge influence on the pregnancy, labour and the postnatal period. (The specific effects of emotions according to TCM (traditional Chinese medicine) were discussed in Ch. 5.) Women with a predisposition to mental and emotional problems in the past may find that these resurface. Any history of physical or sexual abuse can affect the Heart: the Heart is linked to the uterus and the movement of Blood and Qi is affected.

Hormonal system

If a woman understands the important role that hormones play during labour, it can help her significantly, both to recognise what is happening within her body and to ensure that levels of stress and fear are kept as low as possible.

The three hormones that have the most influence are:

- oxytocin
- endorphins
- adrenaline.

Oxytocin

The flow of oxytocin shapes the pattern of contractions. The hormone is released as a result of pressure on the cervix from the baby's head (hence the importance of posture). If the baby's head is well applied to the cervix, contractions will be regular and consistent.

While the membranes remain intact, pressure from the baby's head is cushioned by the bag of forewaters. As long as the head is in a good position and the membranes intact, contractions should be efficient. Once the membranes have ruptured (around the transitional stage), contractions become more painful. As long as there are no problems, I feel that a woman should be encouraged to keep her membranes intact.

Oxytocin continues to be released as the baby's head descends during the second stage and as the perineum stretches during crowning. But certain factors may inhibit the release of oxytocin, including: fear and anxiety, anaesthesia or epidural, induction, episiotomy and past attitudes or memories of a previous bad experience. The effect of reduced oxytocin on labour is never helpful, as contractions become further apart, the cervix is slower to dilate, labour is prolonged and labour pains become more extreme.

So reducing fear and stress levels has profound physical as well as emotional effects. A happy, relaxed woman who feels in safe surroundings and in safe hands is likely to progress through her labour more quickly and less painfully than one who is frightened, anxious and out of control.

The pain messages received by the brain during labour stem from the stimulation of the sensory nerve mass in the uterus. As labour progresses, the pain increases and the nature of the contractions change. The amount of pain a woman will feel depends on both physical and psychological factors. Pain can be increased, for example, because of something simple like a full bladder or full bowels or even straightforward fear.

Endorphins

Substances called beta endorphins are known to increase during labour and to peak at delivery. Endorphins are natural substances, similar to opiates, that are released whenever the body is physically stressed.

Endorphins have three main effects:

- they modify pain
- they alter perception of time and space
- they create a sense of well-being.

Once labour begins, the level of endorphins rises, helping the mother to cope with her contractions and to get some rest in between. Bonica reported in 1994 on a phenomenon called pregnancy-induced analgesia or hypalgesia, suggesting that pain tolerance thresholds normally rise at the end of the pregnancy. He suggested that pregnancy-induced hypalgesia results from the activity of dynorphin opiate receptors in the spinal cord, which are capable of lowering the intensity of the pain in labour.

A very relaxed mother, even to the extent of seeming 'spaced out', is a sign that endorphin levels are adequate. As with oxytocin, though, certain factors will inhibit endorphin release, including an epidural anaesthetic and high levels of fear and stress.

Adrenaline

It is important that the acupuncturist understands the effect of fear on labour, and appreciates how simple measures can allay fear. When people are frightened and in pain, the body automatically increases catecholamine levels and releases the hormone adrenaline. This produces the 'fight or flight' syndrome, a pattern of

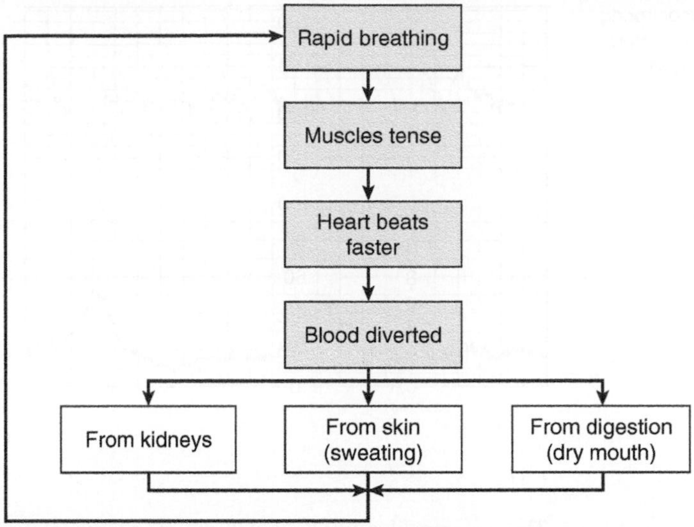

Figure 11.4 Effects of stress.

behaviour intended to rescue them from danger (Fig. 11.4). The cardiac, respiratory, genitourinary, gastrointestinal and skeletal systems are all affected, resulting in an increase in blood sugar, faster heartbeat, raised blood pressure and decreased digestion. This can be caused by any situation where the mother feels threatened, such as during the physiological stress of labour (Simkin 1989).

In labour these processes can manifest as:

- restlessness and anxiety
- the need to shout
- increased pain
- contractions slowing down as the oxytocin level drops
- falling endorphin levels, which only start to rise again when the source of disturbance is removed
- reorganisation of the blood supply, redirecting blood to the vital organs. This results in a reduced blood flow to the uterus and placenta and the baby can therefore become distressed.

A poor labour environment, unnerving comments and uncomfortable positions can all increase pain and cause anxiety. The mother may become agitated and, as a result, labour may slow down.

Management

The role of the midwife

Fetal monitoring

Monitoring of the fetal heart (Fig. 11.5) is done by the midwife in the first stage of labour, to assess the baby's response to contractions. A marked change to the individual fetal heart pattern is significant and may be a sign of fetal distress. Monitoring is carried out using an ultrasonic heart rate detector, Doppler ultrasound or electronic monitoring, using transducers placed on the abdomen or electrodes applied to the bony part of the fetal skull. A cardiotocograph (CTG) measures and records uterine and fetal heart activity, displaying the findings in the form of a graph.

Techniques for fetal monitoring include the following.

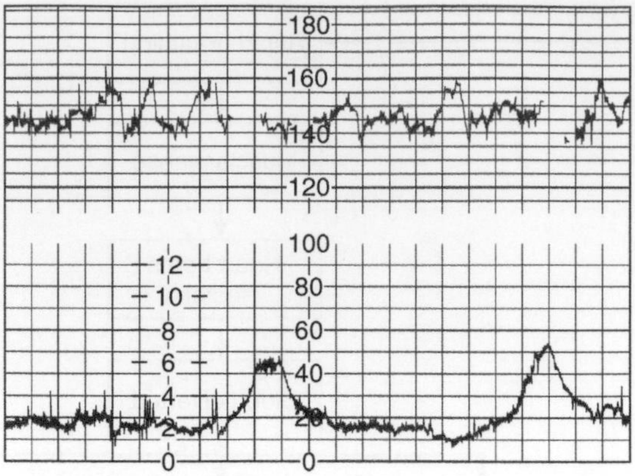

Figure 11.5 Fetal monitoring. (Reproduced with permission from Sweet 1997, p. 225.)

CTG

There is considerable debate about electronic fetal monitoring, because there is no clear evidence that it improves the outcome of the birth. It is associated with higher intervention rates. In its favour, it is argued that it can raise confidence by providing information about the health of the baby but for most women, support from their partner and companions is more helpful.

During labour, the mother will be monitored every couple of hours for 20–30 minutes. Only if there is a problem with the baby's heartbeat will she be advised to have continuous monitoring, when the machine is left on all the time. Modern machines allow the mother to be up and mobile while being monitored.

Intermittent monitoring

The baby's heartbeat can be effectively assessed using less 'high tech' methods. Traditionally the midwife will listen into the baby with a Pinnard's ear trumpet, with which she can hear the heart and count the beats. She can do this with the mother in any position, whether kneeling on all fours, standing or sitting.

Sonic aid or Doppler diagram

This is an ultrasonic device that allows the fetal heartbeat to be heard by the mother too. As with the Pinnard's ear trumpet, a sonic aid gives intermittent monitoring of the baby, which mothers find less intrusive during labour.

Scalp electrode diagram

Late in labour, when the baby's head is visible via the mother's dilating vagina, it is possible to monitor the baby directly with an electrode attached to the scalp. This technique is used if the baby is diagnosed as being at risk and requiring careful monitoring, particularly if the heartbeat is dropping. For accuracy, it should be used in conjunction with a fetal blood sample, and many practitioners consider that it is the best way of ascertaining fetal well-being. Its disadvantage is that it is invasive and painful for the baby, and full mobility is not possible for the mother.

Pain relief in labour

Analgesic drugs may be administered, usually during the first stage of labour, to reduce the level of pain with as few side-effects as possible.

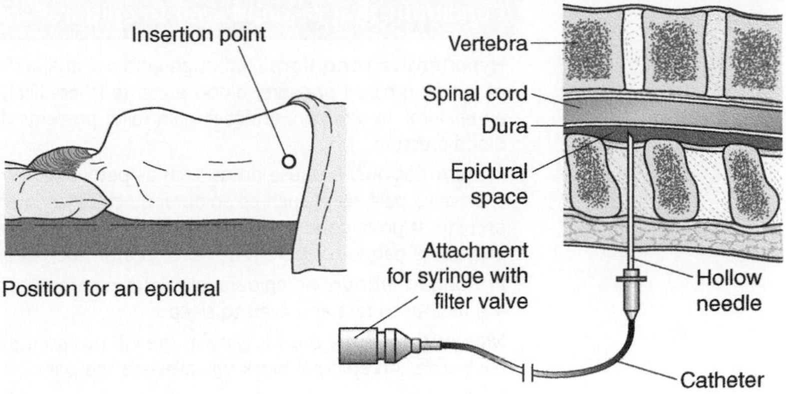

Figure 11.6 An epidural. (Reproduced with permission from Sweet 1997, p. 225.)

Pethidine

Pethidine is one of the most commonly used, as it is effective, rapid acting and relatively safe. It is administered by intramuscular injection and the effects last for about 3–4 hours. The usual dose is 50–200 mg, depending on the weight of the mother, the level of pain she is experiencing and how far she has progressed in her labour.

Possible side-effects include nausea, reduced blood pressure and sweating in the mother and respiratory depression in the fetus and the newborn.

Inhalation analgesia

Inhalation analgesia gives partial relief of pain but no anaesthesia.

Entonox is a mixture of equal parts of nitrous oxide and oxygen (the oxygen helps fetal oxygenation). It is administered from a premixed cylinder by the mother herself, by means of a face mask or mouthpiece.

Entonox is effective only while it is being breathed in, plus about 15 seconds. Deep breathing is required to activate the machine, which makes a gurgling noise. The mother is instructed to start using the mask as soon as the contraction can be felt, so as to achieve maximum analgesia while the contraction is at its height. The mask is usually taken off in between contractions.

It is an effective form of pain relief for long and strong contractions and may also be used during the second stage of labour and during suturing. Its disadvantage is that it may make the mother feel a little nauseous and drowsy.

Epidural analgesia

Epidural analgesia is an invasive procedure to introduce local anaesthetic into the epidural space (Fig. 11.6). It must be performed by an experienced anaesthetist.

Epidural *pudenda block* is an injection of local anaesthetic into the epidural space around the spinal cord between the third and fourth lumbar vertebrae. It numbs the body below the injection site and thus relieves the pain from contractions. It is administered as a single dose or as a continuous technique, giving further doses via a catheter. It gives good pain relief to women in labour and is often used as a form of anaesthetic for caesarean section.

Most hospitals now offer a 24-hour epidural service, making epidural analgesia available to women in labour on request.

Conditions that respond well to epidural anaesthesia

Hypertensive conditions. Although epidural analgesia is not considered to be a means of lowering blood pressure, blood pressure is less likely to rise (and may fall) as a result of an epidural. In addition, effective pain relief prevents distress which could cause a rise in blood pressure.

Preterm labour. Because drugs such as pethidine repress the baby's respiratory centre, alternative pain relief such as epidural block offers many advantages when labour is preterm. It gives good analgesia in a forceps delivery, which is often necessary for premature babies to prevent any pressure on the head.

Prolonged labour. An epidural alleviates pain and can prevent exhaustion by enabling the mother to rest and even to sleep.

Malposition. If the baby is lying in the OP position, the mother is likely to get a lot of back ache. An epidural block will alleviate the pain.

Multiple pregnancy. An epidural allows any manipulation of the twins that the obstetrician may need to do. Second and subsequent babies can therefore be delivered more promptly.

Complications that may result from epidural anaesthesia

Hypotension. This is the most common form of complication and occurs in about 5% of women. Prevention is helped by maintaining an adequate volume of circulating fluid and by turning the mother on to her left side.

Dural tap. This occurs if the dura in the spinal cord is punctured and causes a leakage of cerebral spinal fluid. It happens in around 1% of cases. The mother is likely to develop a severe headache within 1–3 days, which can last for up to a week.

Toxic reaction to anaesthetic. This may be caused by a high dose of local anaesthetic. A mild toxic reaction may give rise to restlessness, dizziness and drowsiness, while a serious toxic reaction can cause convulsions.

Retention of urine. As the epidural block masks the sensation of needing to empty the bladder, the mother should be encouraged to pass urine every 2 hours in labour.

Inadequate epidural block. For various reasons, analgesia may occur down only one side. This situation can be very distressing for the woman but can be remedied by a further injection of local anaesthetic.

Infection. This is a rare complication since a strict aseptic technique is used.

Sense of deprivation. Mothers who have emotionally prepared themselves for pain may feel deprived and unfulfilled if they have a pain-free labour with epidural analgesia. On the other hand, women who choose epidural and who do not have the complete pain relief that they expect can be both disappointed and angry.

Interventions

Augmentation

Augmentation is the enhancement of the strength and frequency of uterine contractions by means of a Syntocinon infusion, administered intravenously. It may be used in a prolonged labour if the condition of mother and baby is good. More effective methods of pain relief may be required as a result.

Syntocinon is a drug used to sustain contractions artificially and is usually administered through an electronic infusion pump, which delivers the drug at a regular rate and volume. It is administered slowly, starting off at 10 units diluted in 500 ml of saline solution, at a rate of 4 milliunits per minute. The dosage is increased every 15 minutes according to the practice of the particular hospital. Syntocinon

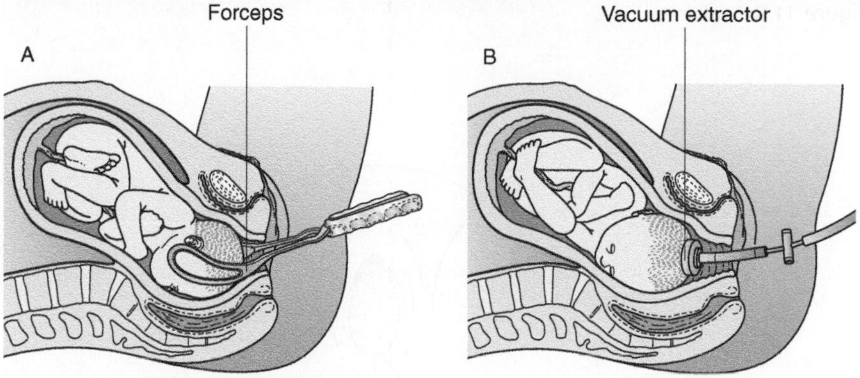

Figure 11.7 A Forceps; B vacuum extraction.

makes the uterus contract, which will help the cervix to dilate. It is used if a woman becomes exhausted and her contractions slow down (Lamont 1990).

Forceps

Forceps (Fig. 11.7A) are a specially designed obstetric instrument, used to expedite the baby's delivery. They may be used if: there is delay in the second stage of labour; the baby is in an OP position; there is fetal or maternal distress; in cases of severe pre-eclampsia, hypertension, heart disease or tuberculosis, to spare the mother muscular effort; or delivery is preterm or breech, in order to protect the infant.

Vacuum extraction

Vacuum extraction (Fig. 11.7B) is an alternative method of instrumental delivery that might be preferred in certain circumstances, such as where the cord is prolapsed and the cervix is more than 7 cm dilated, or for delivery of a second twin. The instrument consists of a suction cap made of metal or rubber (also known as a ventouse). It is placed on the baby's head and suction is applied through an attached tube and vacuum pump. The baby can then be gently pulled out.

Caesarean section

A caesarean section may be carried out at any time during the first stage of labour, or in unusual circumstances during the second stage. Its most common uses are for: fetal distress, failed induction of labour, malpresentation/shoulder dystocia, undiagnosed breech or high-risk pregnancies (e.g. diabetes).

Procedure in a caesarean section

1. The pubic hair may be shaved.
2. A catheter will be inserted into the woman's bladder to empty it prior to theatre.
3. An intravenous infusion will be set up in her hand.
4. General anaesthetic will be given.
5. Once she is unconscious an incision will be made in the lower abdomen on the bikini line. The uterus is then opened, the amniotic fluid surrounding the baby is sucked away, and the baby is lifted out, wrapped and taken to a resuscitaire in the same room for the paediatrician to examine the baby.
6. Following delivery, the layers of uterus and muscle are sutured.

Figure 11.8 Episiotomy.

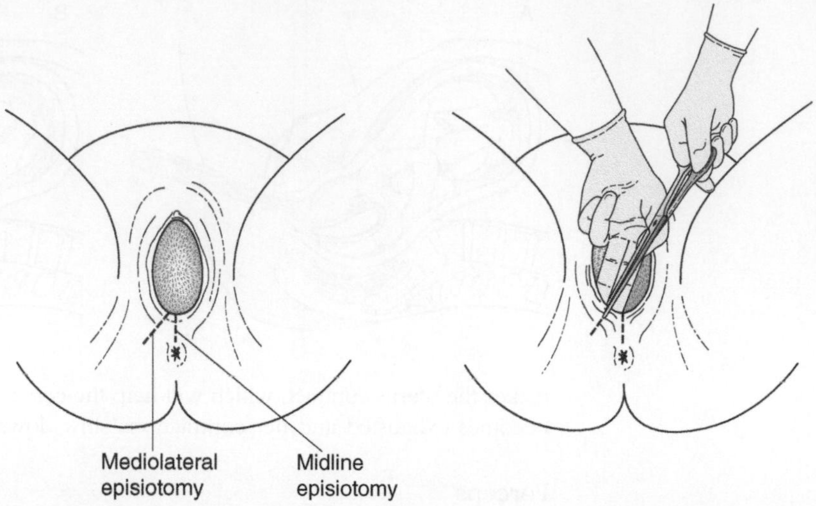

Advantages of caesarean section

These include: safe delivery of a healthy baby, and that the operation can be performed very quickly.

Disadvantages

Because it is major abdominal surgery the recovery takes a long time, it can take longer to establish breastfeeding, and babies have higher rate of respiratory problems.

In recent years there has been an increased use of caesarean section, and the rate varies enormously between countries. The availability of the operation is encouraging some women to elect to have a caesarean section just to fit in with their diaries, in spite of the clear disadvantages involved when it is obstetrically unnecessary.

Episiotomy

Episiotomy (Fig. 11.8) is an incision through the perineum and perineal body. This is performed to enlarge the perineal opening to allow the baby to be born. It is done with special scissors just before the birth. Although used in more than 50% of deliveries in the 1970s and 1980s (Lamont 1990, Sleep 1984), there is no evidence that a clean cut heals better than an uncontrolled tear, and it is now recommended that its use be restricted to fetal indications only:

- to speed delivery when the baby's head is on the perineum and there is evidence of fetal distress
- to reduce the risk of intercranial damage to the fetus in preterm labour and breech delivery.

The role of the acupuncturist

The acupuncturist's best contribution is likely to be in pain relief and relaxation. In an OP position, acupuncture can also be utilised to cope with the back ache, and in these cases both electroacupuncture and V-TENS can be very effective. Ear points are often the most accessible and least intrusive during labour.

Acupuncture treatment in labour

Prior to labour

Acupuncture prior to labour should deal with rebalancing some of the following points. (The effects of different emotions on the Qi were detailed in Ch. 5 and only a summary is given here.)

Worry. This leads to stagnation of Qi and causes the Qi to knot in the Heart, Spleen and Lung.

Anger. This causes Liver Qi stagnation.

Fear. Shock depletes the Heart, Spleen and Kidney and can result from a bad experience, memories of a prior delivery, a precipate delivery or anxiety about any abnormality detected during the pregnancy.

Overwork. Women who work long hours, and who keep working until shortly before the time of their delivery, enter labour exhausted. Overwork and lack of rest can cause Kidney deficiency. They are also mentally unprepared, although it is very hard to forewarn somebody of how difficult coping with a baby can be.

Overexercising. This weakens the Spleen and in pregnancy affects the Penetrating and Directing Vessels.

IVF (in vitro fertilisation) pregnancies. These often cause Kidney deficiency. Such women are also at risk of complications and of not going to full term (see Ch. 8).

OP position

Acupuncture should be aimed at dealing with the back ache (Martoudis & Christofides 1990). I use electroacupuncture with my V-TENS machine on BL-31 and 32 to help ease it. It can be very difficult to use certain points when the mother is in pain. She may tend to curl up around her bump, so that the acupuncturist can gain access only to her back. In this position it can help a great deal to give massage at the site of the pain.

Ear points

- Bladder point of the ear, with electroacupuncture or just left in situ.
- Shenmen, with electroacupuncture or just left in; if the ear is stimulated with electroacupuncture you get a much better endorphin release.

Keep the patient well hydrated and try to encourage sleep if she has any respite from the pain.

POINTS TO TREAT

- **BL-67: tonify and take the needle out; this may help to regulate the contractions but is painful to do and quite difficult, depending on the position of the mother.**
- **BL-60: again, tonify and take the needles out.**

CASE STUDY 11.1 OP POSITION

Maddie was 38 weeks pregnant with her first baby, had been up all night with contractions, and felt she was going into labour. She phoned me at 7.30 a.m. because she felt things were moving. I had a day's clinic to do, so I phoned her during the day to see how she was progressing. As it was her first baby I knew it would not be quick.

I visited her at home at 7.00 p.m., after she had been contracting on and off throughout day. She had also been experiencing a lot of back pain. She was excited and positive because she thought it was all happening, and she was trying to breathe through her contractions. I used electroacupuncture on her BL-31 and 32 at a setting of 200 pulse rate and 2.5 pulse width on the V-TENS machine. I also needled BL-60 for her backache every 15 minutes, removing the needle in between, and used Shenmen in the ear with a quarter-inch (0.6 cm) needle.

At 9.00 p.m. she was still contracting and the pain was getting worse in her back. I took the needles out and she got in the bath, hoping that the warmth of the water would soothe her. At 11.00 p.m. I told her I thought she should go to the hospital. There was a limit to the pain relief and general medical attention that I could give her at home. I felt that she was not progressing as well as she thought and would only be about 2 cm when she got there. I was concerned that this would be a huge blow to her confidence, as she was probably thinking she was well on the way. Her contractions were quite strong and painful, but they were still very irregular and most of the pain was in her back.

In the hospital she was given a sedative (this practice is no longer undertaken) and slept for 4 hours. The next day I had other duties and got back to her at 2.00 p.m. She was out of bed but still labouring and struggling with the pain. At 5.00 p.m. she was allowed into the water pool as she was now 5 cm, but she was exhausted and not really coping with the pain.

She came out of the water at 8.00 p.m. and felt quite refreshed but still exhausted. On examination, she was 8 cm. I stimulated ST-36, LI-4 and SP-6 but by now she did not want acupuncture. At 10.00 p.m. she was still only 8 cm and the hospital staff decided to break her waters. I was not keen on this, as I knew she would feel the pain even more, but the fetal heart was getting tired and so was she, so I understood why the decision was made. She also decided to have an epidural, which was completed at 11.00 p.m., and for the first time she was out of pain.

Too exhausted to push, she delivered by forceps at 2.00 a.m. – a little boy.

Maddie's example illustrates the physical stresses that an OP position can impose on the mother and fetus. As a midwife, I knew what the outcome was likely to be as soon as the OP was apparent 24 hours before the birth, but I was still disappointed that the delivery ended with an epidural and forceps. Acupuncture was of some help in pain relief and emotional support but the physical exhaustion of a long labour was in the end the overwhelming issue. The process could have been speeded up with earlier use of an epidural, but Maddie was adamant that she did not want to use that option as long as she felt the labour might improve.

In consolation, 3 years later she had a little girl who I delivered using acupuncture and water labour.

Summary

- Problems in labour include: OP position, pain, fetal distress and complications.

- Obstetric interventions include: augmentation, forceps, vacuum extraction, caesarian section and episiotomy.
- Acupuncture points to use during labour include:
  - *OP position:* BL-31 and 32
  - *ear points:* Bladder and Shenmen.

References

Bonica JJ 1994 Labour pain. In: Wall PD, Melzack R (eds) Textbook of pain. Churchill Livingstone, New York

Lamont R F 1990 Induction of labour. Obstetrics and Gynecology 2: 16–20

Martoudis S, Christofides K 1990 Electroacupuncture for pain relief in labour. Acupuncture in Medicine 8(2): 51–52

Simkin P 1989 Stress, pain and catecholamines in labour, part one: a review. Birth 13(4): 186

Sleep J 1984 Episiotomy and normal delivery. Nursing Times 80(47): 29–30

Sweet BR (ed.) 1997 Mayes' midwifery, 12th edn. Baillière Tindall, New York

Further reading

Dunn P, Rogers D, Halford K 1989 Transcutaneous electric stimulation at acupuncture points in the induction of uterine contractions. Obstetrics and Gynecology 73: 286

12 First stage of labour

Chapter outline

The use of complementary therapies is growing faster than ever and midwifery is one of the key areas. Women are increasingly keen to know about remedies for the common ailments of pregnancy and particularly for pain relief in labour. They are understandably reluctant to take drugs during pregnancy, and acupuncture is an obvious drug-free alternative, with no unwanted side-effects (Pei & Huang 1985).

Effective acupuncture requires the practitioner to have a detailed understanding of the points used in pregnancy, and to needle them accurately. However, I firmly believe that it is not only the use of appropriate acupuncture points that has such good effect; also vital is the acupuncturist's understanding of the mother's behavioural patterns and emotional needs. Insight into the mother's emotions helps to guide the acupuncturist in determining which points to use.

Although acupuncture is not commonly used to relieve the pain of labour in China, it has been used in Europe since the 1970s.

Labour terms explained

These are some terms you may hear on a labour ward during the first stage of labour.

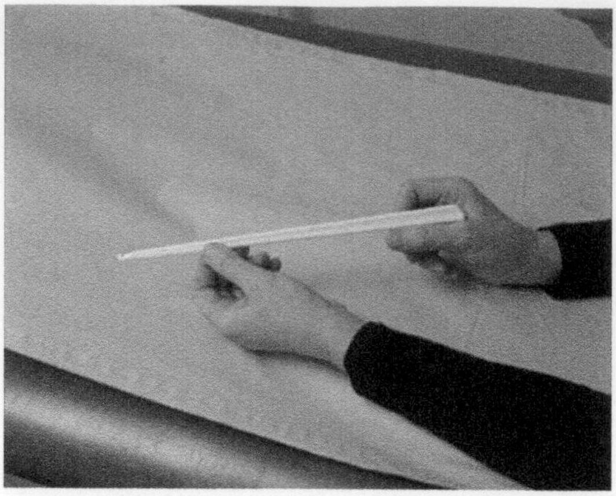

Figure 12.1 Amni hook used to rupture membrane.

Acceleration and deceleration pattern. Accelerations of the fetal heart of 15 bpm from the baseline are regarded as a positive sign of fetal health. Decelerations are a cause for concern; they may be *early* or *late* (see Fig. 12.8).

ARM (artificial rupture of membranes). This may be done during the first stage of labour using amni hooks. These are small plastic hooks that nick the membrane to allow fluid out (Fig. 12.1); it is not a painful process.

Baseline variability. This is the variation in heart rate of 5–15 bpm over a time base of 10–20 seconds. Good variability is an important sign of fetal well-being.

CTG (cardiotocograph). This is a machine that monitors the baby's heartbeat (see Fig. 11.5). It is attached on to the mother's abdomen in two places, one to monitor the contractions and one to monitor the baby's heartbeat. The normal fetal heart rate is between 120 and 160 bleeps per minute.

Effacement of the cervix (Fig. 12.2). This is the term for the thinning out and dilating of the cervix.

IVU. Intravenous infusion, or drip.

Pain relief. When offered during the first stage of labour, this may be injections of pethidine, an epidural or sometimes Entonox, which is a mixture of gas and air (described in Ch. 11).

Partogram. This is a chart which the midwife fills in to measure contractions and to record blood pressure and the descent and position of the baby's head (i.e. occipito-posterior (OP) or occipito-anterior (OA)) (Fig. 12.3).

Vaginal examination (VE). Two fingers are inserted into the vagina to see how much the cervix is dilating and to assess the progress of the labour.

Characteristics of the first stage of labour

Phases in the onset of labour

Signs of the first stage of labour are the thinning and opening of the cervix, the start of rhythmic contractions of the uterus, the dilation of the cervix, and sometimes a 'show'. This can happen at any time after 37 weeks.

The average length of the first stage of labour with a first baby is 12–14 hours. The first stage can be divided into three parts:

1. early labour
2. accelerated labour
3. transition.

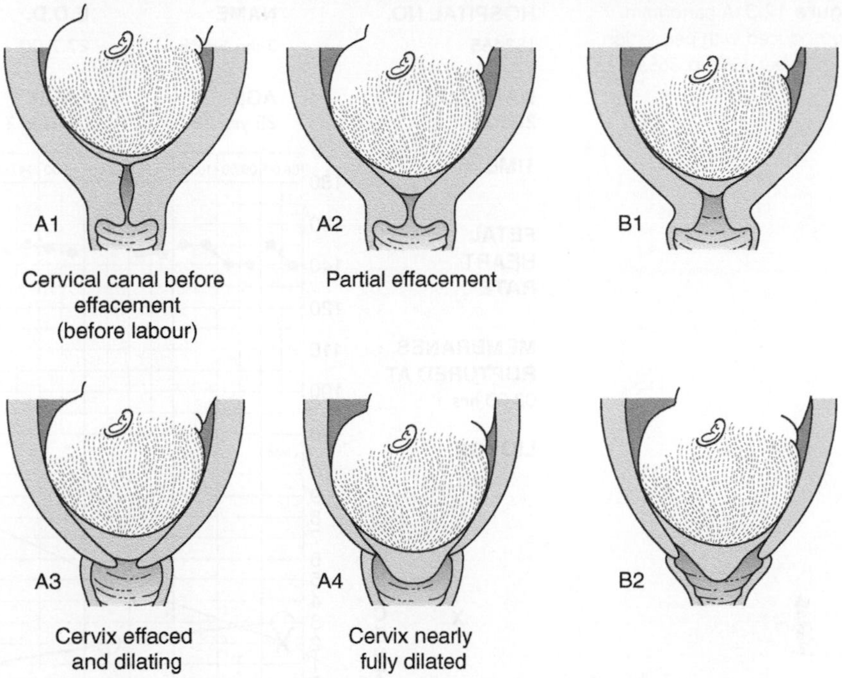

Figure 12.2 Effacement and dilation of the cervix. (Reproduced with permission from Sweet 1997, p. 358.)

Early labour

During this stage, the cervix dilates from closed to open, expanding from 0 to 4 cm. The baby moves deep down into the pelvis and the face gradually turns towards the mother's back.

Labour begins with regular contractions, which the mother feels in the groin or low in the abdomen or back, and the uterus can be felt hardening. Contractions in the early stages of labour last 50–60 seconds and can be 5–10 minutes or more apart. How bearable they are depends on the position of the baby and the mother's pain threshold. Sometimes there is constant back ache, and sometimes the waters may leak.

Accelerated phase

Labour is now established. The cervix is dilated to 4–8 cm. Contractions will now be 2–3 minutes apart, lasting 45–60 seconds, and they will be stronger and more intense. They may become more frequent.

Transition

Transition occurs at between 8 and 10 cm dilation of the cervix. Physiologically the cervix is changing from the opening out phase to the bearing down phase. Contractions will be at their strongest, 1–3 minutes apart, lasting 45–90 seconds.

Labour pain

The physiology of labour pain

The location and sensation of pain are constantly changing in duration, degree and frequency throughout labour (Fig. 12.4). Initally, in the early stages, the pain

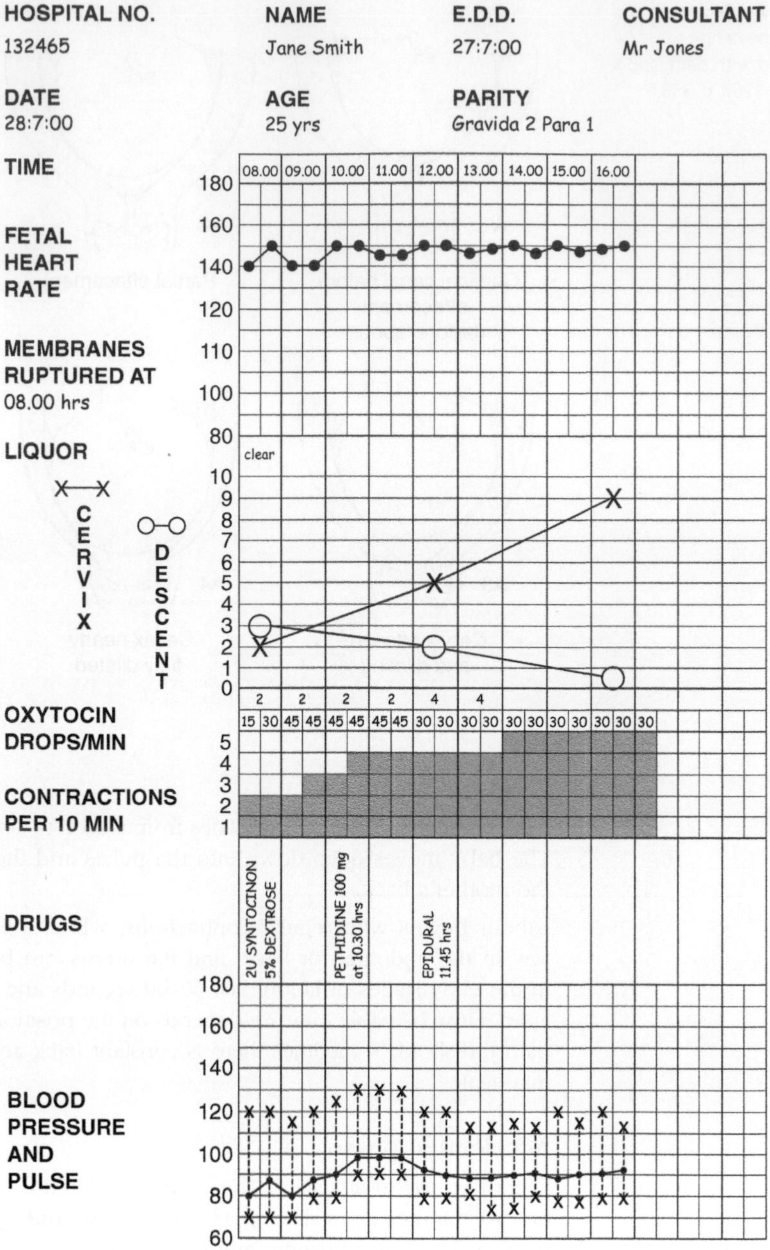

Figure 12.3 A partogram. (Reproduced with permission from Sweet 1997, p. 365.)

enables the mother to stop, think, slow down and find somewhere safe to prepare to have her baby.

Pain in the first stage of labour

Pain in the first stage of labour is due to dilation of the cervix and to stretching of the lower segment of the uterus (Bonica 1994) (Fig. 12.5).

The spinal cord is composed of nerve cells of grey matter, which relay these pain signals to the brain, and nerve axons of white matter. It runs inside the vertebral column, branching out in pairs through openings called intervertebral foramina.

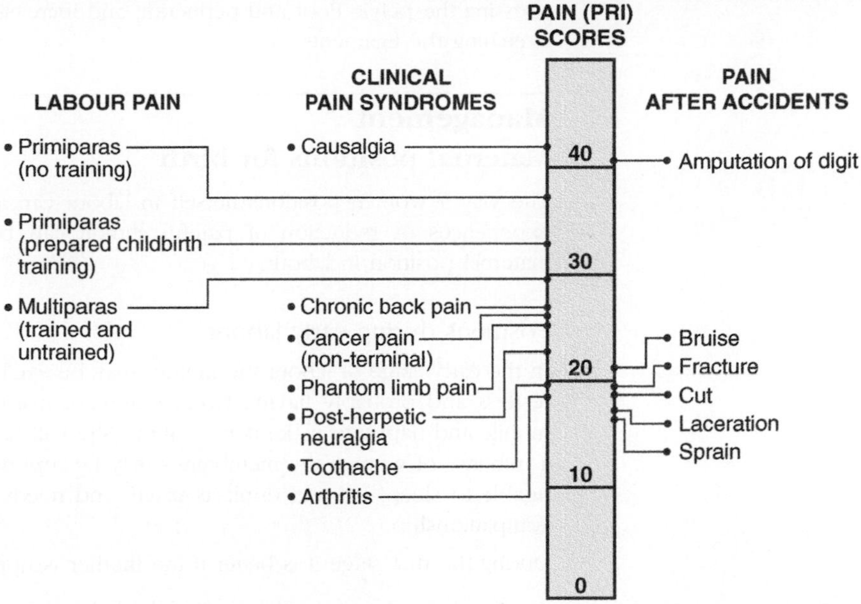

Figure 12.4 Pain scores. (Reproduced with permission from Moore 1997, p. 4.)

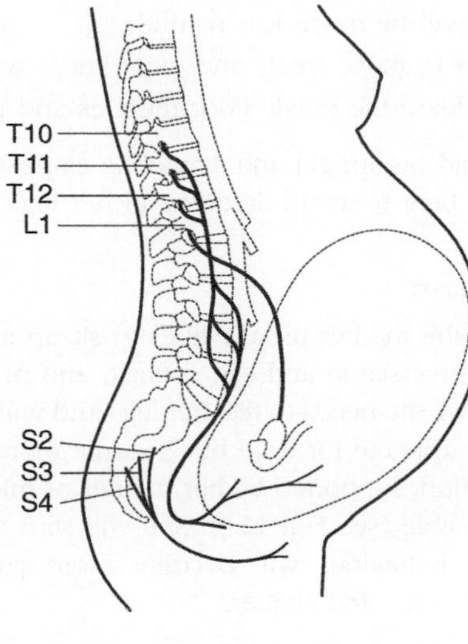

Figure 12.5 Neural pathways supplying the uterus, cervix and perineal structures. (Reproduced with permission from Moore 1997, p. 41.)

There are over 30 such pairs of spinal nerves, named according to their source; for example, cervical nerves arise from the neck and thoracic nerves from the thorax. Bonica (1994) reported that nerves T10, T11, T12 and L1 (corresponding to the respective thoracic and lumbar vertebrae) supply the lower segment of the uterus and the cervix (although this is contradicted by some texts that consider that the cervix is supplied by sacral nerves). Labour pain is felt over the areas of the back (dermatomes), which are supplied from these spinal nerves. In the first stage of labour the area affected relates to T11 and T12.

Pain in the second and third stage of labour

Pain in the later stages is different from that in the first stage of labour. The cervix is now fully dilated as the head of the baby progresses through the birth canal, stressing the pelvic floor and perineum, and increasing the pain to those areas by stretching the ligaments.

Management

Maternal positions for birth

The way a woman positions herself in labour can affect the amount of pain she experiences. A reduction of painful stimuli can be achieved by changing the maternal position in labour.

Positions during early labour

In the early stage of labour the mother may be excited, nervous with anticipation, restless and probably having twinges and inconsistent contractions. She will be mobile and happy to make conversation. She will have a mucus discharge, and in a minority of women the membranes may be ruptured. She makes eye contact, is unable to sleep, eat and drink as usual, and needs conversation, distraction and companionship.

During the first stage it is better if the mother is upright:

- it enables the presenting part of the baby to be well applied to the cervix, which helps to trigger oxytocin and maintain contractions
- contractions will be much less painful
- it enables her to move freely and experiment with different positions
- it helps to release the pelvic floor muscles and protect the perineum.

The mother should be upright and as mobile as possible, fully supported, and her knees should be bent to avoid tiredness in her legs (Fig. 12.6).

Accelerated phase

During this time the mother usually likes to sit up and rest between contractions. She will avoid conversation and eye contact, and probably will rest her head and arms on the pillow. She needs to rest her legs and will be more comfortable upright. She will lose her appetite for food but become more thirsty. Let her find her own comfortable position, supported by her partner or midwife on pillows, but keeping as upright as possible (see Fig. 12.6). She will start to develop her own breathing pattern and her behaviour will become more passive. She needs a lack of disruption; avoid noise and chatter.

Transition phase

The mother's endorphin level now rises in response to pain, and she may suddenly change the behaviour patterns that were previously established. She may be irrational and irritable, feel out of control and unable to manage, and may be restless and needing to move. Try different levels of comfort. She may be noisy – don't take any abuse she gives personally! Her membranes may rupture, and it is very common during this stage for her to be shaking and vomiting.

Standing or sitting will help ease much of the pain, especially towards the end of the first stage. It is easier for the mother to rest if she is well supported on pillows or a bean bag. Wet towels and back massage are helpful.

The mother may wish to push before she is fully dilated. Frequently the anterior lip of the cervix will impede full dilation; this happens when the cervix is almost,

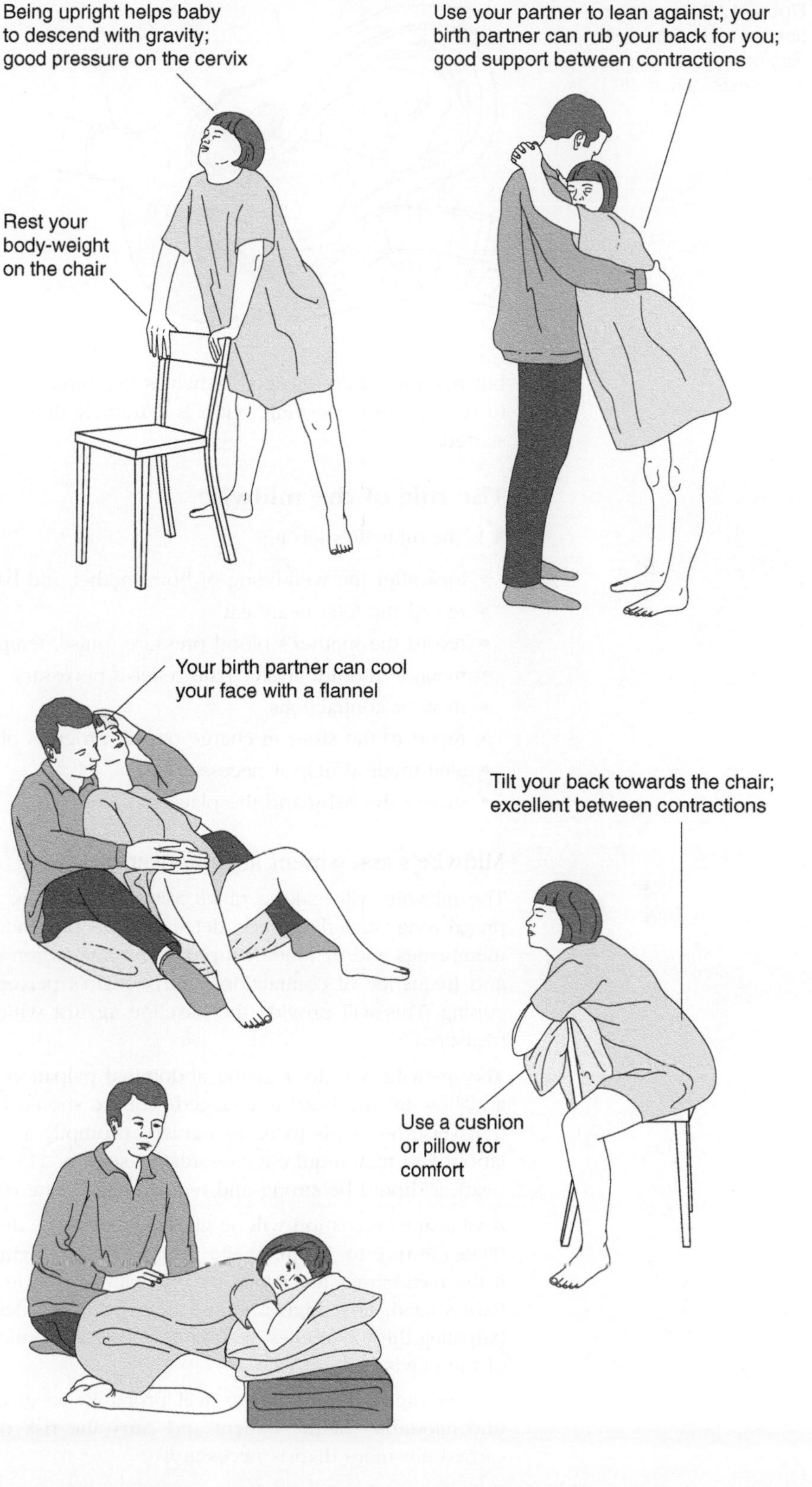
Being upright helps baby to descend with gravity; good pressure on the cervix
Use your partner to lean against; your birth partner can rub your back for you; good support between contractions
Rest your body-weight on the chair
Your birth partner can cool your face with a flannel
Tilt your back towards the chair; excellent between contractions
Use a cushion or pillow for comfort

Figure 12.6 Positions for the first stage of labour.

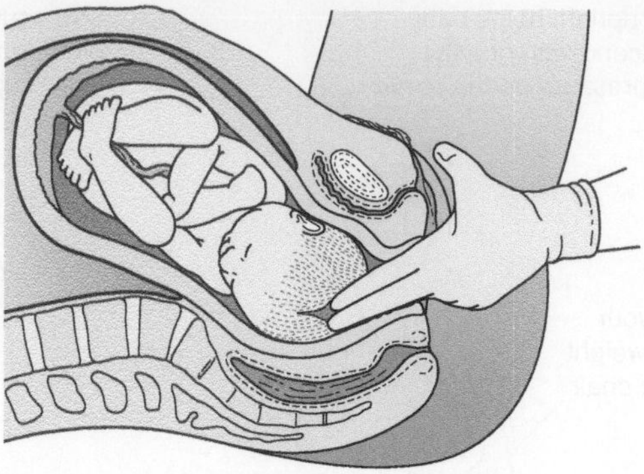

Figure 12.7 Palpating the position of the fetal skull. (Reproduced with permission from Sweet 1997, p. 381.)

but not quite, fully dilated. Midwives frequently lie the woman on her side to try to stop her from pushing, but it is extremely difficult to resist the urge once it has started.

The role of the midwife

It is the midwife's job to:

- look after the well-being of both mother and baby
- record the fetal heartbeat
- record the mother's blood pressure, pulse, temperature and bladder output
- monitor and administer pain relief if necessary
- monitor contractions
- report to the sister in charge on the progress of the labour
- alert medical help if necessary
- deliver the baby and the placenta.

Midwife's assessment at the onset of labour

The midwife will make a quick assessment of the stage of labour and how it is progressing, including such details as the presence of a show, the state of the membranes and/or time of rupture, the time when contractions began, the length and frequency of contractions, the woman's perception of pain and how she is coping. This will provide the baseline against which further assessments can be measured.

The midwife will do a gentle abdominal palpation to see how the baby is lying and how far the head is engaged. The lie should be longitudinal (an oblique or transverse lie needs to be recognised promptly as it could lead to an obstructed labour and may require a caesarean – see Ch. 11). She will also listen to the fetal heart; it should be strong and regular with a rate of between 110 and 150 bpm.

A vaginal examination will be given to assess the dilation of the cervix. The cervix dilates from 0 to 10 cm, at the rate of roughly 1 cm an hour. As well as showing if the membranes are intact, the VE will give an indication of the position of the baby's head, how high it is and how far it has descended. The midwife will be palpating the fontanelles, feeling the posterior fontanelle towards the anterior part of the pelvis (Fig. 12.7).

Further vaginal examinations will probably be given every 4–5 hours. They are uncomfortable for the patient and carry the risk of infection, so should not be carried out more than is necessary.

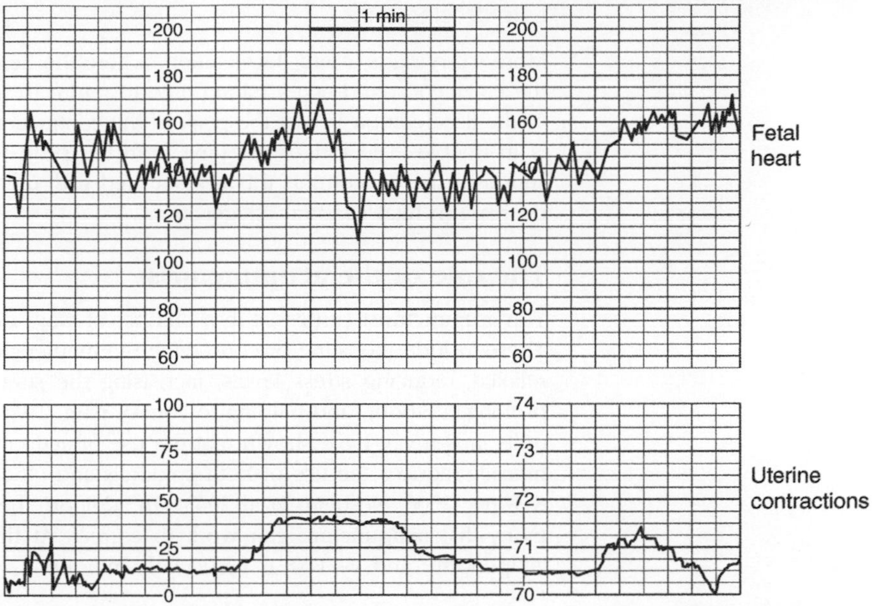

Figure 12.8 Normal cardiotocograph: the fetal heart rate is normal and reactive. (Courtesy of JA Jordan, Birmingham Maternity Hospital; from Sweet 1997, p. 372.)

All the midwife's findings will be plotted on a partogram, which will also include details of the patient's temperature, pulse rate, blood pressure, urinalysis and any oedema.

Assessing the condition of the fetus

There is huge controversy about the value of this, and no clear evidence that electronic monitoring improves the outcome of labour. Clinical tests such as ultrasound or CTG (see Ch. 11) are only tools to help the practitioner, and the most effective way of monitoring the well-being of both mother and baby is for the same midwife to attend throughout labour. Certainly for the women themselves, methods of monitoring are far less important than the support they get from the hospital staff and from their birthing partners.

To determine the baby's response to the stress of labour, the fetal heart rate is assessed. This is usually done manually by a hand-held stethoscope or electronically by a CTG machine, which also monitors the strength of the contractions. A continuous trace of the heartbeat allows the midwife to see how the baby is reacting to the contractions (Fig. 12.8).

The normal fetal heartbeat is 100–150 bpm. This baseline rate refers to the heart rate between periods of acceleration and deceleration.

Baseline variability

Baseline variability is the variation in heart rate of 5–15 bpm which occurs over a time base of 10–15 seconds. The presence of good variability is an important sign of fetal well-being.

Early decelerations

Early deceleration is when the fetal heart rate drops by more than 15 bpm synchronous with a contraction and then returns to the baseline after the contraction has finished.

Late decelerations

More worrying is a late deceleration, where the heart rate slows after the start of the contraction and takes a long time to return to the baseline. The lowest point of the deceleration is past the peak of the contraction. This indicates that the fetus is in trouble. The longer the time from the peak to the lowest point, the more serious is the concern, as this is associated with uteroplacental insufficiency and a decrease in fetal cerebral oxygenation.

The role of the acupuncturist

The acupuncturist can assist in a number of ways during the first stage of labour. These include: boosting or conserving the mother's energy, keeping her calm and relaxed, reducing stress levels, increasing the strength of contractions to avoid prolonged labour, and helping to control pain. Two recent studies from maternity units in Norway have shown that the use of acupuncture as labour analgesia significally reduces the use of both epidurals and other Western analgesia (Nesheim & Kinge 2006, Nesheim et al 2003). In addition, there may be patterns of disharmony that acupuncture can work to correct. At this stage, the use of auricular acupuncture and V-TENS is particularly indicated.

Acupuncture treatment during the first stage of labour

Preparation

Most treatments that an acupuncturist gives are in the well-controlled conditions of a consulting room with a co-operative and responsive patient. In labour the level of discomfort and strength of reflexes that the mother experiences create quite different circumstances, and you have to be ready to work in whatever position she adopts for her own comfort. The points that you would ideally like to use (e.g. on the patient's back) might not be accessible, but normal labour follows a generally typical pattern of behaviour, and this chapter sets that out.

Before going into the labour room with the mother, be aware of the importance of the following factors.

Creating a pleasant environment

Talk to the mother before she goes into labour to find out what would help her to feel relaxed. Get her to bring her own tapes, bean bags, cushions, chairs – anything she feels that would make her more comfortable. It is very important to allay fear. Arranging her surroundings and subduing the lighting, for example, can help her to feel quiet and calm.

Decide who will give instructions to the mother – too many people advising can be distracting and confusing.

Establishing a rapport with the midwives and other staff

Communicate your needs and intentions to the midwives, so that there is no breakdown in communications. Keep in contact with the midwives about the progress of labour, for example, dilation of the cervix.

Explain what you intend to do, such as where you intend to put the acupuncture needles. Explain the uses of acupuncture for labour and what you feel you can help with realistically – for example, increasing the strength of contractions or reducing stress levels.

Shift changes might happen three times while you are there. Give a report at the end of each shift to the staff, explaining how you are progressing with the treatment.

Chinese and Western viewpoints compared

Western concepts

According to these:

- labour starts at the end of 10 lunar months
- the precise mechanism that starts labour is unknown
- oestrogen rises
- progesterone declines
- muscular tension increases contractions in the uterus.

Chinese concepts

According to TCM (traditional Chinese medicine), labour starts when two conditions are fulfilled:

- there is a shift from Yin to Yang
- Yang expels Yin.

Patterns of disharmony for labour

There are four major patterns.

1. *Deficiency of Qi and Blood:* this may be due to the premature rupture of membranes prior to labour or it can be the result of heavy periods or heavy blood loss following previous deliveries.
2. *Kidney deficiency:* this may be due to multiple pregnancies or IVF pregnancies; short gaps between pregnancies deplete the Kidney energy.
3. *Spleen and Stomach deficiency:* this may be due to a lack of proper nourishment prior to labour.
4. *Ki and Blood stagnation (Liver Qi stagnation):* this is due to emotional problems or bad premenstrual tension prior to pregnancy.

Acupuncture in early labour

The acupuncturist will be using various acupuncture points, keeping close to the mother if she wants to be up and mobile.

Give the mother regular drinks to keep her blood sugar up and make sure she is managing to find a comfortable position for labour.

Ear acupuncture

I have increasingly found ear points to be effective in pregnancy and in labour. Ear points are particularly good for the first stage (Fig. 12.9), as follows.

- Uterus: to stimulate uterine contractions.
- Shenmen: for general analgesia.
- Endocrine: to stimulate uterine contractions.

The use of ear points in labour can, in my opinion, help with the 'spaced-out' state that often ensues as labour progresses. The most effective ear points to use here are Uterus and Shenmen. You can also add Endocrine to the above (Pei & Huang 1985).

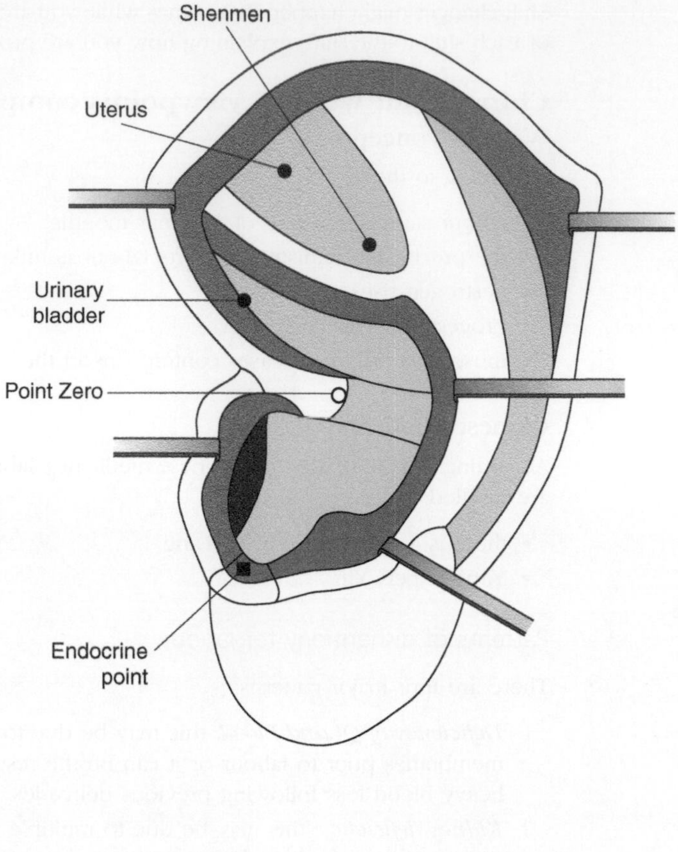

Figure 12.9 Needles inserted into ear points for labour.

Use quarter inch (0.6 cm) needles on the points in one ear. The needles are small enough to support themselves, but it is always a good idea to use some micropore tape to hold them in position. Insert the needles into the points as far as they will go, and tape them into position (see Fig. 12.9). You can also attach the needles to an electroacupuncture machine, using the crocodile clips supplied with the machine. (I use a V-TENS: see Martoudis & Christofides 1990.)

The machine should be set at a pulse width of 200 and a pulse rate of 2.5. This has an effect similar to acupuncture, giving a high endorphin release whilst still being comfortable for the patient, who can control and adjust the frequency herself. The typical sensation is a warm thudding in the ear. It takes 30–40 minutes to build up the endorphin level sufficiently to give a therapeutic effect.

Ear points can be positioned in early labour and left in place for the whole labour. I have found them to be highly advantageous for women who are being induced. Starting contractions artificially does not promote the natural build-up of endorphins, with the result that induced labours can be more painful. Many women find themselves unable to bear the pain quite early in the labour and frequently end up with an epidural. Ear acupuncture during the early phase of labour helps to get them through it.

The advantage of ear acupuncture over other points on the body (such as LI-4 and SP-6, points specified in the ancient texts) is that it enables the patient to move and walk around. The box can be clipped onto clothes and doesn't interfere with monitoring of the baby and contractions. Contractions are also likely to be better if the mother is up and about.

The disadvantages are few: sometimes the needles fall out and occasionally the ear may bleed, but such problems are not unique to electroacupuncture needles. (Remember that if the mother chooses a water birth, both electro- and standard acupuncture needles will have to be removed.)

POINTS TO TREAT (see Fig. 12.9)

Shenmen. **Shenmen is considered to be one of the master points; it is also known as Spirit Gate or Divine Gate. The point is located slightly superior and central to the curving tip of the triangular fossa. The function of Shenmen is to tranquillise the mind and allow connection to the spirit. It alleviates stress, pain and tension.**

Endocrine. **The Endocrine point is found on the wall of the intertragic notch. This is a master point that brings endocrine hormones to their appropriate homeostatic levels, either raising or lowering them.**

Uterus. **This point, in the central region of the triangular fossa, stimulates the uterus and helps to keep the contractions going.**

Bladder. **I sometimes use the Bladder point, on the superior concha, instead of the Uterus if there is a lot of back pain.**

Point Zero (also called Point of Support, Umbilical Cord or Solar Plexus Point). **The point is found in a notch on the helix root, as it arises from the concha ridge. It is a master point, which is said to bring the whole body to a homeostatic balance of energy, hormones and brain activity. It supports the actions of other auricular points and is located where the umbilical cord would rise from the abdomen of the inverted fetus pattern found on the ear.**

Weak/slow contractions

One of the most common reasons for considering the use of acupuncture in labour is to improve weak or slow contractions.

Contractions can become weak and slow for a number of reasons. In Chinese terms there is usually deficiency of Qi and Blood, and using acupuncture to boost the mother's Qi in such a case can be invaluable. If contractions do become weak and slow, the labour is likely to be prolonged, as the cervix cannot dilate without good contractions.

POINTS TO TREAT

- **BL-31 and 32.**

I find these to be the key points for getting contractions going and I use them frequently for induction of labour. They initiate contractions because they are needled straight into the sacral plexus. They are also good for a poorly dilating cervix.

The easiest way to use them in labour is to get the mother to straddle a chair, facing the back, with a cushion to support her bump and the back of the chair for her to lean on. This gives you full access to her back and makes it easy to locate the points, which can be difficult to find. I use $1^1/_2$-inch (3.8 cm) needles bilaterally, inserted directly perpendicularly into the foramen. They do not need to be taped in place because they are inserted all the way in and will support themselves. Stimulate all four very strongly. It is best to do this manually for about 10 minutes, but avoid doing so when the mother is having a contraction, since it can be too painful for her.

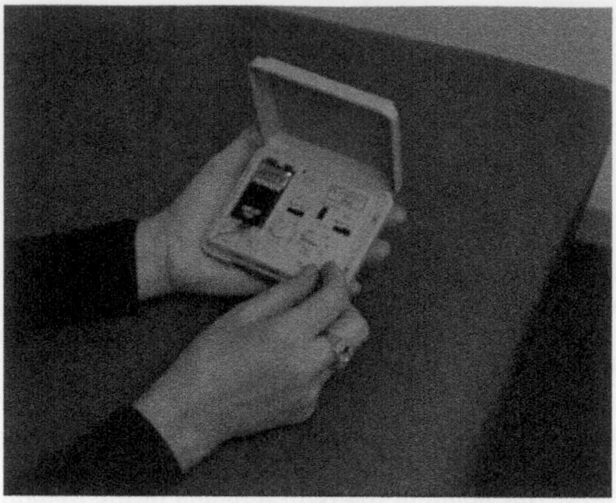

Figure 12.10 A TENS machine.

POINTS TO TREAT

- **LI-4 and SP-6 can also be used for weak contractions in addition to BL-31 and 32, but they are more difficult if the mother is moving around; angle the needles toward the uterus.**
- **Other points that can be added once these are in place are LI-4 and LR-3.**

Stimulate each in turn. After 10–15 minutes the patient will probably become uncomfortable on the chair, so LI-4 and SP-6 can be removed. But leave the others (BL-31 and 32) in, and the woman can walk around while you stimulate them accordingly. Depending on the position the mother has adopted, you can also needle BL-67 to get the contractions going again.

Establishing where the pain is

Back ache could mean that the baby is in a posterior position, which can be quite painful.

POINTS TO TREAT

- **Use BL-31 and 32, leaving the needles in without stimulation; you can also use a TENS machine (Fig. 12.10) with rubber electrodes over these points.**
- **BL-60 is useful but difficult to get at, as the mother is unlikely to be able to keep still enough if she is having this sort of pain.**
- **For abdominal pain, LR-3 in conjunction with GB-34 can help, if you have easy access to the points; the chair position is helpful for this.**

Acupuncture in the accelerated phase

The acupuncturist should concentrate on conserving the mother's energy, helping her to find positions where she can relax fully, supported both between and during contractions. Keeping the mother's energy up during labour is very important and helps to prevent a prolonged labour. Give minimal needling if possible and keep her drinking fluids. A lot of back massage is very helpful here, using strong pressure right into the sacroiliac. Encourage her to have a bath to help her to relax, and to keep changing positions until she finds something that is comfortable.

POINTS TO TREAT

If labour is progressing well then ear points (see above) should be sufficient. It is important to assess constantly where the pain is and to insert the needles accordingly, as mentioned in the section on early labour. Other acupuncture points can be added accordingly, in order to boost the mother's energy. I find tonifying the Back Shu points is the easiest and most accessible:

- **BL-20**
- **BL-21 to tonify the Stomach and Spleen**
- **ST-36 to tonify Qi generally.**

Acupuncture in the transition phase

This is very often the most difficult part of the labour unless the mother maintains control throughout. At this stage the ear point can frequently become dislodged as the mother thrashes around. Her pain at his point will be of a different kind and as the contractions get stronger, she will want to push in response. She will experience the pain differently, so the aim of acupuncture moves from providing pain relief to calming her. Keep the mother calm and relaxed. Be firm with her if she starts to lose control.

POINTS TO TREAT

Depending on the position the mother adopts for this stage, useful acupuncture points are:

- **BL-31 and 32, needled on the side where the cervix is still present; this can be ascertained only by vaginal examination, so ask the midwife whether it is left or right. It will be possible to use these points only if the mother is kneeling and not on her back or being monitored**
- **if she is on her back, LR-3 and GB-34 used together will help; GB-34 is the point for sinews and will help the cervix to dilate.**

The use of electroacupuncture

As well as having the ear points in situ, application of Acu-TENS or TENS over T11 and T12 may help, or Acu-TENS on BL-31 and 32. It is good to have a couple of pads on both sides of the back, in the location of T11 and T12, as this is pain felt over the dermatomes supplied by the spinal cord segment that receives stimulation from the uterus and cervix. (Needles could be inserted as previously mentioned, but pads are easier for most women.)

Use of TENS machines and electroacupuncture machines

TENS stands for transcutaneous electrical nerve stimulation. The technique involves the application of electrical stimulation to the skin via electrodes to stimulate the afferent nerves to bring about pain relief (see Fig. 12.10).

In 1967 Shealy, a prominent neurophysiologist, considered that direct stimulation by TENS of the dorsal column of the spinal cord could inhibit the transmission of pain to the higher pain perception centres of the brain (Shealy et al 1967). The discovery in 1975 of morphine-like peptides known as endorphins (Hughes et al 1975) was followed closely by the discovery of opiate receptors distributed throughout the central nervous system and the release of endogenous opioid by acupuncture (Sjölund & Eriksson 1979). When released, endorphins travel and attach themselves to these receptors: this action increases pain tolerance.

TENS produces analgesia by blocking pain impulses to the brain and stimulating endorphins.

Today many women hire TENS machines: pregnant women usually get them a month before their labour is due.

The intensity of direct electrical current is measured in milliamperes (mA) or volts (V). The frequency of the electrical pulses is measured in hertz (Hz, i.e. the number of pulses per second).

All electrical pulses that stimulate nerve tissues are TENS. The majority of TENS units have a variety of pulse widths, frequencies and intensities. The duration of the pulse width can be between 0.02 and 0.04 milliseconds, although in the majority of TENS units the pulse duration is fixed.

The frequency of the TENS machines ranges from 0 to 200 Hz. TENS can be applied at any time during labour but will work better in the early stages. In maternity units, specifically designed obstetric TENS are commonly used. They vary in intensity; some are set at a fixed frequency and others at a fixed pulse width.

TENS safety

TENS must not be used by anybody with a pacemaker and must never be placed over the carotid artery. They should not be placed over the eyes, near the heart or over cuts. In pregnancy, they must not be used in the first trimester; most are safe to use after 36 weeks.

Conventional TENS use higher frequencies, 50–150 Hz, and have shorter pulse duration (Box 12.1). I prefer to use a V-TENS machine because it is biphasic and will not give shocks.

Treatment parameters

Most of the TENS treatments I give are for labour. I use my machine for back ache during pregnancy and towards the end of pregnancy, and I may use it for pubic pain.

Using a V-TENS machine

For labour pain I use my V-TENS machine (see Fig. 12,10), setting the pulse width at 200 and the pulse rate at 2.5 Hz (Box 12.2). I use it on a continuous setting and allow the patient to set the intensity herself so that she can turn it up to a bearable level. I may use pads on the back with one set of electrodes on BL-31 and 32 (Fig. 12.11), and then with the other electrodes in the ear attached by clips to the Uterus and Shenmen acupuncture points. This setting produces the maximum endorphin release and most ease for the patient.

Using a conventional TENS machine

The conventional TENS machine is the type that women are most likely to hire, and they can be instructed in the following method to apply to themselves. Clean and dry the skin before use. Remove the electrodes from their backing sheet and apply them carefully, pressing firmly to ensure complete contact.

The top pair of electrodes must be positioned each side of the spine between T10 BL-17 and T12 BL-23, and the second pair each side at S2 and S4.

Case study 12.1 illustrates the use of acupuncture in the first stage of labour.

Box 12.1 Comparison of the two methods of TENS

Conventional TENS	Acupuncture-like TENS
High frequency, low intensity, gate control theory mechanism	Low frequency, high intensity, Deqi mechanism
Low intensity activates large muscle (type I) and large skin (A-beta) nerves for gate effect	High-intensity pulses produce (type III) Deqi via small muscle nerves to release endorphins
Segmental effects based on gate theory: large-diameter fibres inhibit pain from small fibres	Non-segmental and segmental effects: small fibres act on three sites: spine, brainstem and pituitary
High intensity of most TENS devices causes burning from skin but no Deqi from muscle	High intensity of some TENS devices activates small muscle (type III) nerves producing Deqi
Pads are placed near the site of pain as large-diameter fibres are widely distributed	Pads placed on acupuncture points as these are over small-diameter afferent nerves (type III) in muscle
High frequency (50–200 Hz) produces best presynaptic inhibition at low intensity (for gate) but produces spasm at high intensity	Low frequency (1–4 Hz) produces no muscle spasm at high intensity and hence allows strong stimulation needed for Deqi
Pulse trains maximise comfort of low-intensity, high-frequency stimulation	Pulse trains cause muscle spasms at high intensity and do not permit adequate intensities for Deqi
Analgesia has rapid onset and short duration, requiring continuous treatment all day long	Analgesia has slow onset and long duration; needs only 30 minutes of therapy for prolonged effects
Tolerance develops from continuous therapy	No tolerance from short, 30-minute treatments

From Pomeranz & Stux (1995)

Box 12.2 Frequency windows

0.5–3 Hz (delta): this band is associated with deep sleep, meditative and subconscious states; analgesia produced using these frequencies appears to be blocked by naloxone, implicating beta-endorphin production. Virtually any frequency within this band is capable of producing fast relaxation, treating insomnia and providing good pain relief. This band is recommended for high-intensity electroacupuncture, neuroelectric acupuncture or acupuncture-like TENS.

3–7 Hz (theta): this band is associated with conceptual thought, REM sleep, artistic, creative and intellectual thought processes, some cases of epilepsy, psychopathy and other mental disturbances. This frequency can cause mental disturbance in a proportion of patients and should be avoided. The lower end of this frequency window appears safer but frequencies in this octave should not be used without testing first on the patient. Aspirin will increase both delta and theta activity.

7–12 Hz (alpha): this band is associated with the relaxed waking state, with conscious physical relaxation; with the second stage of sleep. A frequency around 10 Hz is the safest frequency in the whole spectrum. It acts both as an analgesic and as a tonic and exerts a stabilising influence. Yoga and Zen meditation increase alpha activity. If in doubt, use 10 Hz.

12–30 Hz (beta): this band is associated with mental activities involving thought, deduction, worry, autonomic processes, emotional states, etc. It is not generally suitable for pain control but may be used in patients who are overtired – with care. Smoking marijuana increases beta activity.

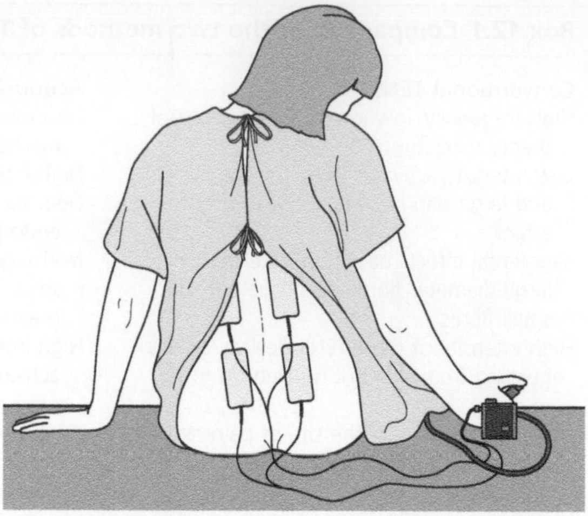

Figure 12.11 Using a TENS machine.

30–60 Hz (gamma): this band is associated with tense alert states and with problem solving in fear situations.

60–120 Hz (lambda): this band is associated with psychological states and peak production of 5-HT; if this is combined with a delta frequency (or pulse bursts at 1-second intervals) both 5-HT and beta-endorphin will be produced for maximum pain control. Frequencies in this band are usually recommended for low-intensity TENS therapy with or without a pulse burst modality.

CASE STUDY 12.1

Mandy was 29 years old and 39 weeks' pregnant with her second baby. Her previous hospital experiences had not been good and she was more than a little apprehensive and nervous about this delivery.

I first met Mandy and her husband when I came on duty for a routine shift at 7.30 one morning. She had been having Braxton Hicks contractions for a couple of days at home, followed by period-type pains, back ache and then regular contractions every 2–3 minutes, each one lasting about a minute. She had also had a show. But when she arrived at the hospital at 5 a.m. everything stopped, as is so often the case.

When given a vaginal examination by the night staff, she was found to be 2–3 cm dilated. Her membranes were present (or intact, as the midwife would say) and the baby was lying in the favourable OA position.

Mandy was placed on a fetal monitor for 20 minutes to measure the strength of her contractions and to check the fetal heart. After breakfast, if nothing was happening, she was going to decide whether or not to go home. At 8.30 a.m. I asked her if she was interested in having some acupuncture, to see whether we could get the contractions going again. She agreed.

With her sitting upright on the bed, I began by using four plain $1\frac{1}{2}$-inch (3.8 cm) needles in BL-31 and 32, and really stimulated them. Then I put needles bilaterally in LI-4 and SP-6, and kept that up for about 40 minutes. The contractions definitely started to become stronger and more regular.

At 9.30 a.m. I took the needles out and placed three small quarter-inch (0.6 cm) needles into Mandy's right ear (either ear would be equally effective). I put them into Uterus, Shenmen and Endocrine, taped them down with some microprobe tape, and attached them by crocodile clips to my Acu-TENS machine. I clipped this to her dressing gown pocket and encouraged her to walk along the corridors for 20 minutes or so, stopping whenever she was having a contraction. It is always better to keep moving so that contractions continue and the fetal head is well applied to the cervix, encouraging it to dilate more efficiently.

After 20 minutes she rested and felt that the TENS was starting to kick in. The contractions were definitely getting stronger. At around 10.30 a.m. I placed some pillows on a chair and suggested Mandy straddle the chair, leaning against the pillows on to the back of the chair. This helped support her during the contractions.

She was experiencing quite a lot of back ache, even though the baby was in the correct OA position. So, still keeping the needles in her ears and with her still straddling the chair, I asked her to point to where the back ache was most intense. Using the second output on my machine, I put two pads low down on either side of her spine, keeping the same frequency on the machine.

Her waters were still intact (this is always preferable, as I feel women suffer far less pain when the membrane is allowed to rupture naturally). As part of my duties as a midwife, I recorded her partogram (labour chart) and checked that she had passed urine, enabling the baby's head to descend. She was still happy to chat and eat and drink. Her back ache was quite severe during contractions but she seemed to be coping well with the pain, sitting on the chair during each contraction.

At 11.30 a.m. Mandy's ear needles fell out and had to be reinserted. She was still coping but feeling less inclined to get up and walk around and decided that she would like to have a rest on the bed. Her contractions were now coming every 3–4 minutes and lasting for about a minute. The back ache was still bad, even with the TENS machine in place, and she was finding it hard to find a comfortable position. At this stage it was quite difficult to help her, as each time we tried, a contraction would come. She needed firm yet gentle guiding, but her poor husband could do nothing right!

Mandy then decided she wanted to use the birthing pool. Unfortunately this was already in use, so I got her to kneel on the bed with a bean bag to support her bump and lots of pillows. I also gave her some Entonox (gas and air), and in about 15 minutes she was comfortable and calm again, in a position in which she felt happy and at ease.

It is usually around this point that women ask for pain relief. Mandy was now probably about 5 cm dilated. Her behaviour was very different, much quieter and more passive. She didn't want any contact in between contractions but needed to feel by herself with her own thoughts. The worst thing you can do at this stage is to ask irrelevant questions.

By 1.00 p.m. Mandy was still doing well but asking for something stronger to help with the pain. Having stayed on the bed for 45 minutes, she was now straddling a chair again. She was still using the Entonox between contractions, and the TENS and the needles were still in place.

I gave her a vaginal examination and found she was now 6–7 cm dilated – only three more to go. After the VE she became quite distressed – it is often the case that the contractions feel worse after an examination. By now she was asking for an epidural but I told her how well she was doing and that by the time the epidural came, it would be time to have her baby. I suggested that, as the birthing pool was now free, we should have a go at getting her into the water. I took the TENS and the ear crocodile clips off but kept the ear needles in, and we got her into the water and made her comfortable. It is amazing how quickly women relax once they're in the bath. Mandy kept using the Entonox and seemed to be coping with the pain. The fetal heart was still good.

At around 2.30 p.m. she became very restless and uncomfortable and started to thrash around in the water. She wanted pain relief and felt that she wanted to open her bowels – all typical signs of transition at 10 cm dilated. Because she did not want to deliver in the water, she got out of the pool and on to the bed again. It was difficult to manoeuvre her, as the contractions were very strong and lasting 45–90 seconds.

By 3.30 p.m., she was on the bed and using the Entonox. The needles had now fallen out so I let them be and used no more acupuncture. Mandy was still bearing down and wanting to push. It took about 30 minutes to settle her and reassure her, but the water had refreshed her amazingly. She wanted to stay on the bed, so we helped her to sit upright. By now she was starting to have a much longer break in between contractions and was getting her second wind. She was very relaxed and calm, again indicating that she was almost in the second stage. The baby's heartbeat was fine.

At around 4.00 pm, she began bearing down under her own steam, doing what felt natural to her. After about 15 minutes, her membranes ruptured. The waters were all clear. Although it is normal for there to be a longer gap between contractions at this stage, by 4.30 p.m. I was starting to get concerned that the gap was a bit too long and that she was getting very tired. (As an acupuncturist you can suggest to the midwife alternatives that can help at this stage.) For me the choice was either to use BL-31 and 32 to get things going again (but I didn't want to mess her around and move her off her back) or I could use GB-21 (but again it was a difficult point to get to). I decided to stand her up so that gravity could help and to needle the Bladder and Uterus points in the ear. Was it the acupuncture that got her going again or was it standing her up to allow gravity to work? We will never know.

At 5.10 p.m. she delivered a lovely baby girl. At 5.15 p.m. the placenta and membranes were delivered. At 5.30 p.m. I examined her. She had a slight tear that would require a stitch. At 6.00 p.m., when she had had time for a breathing space, I needled BL-17 for blood bilaterally. I also tonified HT-7 for shock.

What to expect if a woman is having a water birth

In hospital the emphasis in the poolrooms is on privacy and calm; they are usually appropriately decorated with murals with amenities such as a tape recorder, aromatherapy burners and lowered lighting. The pool is filled to the level of the mother's breasts when sitting. The pool temperature is recorded using a digital thermometer at each stage of labour. The water is kept at the most comfortable temperature for the mother and her baby. Observations are carried out as normal and vaginal examinations are made in the water if required. The baby is monitored with a waterproof sonic aid, so that the midwife can listen to the heartbeat. The pool is kept free from blood clots or faecal matter by filtering the water. When the mother feels she needs pain relief, she can use Entonox.

Second stage

In the pool the woman pushes when she feels the urge to. Traditionally the midwife controls the delivery with her hand on the baby's head. Because of the support provided by the water, this is not considered necessary and the midwife will give verbal guidance to the mother.

Third stage

The third stage is managed without getting the mother out of the pool. The mother holds the baby with its head level with the water surface and the rest of the body below. In the water, the cord remains unclipped. The placenta is delivered underwater. If there is excess blood loss the mother is helped out of the pool and necessary action taken.

Pain relief in a water bath

It is suggested that the buoyancy and weightlessness provided by the water allow the mother to move easily. In the first stage of labour, it reduces the intensity of the uterine contractions and helps the cervix to dilate. I have seen many women who dilate very quickly once they are in the water. The water bath lowers blood pressure, which reduces perineal trauma.

There is some risk of infection to the newborn; if the labour is in hospital, the midwife will assess when it is appropriate for the mother to go into the water.

Nutrition in labour

Views vary on eating and drinking in labour. In many developed countries there is a fear that the contents of the stomach will aspirate during anaesthesia; this is called Mendelson's syndrome (Moir & Thorburn 1986). Since at the beginning of labour the possibility of anaesthesia cannot be entirely ruled out, food and drink are often withheld. However, to date there have been no randomised controlled trials on the wider effects of withholding food and drink during labour.

Labour requires enormous amounts of energy. As the length of a labour cannot be predicted, restriction of fluids can lead to dehydration and ketosis (Ludka 1993). Lack of energy during labour may slow it down and make intervention more likely. Feeling hungry and thirsty can be unpleasant and add extra stress.

During exercise, muscles contract, using glycogen converted from carbohydrates. Where there is insufficient dietary carbohydrate, body fat will be used as an alternative source, releasing fatty acids into the blood. Ketone bodies are a product of this process and any excess is built up in the blood and then excreted in the urine. Build-up of ketones is associated with increased acidity of the blood: as the blood becomes more acid, it becomes less able to carry oxygen efficiently. If this starts to happen in labour, intravenous infusions are used.

There are drinks on the market that can help overcome these kinds of problems in labour. They provide a combination of sugars for both sustained energy release (maltodextrin and fructose) and instant availability (glucose), to help deal with both immediate demands and the prospect of labour through the long hours ahead.

Summary

- The first stage of labour is divided into three phases: early labour, accelerated labour and the transition stage.
- Problems in the first stage of labour include: pain due to dilation of the cervix and stretching the lower part of the uterus, fear and fetal distress.
- Different maternal positions are appropriate for each phase and stage of labour.

- Problems in labour may be due to: deficiency of Qi and Blood, Kidney deficiency, Spleen and Stomach deficiency, or Qi and Blood stagnation.
- Acupuncture points used during the first stage of labour include:
  - *ear points:* Shenmen, Endocrine, Uterus, Bladder; plus Point Zero (to balance the mother)
  - *weak/slow contractions:* BL-31 and 32 (if access to the back), also LI-4, LR-3 and SP-6, or BL-67, Bladder point of ear
  - *back ache:* BL-31 and 32, also BL-60
  - *fear and anxiety:* PC-6
  - *cervix not dilating:* BL-31 and 32
  - *anterior lip to cervix:* BL-31 and 32, and GB-34
  - *abdominal pain:* LR-3 and GB-34
  - *boosting the mother's energy:* BL-20 and 21, and ST-36
  - *transition phase:* BL-31 and 32, or LR-3 and GB-34.

References

Bonica J 1994 Labour pain. In: Wall PD, Melzack R (eds) A textbook of pain. Churchill Livingstone, New York

Hughes J, Smith TW, Kosterlitz HW, Fothergill LA, Morgan BA, Morris HR 1975 Identification of two related pentapeptides from the brain with potent opiate agonist activity. Nature 258: 577–579

Ludka R 1993 Eating and drinking in labour: a literature review. Nurse Midwifery 38(4): 199–207

Martoudis S, Christofides K 1990 Electroacupuncture for pain relief in labour. Acupuncture in Medicine 8: 52

Moir D, Thorburn J 1986 Obstetric anaesthesia and analgesia, 3rd edn. Baillière Tindall, New York

Moore S 1997 Understanding pain and its relief in labour. Churchill Livingstone, Edinburgh

Nesheim BI, Kinge R 2006 Performance of acupuncture as labour analgesia in the clinical setting. Acta Obstetrica et Gynecologica Scandinavica 85(4): 441–443

Nesheim BI, Kinge R, Berg B et al 2003 Acupuncture during labour can reduce the use of meperidine: a controlled clinical study. Clinical Journal of Pain 19(3):187–191

Pei D, Huang Y 1985 Use of acupuncture in childbirth. Journal of Traditional Medicine 5: 253–255

Pomeranz B, Stux G 1995 The scientific basis of acupuncture. Springer-Verlag, Berlin

Shealy CN, Mortimer JT, Reswick JB 1967 Electrical inhibition of pain by stimulation of the dorsal column: preliminary clinical reports. Anesthesia and Analgesia 46: 489–491

Sjölund BH, Eriksson MBE 1979 The influence of naloxone on analgesia produced by peripheral conditioning stimulation. Brain Reviews 173: 295–301

Sweet BR (ed.) 1997 Mayes' midwifery, 12th edn. Baillière Tindall, New York, pp 358, 372–377, 381

Further reading

Robson A 1997 Empowering women. Ace Graphics, Sevenoaks, Kent

Simkin P 1989 Stress pain and catecholamines in labour, part one: a review. Birth 13(4): 186

Wall PD, Melzack R 1967 The laminar organisation of the dorsal horn and effects of descending impulses. Journal of Physiology 188: 403

Wall PD, Melzack R (eds) 1994 A textbook of pain. Churchill Livingstone, New York

13 Second stage of labour

Chapter outline

The second stage of labour covers the period from full dilation of the cervix to the birth of the baby. The defining physiological process during this stage is the descent of the baby's head. The transition phase (see Ch. 12) stimulates a surge of endorphins, helping to give the mother 'second wind'.

It used to be said that a set time of an hour or so should be allowed for the mother to complete the second stage, but evidence from research suggests that such a rigid approach is not appropriate. It is now generally accepted that if there are good contractions and progress, and the condition of mother and fetus is fine, then intervention is not necessary.

Common terms used in the second stage

Anterior lip of cervix. Part of the cervix is still present over the baby's head.

Fully dilated. The cervix has dilated to 10 cm.

Meconium. A black sticky substance which, if present in the amniotic fluid, indicates that the baby has opened its bowels and may be in distress.

Characteristics of the second stage of labour

Pain in the second stage

The pain at this stage of labour has a different quality, as the cervix is now fully dilated (Figs 13.1, 13.2). It is often described as 'cramping' or 'burning'.

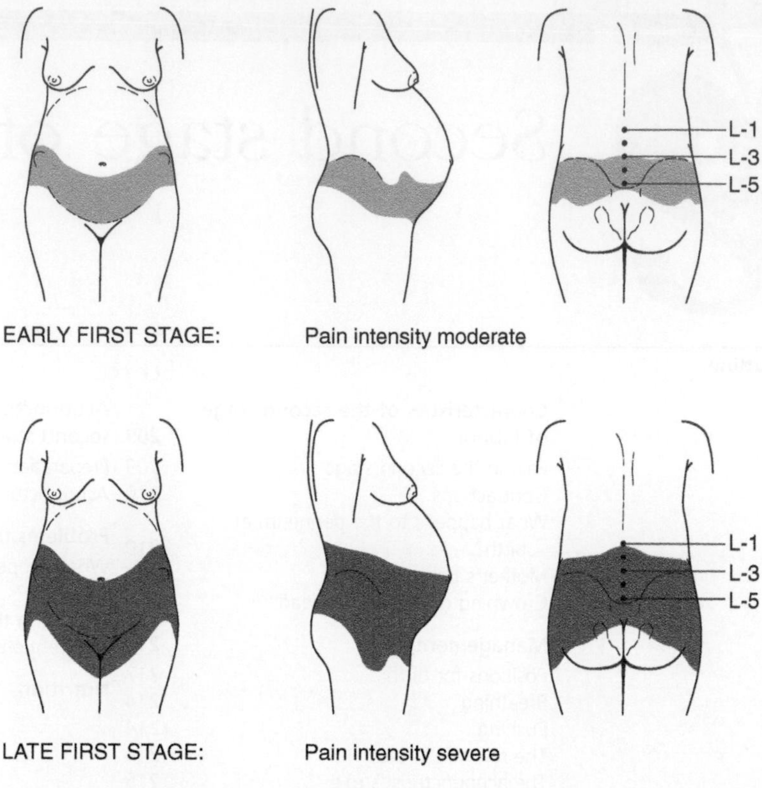

Figure 13.1 Pain intensity and distribution in relation to dermatomes in (above) the early and (below) late first stage of labour.

Contractions

The character of contractions in the second stage of labour is different from those in the first stage. Contractions become slower, and may stop altogether, to allow the mother a rest. When they occur, they are shorter and more widely spaced. In addition to the contractions, the mother will feel a strong urge to bear down, and this urge to push can be regarded as an indication that the second stage is under way.

What happens to the perineum at birth?

At the end of the first stage of labour, the cervix has thinned out and opened up, so that the uterus and birth canal become one opening ready for the baby to start its descent. As the second stage begins, the woman feels an overwhelming urge to push or bear down. This action is irresistible and with each pushing action, the baby moves down through the birth canal. As the head presses down, pressure is first felt on the rectum and then, as the baby continues to descend, the head presses on the perineum and the vaginal tissues open up. A burning sensation will develop as the skin of the perineum stretches to its full capacity; it may feel to the woman as though she is going to tear completely. This is a signal to push gently as the baby's head crowns, to allow the skin of the perineum to stretch gently, easing it over the baby's face. The sensation is relatively shorlived.

Mother's behaviour

A number of features are typical of the mother's behaviour during the second stage:

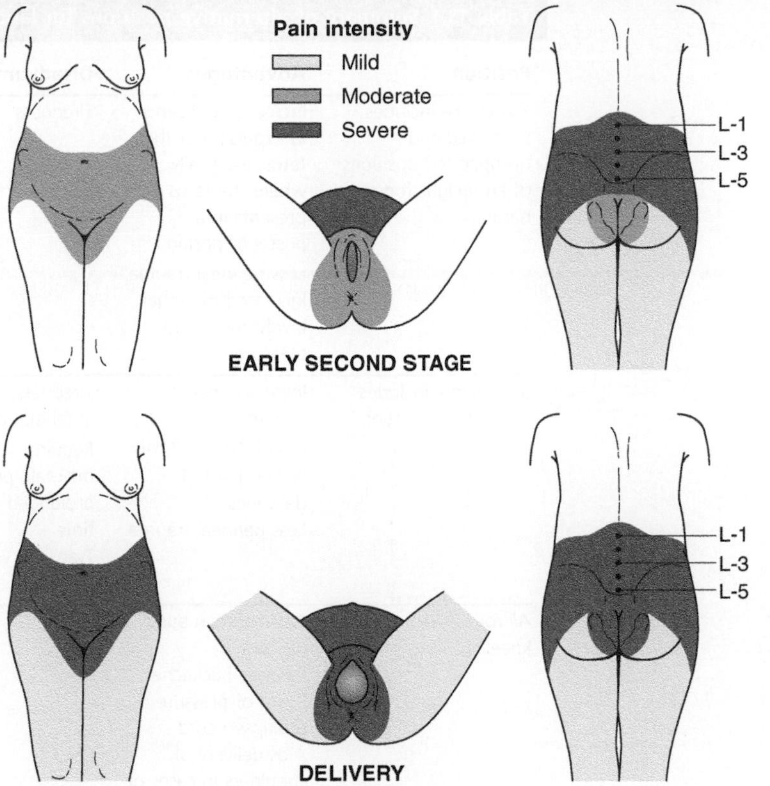

Figure 13.2 Pain intensity and distribution in relation to dermatomes in (above) the early second stage of labour and at delivery (below).

- she may feel a spurt of energy or 'second wind'
- she is likely to feel calmer, and the sense of purpose that she may have experienced earlier may return
- she will need physical help and support
- she may make grunting noises
- her membranes may rupture
- she may panic about needing to open her bowels at this stage and may need reassurance
- she will become more energised and focused
- as the pushing urge develops, she may become introspective
- many mothers close their eyes and withdraw, to concentrate on the effort of giving birth
- the mother may experience the sensation of the baby's head descending through the birth canal as a tight burning sensation, as the perineum begins to stretch. The pain from the perineum is nature's way of signalling the mother to hold back from pushing, allowing the perineum to stretch without tearing.

Crowning of the baby's head

When the full diameter of the baby's head has emerged under the pubic arch, it is said to have crowned. Prior to this, it will slip back between contractions. It is a time of great anticipation; the mother becomes much quieter and the atmosphere in the delivery room should be calm and unhurried.

Table 13.1 Summary of alternative positions for labour and delivery

Position	Advantages	Disadvantages	Comments
Standing – includes supported and unsupported positions of an upright forward nature	Increased efficiency in expulsion of the fetus, especially where the fetus presents in a posterior position Less perineal trauma Increased maternal involvement and pleasure	Tiredness	For the comfort of the mother, use of a thinner mattress on the floor
Squatting – includes supported squatting	Increased pelvic diameters Aids force of gravity Fewer assisted deliveries Less perineal trauma	Tiredness, needs antenatal preparation Requires support to maintain position for prolonged periods of time Transient vulval oedema	Need to discuss in antenatal period Adaptation of equipment in a labour ward
All fours – includes kneeling	Aids rotation and descent Relieves backache Relief of pressure on prolapsed cord Aids delivery of shoulders in cases of shoulder dystocia Less perineal trauma		Aids required for support and comfort of the woman
Birthing chair	Facilitates upright maternal position without other aids or people giving support	Increased risk of postpartum haemorrhage	

Adapted from table supplied by Patricia Simcock, PGCEA Student, University of Surrey, 1995.

Management

Positions for birth

The midwife will work with the mother to find a position that will be comfortable for her. Many options are available to women (Fig. 13.3, Table 13.1) but it is still the most common practice in Britain to give birth on a bed. Whatever the position chosen, the acupuncturist must remember that the mother needs physical support and to be upright. Pillows are invaluable.

Squatting position

This is still the most common position for birth in the developing world. My own experience working with village people in the Middle East is that women do this almost instinctively and with ease.

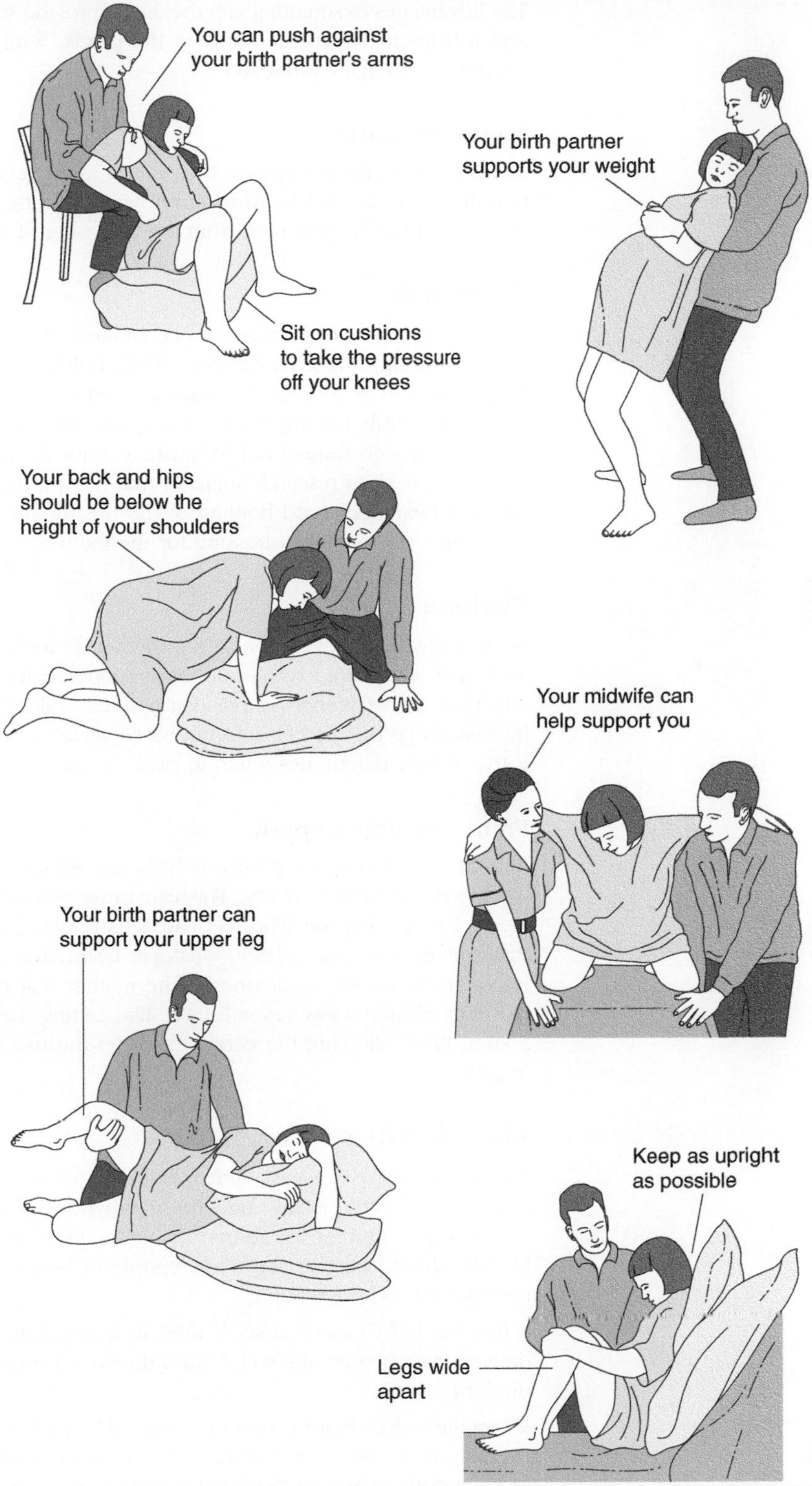
You can push against
your birth partner's arms
Sit on cushions
to take the pressure
off your knees
Your birth partner
supports your weight
Your back and hips
should be below the
height of your shoulders
Your midwife can
help support you
Your birth partner can
support your upper leg
Keep as upright
as possible
Legs wide
apart

Figure 13.3 Positions for the second stage of labour.

The advantages to squatting are: the thighs provide support for the heavy abdomen, and it helps to widen the outlet of the pelvis. While squatting, the mother needs support with each contraction.

Hands and knees

Some women favour being on their hands and knees. The advantages to this position are: it gives relief to women who are suffering with back pain, and it causes less trauma to the perineum from the crowning of the baby's head.

Breathing

You may come across a practice encouraged by some midwives of organised sustained pushing during contractions while holding the breath. When the mother is fully dilated, it is sometimes suggested that she place her chin on her chest and bear down while holding her breath, in the belief that this will shorten the second stage. She is encouraged not to 'waste' contractions by failing to push in this way. However, modern research suggests that this practice can lead to difficulties with the fetal heart. Enforced holding of the breath can affect the oxygen level in the brain and can also be distressing for the mother.

Pushing

Some midwives offer advice to the mother about when to push down. However, most now encourage women to push spontaneously, and mothers frequently fall into their own patterns for pushing naturally (Sleep et al 1989). In any case, it is important that the mother does not waste valuable energy, and this is best achieved if the mother determines when to push herself.

Premature urge to push

The danger of pushing prematurely is that excessive pressure will be applied to the cervix before it is ready. This can cause it to swell, creating greater difficulty in the labour. Anyone who has had a baby will know that the urge is so strong that nothing can hold it back, whatever instruction or advice is given, so that it is important to create conditions for the mother that do not unnecessarily stimulate its onset. Simple measures will help, like getting the mother to lie on her side for a short time, allowing the cervix to dilate; the use of Entonox will also help her to relax.

The midwife's role

The second stage is a very demanding time for both the mother and the baby; for example, this is the riskiest time for fetal hypoxia (Sweet 1997). Careful monitoring is necessary, and observations are taken at 15-minute intervals. The mother's bladder should be emptied every couple of hours, as a full bladder can prevent the baby's head descending.

When the baby's head is seen, then in hospital the midwife will start to get her delivery pack ready. She will control the advance of the baby's head as necessary, until it crowns.

When the baby's head is born, the midwife checks whether the cord is present by slipping her finger over the head and around the neck to feel for it. It is essential that the cord is free so that, if she finds it, she will slip it over the head and cut it, first clamping it with two pairs of artery forceps. Usually the next contraction pushes the baby's body out. The midwife controls this by placing her hands on the baby's head and then, with the contraction, uses a gentle downward movement to deliver the anterior shoulder. When the body is delivered, the cord is clamped, if the midwife has not done so already, and an injection of syntometrine is given to the mother (see Ch. 14). Depending on the mother's wishes, she can then hold and suckle the baby for the first time.

The acupuncturist's role

During this stage, acupuncture is particularly useful when contractions stop or the period between them becomes too great, which can happen if the mother is becoming exhausted. There is no need to use acupuncture when the mother is pushing *unless* her contractions start to slow.

Acupuncture treatment in the second stage of labour

During this phase, it can be difficult to give acupuncture because the mother is likely to be disturbed and thrashing around in pain. Needles in the ear are less of a problem but, even so, I usually take these out at the transition phase, the time when the mother's level of agitation is likely to become high. Remember, too, that if the mother is using a birthing pool, you cannot use electrical stimulation in the water.

Preparation

It is important to create an atmosphere which is appropriate to this stage of the mother's labour, in particular avoiding pressurising or confusing influences. Place no time limits on the mother. Do not worry if things are taking a long time, provided that the condition of the fetal heart and the mother is satisfactory.

Encourage her to choose a safe position. Give her no directions, avoid instruction. Also avoid eye contact, chatter and unnecessary interruptions by other people, which could break her concentration.

Sips of iced water may be welcome if the woman is very thirsty, as may sponging of her face and hands. This should be left to the woman's personal choice.

Acupuncture for augmentation

The acupuncture points are exactly the same as for induction of labour (Dunn et al 1989, Kubista et al 1975), and should all be used with heavy stimulation.

It is natural during the second stage for contractions to become less frequent, which allows the mother to get her second wind. However, sometimes the midwife may feel that there is too long a gap between contractions. In this case I find it useful to get the mother to stand up between her contractions and to needle the ear point for the bladder, using a quarter-inch needle in one ear and leaving it in position.

POINTS TO TREAT

- **The Bladder point in the ear has a good effect, and I would generally try this as my first choice.**
- **If the patient is sitting, you can also use needles in BL-31 or 32 and stimulate.**

Other useful points at this stage are:

- **GB-21: this has a strong downward movement which will get the contractions going again.**
- **BL-67: this also has a strong downward movement.**

Problems that may be experienced

What happens if the perineum doesn't stretch?

Most midwives try hard to deliver a baby so that a cut or tear is avoided. If damage to the perineum is inevitable, a tear is preferable to a cut because it will follow a natural stress line and will not cut into muscle. The perineum will heal more easily and more comfortably.

Reasons why tearing might occur

First, the baby may be large; the baby's face might touch the perineum first instead of the back of its head, causing a tear. Second, the perineum may be tight and inflexible, unable to stretch to accommodate the head. Third, in a fast delivery the baby's shoulders might tear the perineum.

Tears cannot always be avoided, but the extent of the damage can often be minimised by the skill of the midwife. Encourage the woman to listen to her and trust her advice as she is pushing her baby out.

Classification of tears

First-degree tear. This is very superficial. It only affects the skin and does not require suturing.

Second-degree tear. Most tears that occur are second degree and involve the skin and muscle layer. Whether it is stitched or not will depend on the extent of the tear. A small tear may be left to heal naturally, but usually some stitches are required.

Third-degree tear. This involves the muscle and extends to the rectum. It is a rare event and can usually be avoided by careful management.

Protecting the perineum

These guidelines will help minimise the risks of having stitches.

- Encourage the woman to relax and stay in control of what is happening to her. The state of mind at the time of birth is very important. The states of labour are controlled by hormones that the body produces naturally. They both affect the mood and are affected by it. For example, when the baby's head reaches the perineum there is a surge of the hormone oxytocin, which helps to maintain contractions. Fear and anxiety inhibit its production and can therefore prolong the labour.

  Endorphins are another natural substance produced by the body (see Ch. 11) whenever the body is stressed beyond its normal limits. They modify pain and help to create a sense of well-being. Levels rise as the labour progresses but if the woman becomes frightened, adrenaline is produced to counter the endorphins. Endorphin levels then fall and labour may again be prolonged.
- Choose an upright position. This will get gravity working with you and will enhance the contractions. It will also help the pelvic floor muscles and reduce stress on the perineal tissue to prevent tearing.
- The woman should push only as her body indicates. The urge to push builds up gradually. The burning sensation of the baby's head on the perineum is another signal from the body, designed to make her hold the pushing back, allowing the perineum to stretch without tearing.

- It is important that the woman takes time and doesn't feel rushed to have her baby.

Interventions and emergencies

Chapter 10 discusses obstetric interventions used in emergencies and developments that can delay labour at this stage. Some common problems are described here.

Use of forceps and vacuum extraction

If the mother has been in the second stage for a long time and is becoming exhausted, forceps may be used to lift the baby out. Delay in second-stage labour is the most common reason to use forceps. This may happen if:

- the baby's head is not descending as it should
- the baby is in an occipito-posterior (OP) position
- fetal distress.

To be able to use forceps, the cervix must be fully dilated, the membranes ruptured and there must be no obstruction below the head. A paediatrician will be called in case the baby is distressed when delivered and needs resuscitation. The mother will be given an analgesic via a pudendal nerve block to numb the whole area before the forceps are used. If she has had an epidural for pain relief, it will be topped up instead. Her legs will be elevated in stirrups. Occasionally the forceps leave marks on the baby's face, but they will disappear after a few days.

An alternative is to use vacuum extraction. This process can be used before the cervix is dilated, and an episiotomy is not normally required.

Episiotomy

Episiotomy may become necessary for a number of reasons:

- if the baby is premature, and its head needs to be protected during birth
- to speed up delivery if the baby is distressed or tired, or if the mother has become very tired and exhausted herself
- if the perineum is rigid and will not stretch
- if a forceps delivery is needed
- to save the tissues inside the vagina where there is evidence of internal tearing.

The woman will always be asked to give her permission before an episiotomy is performed. Usually local anaesthetic is injected into several places close to where the incision is to be made. Sometimes the skin may be numb already from stretching and there may be no need to use anaesthetic until stitches are required.

When the head is crowning, the doctor or midwife will make an incision from the base of the vagina, most commonly out to the side laterally or down towards the midline; sometimes a J-shaped incision will be made. Occasionally an episiotomy may be necessary on both sides – if, for example, the baby is breech or if the head is big.

Caesarean section

The use of caesarean section in the second stage is most likely for emergencies such as:

- fetal distress
- failure of the head to descend
- detachment of the placenta from the uterine wall
- prolapse of the cord.

The need for a caesarean section is frequently associated with obstetric emergency, and the mother will be taken very quickly to where a general anaesthetic will be used. (For an elective caesarean section (see Ch. 10), where there is not an emergency, an epidural will be used.)

An emergency caesarean section during either the first or the second stage is very traumatic to the mother and her partner, particularly because everything happens very quickly, often leaving very little time for explanation.

Nutrition

Good nutrition is essential after delivery. Because of normal blood loss which occurs at delivery, it is all too easy to become deficient in vital nutrients. Blood loss will vary depending on the size of any tear or episiotomy. Specific supplements and their food sources were detailed in Chapter 3. Those nutrients specifically needed at this stage are discussed in Chapter 15.

Summary

- Problems in the second stage of labour include: cramping or burning pain, slowing or stopping of contractions, a premature urge to push, fetal hypoxia and tearing of the perineum.
- Acupuncture points used during the second stage of labour include:
  - *ear points:* Bladder
  - *augmentation:* BL-31 or 32, plus GB-21 and BL-67.

References

Dunn P, Rogers D, Halford K 1989 Transcutaneous electrical stimulation at acupuncture points in induction of uterine contractions. Obstetrics and Gynecology 73: 286–290

Kubista E, Kucera H, Riss P 1975 Initiating contractions of the gravid uterus through electroacupuncture. American Journal of Chinese Medicine 3: 343

Sleep J, Roberts J, Chalmers I 1989 Care during the second stage of labour. In: Chalmers I, Enkin MW, Keirse MJNC (eds) *Effective care in pregnancy and childbirth*. Oxford University Press, Oxford, pp 1136–1141

Sweet BR (ed.) 1997 Mayes' midwifery, 12th edn. Baillière Tindall, New York

Further reading

Melzack R, Wall P 1982 The challenge of pain. Penguin, London

Robson A 1997 Empowering women. Ace Graphics, Sevenoaks, Kent

14 Third stage of labour

Chapter outline

The third stage of labour is the period following the birth of the baby, and includes the expulsion of the placenta and membranes. It is the most hazardous for the mother, because of possible complications such as haemorrhaging. The placenta can take between 5 minutes and an hour to deliver.

In Western medicine delivery of the placenta or afterbirth is often literally an afterthought in the minds of practitioners, midwives and mothers. In traditional or Third World cultures, however, the afterbirth is given more respect. It is seen as a miraculous organ, which has kept the baby healthy and alive.

Common terms used in the third stage

Syntometrine. An injection given when the anterior shoulder of the baby is delivered, to minimise bleeding and reduce the risk of excessive blood loss. It limits the time before the placenta must be delivered, so that the umbilical cord has to be cut immediately at birth, before it has finished pulsating.

Blue baby. A baby born not breathing that looks blue.

Flat baby. A baby born not breathing and possibly in need of resuscitation.

Lacerations. Small tears in the vaginal wall following delivery.

Characteristics of the third stage of labour

Mother's behaviour

The endorphins released during the birth process create a euphoric state in the mother. She has eyes only for her baby and the urge to bond is strong. Typically, she feels elated, sits up to hold her baby and gathers the baby to the breast.

For the same instinctive reasons, this is very often a time when the mother and father would like some peace and quiet, to be alone together with their new baby.

The newborn baby

The transition from fetus to newborn is one of the greatest hazards a baby is likely to go through in its life. With the rapid change from the warmth and shelter of the uterus to the cold uncertainty of the outside world, a number of mechanisms have to be in place in order to assure the survival of the baby through that transition. The baby has to establish certain breathing mechanisms, changes in the cardiovascular system, regulation of the body temperature, processes for absorption of food, and resistance to infection.

The stimulus to take the first breath is triggered at the respiratory system centre (called the medulla). This happens at birth when the cord is clamped with a resultant reduction of oxygen and accumulation of carbon dioxide in the blood. Birthing is also stimulated by sensory stimuli such as touch, the cool air on the skin, light and noise. When the cord is cut certain changes in the cardiovascular system take place to divert blood from the placenta to the lungs, coinciding with the baby's first breath.

Changes in the blood

In utero, the haemoglobin (Hb) of a baby is 17 g compared with the 11–13 of its mother (Sweet 1997). This high concentration is required to increase the oxygen-carrying capacity of the fetal blood. At birth the prothrombin level is low owing to lack of vitamin K, which is required for the activation of several clotting proteins in the blood. A deficiency of vitamin K may result in spontaneous bleeding in the newborn between the third and sixth day of life. The administration of vitamin K can correct this problem (see later in this chapter).

Temperature control after the birth

The newborn has to adjust to a lower environmental temperature but the heat-regulating mechanism in the baby is inefficient and the baby may sustain a significant drop in body temperature unless great care is taken to avoid it getting cold. Heat is lost throughout the skin. A newborn baby cannot shiver as we do when cold, so that the baby's fat stores are utilised for heat production when required. Consequently an adequate food intake is required to replenish fat to keep the baby warm.

Management

Active management

It has become common practice to manage the third stage of labour by giving women an oxytocic drug, which helps the uterus to contract to deliver the placenta. The usual drug is 1 ml of Syntometrine, which is a mixture of oxytocin and ergometrine given as an intramuscular injection into the woman's buttock, as the baby's shoulder presents. This is known as 'active management' of the third stage.

Reasons for using Syntometrine

First, there may be a poor obstetric history, especially if there has been a previous postpartum haemorrhage. Second, there may be low haemoglobin levels, meaning the woman is anaemic. Third, it may be needed following a caesarean section.

Effects on the mother

Advantages

First, the third stage of labour is completed more rapidly. Also, there will be less bleeding after the birth.

Disadvantages

If the placenta does become trapped in the uterus, it may need to be removed manually, under anaesthetic. While oxytocin has benefits, its routine use has been the subject of much debate regarding its actual usefulness and side-effects. For the mother, these can include nausea, vomiting, headaches and raised blood pressure, quite apart from the painful intrusion of the injection at the climax of the birth process.

Effects on the baby

For the baby, there is the risk of overtransfusion or oversupply of blood in the last minutes of birth before the cord is cut. A normal baby's system is designed to cope with only 120 ml of blood. The effect of the Syntometrine is to push the uterus into overdrive, pumping a greater volume of blood through the umbilical cord into the baby's system. This sets up the dilemma of when to cut or tie the cord. If it is cut early, there may not be enough blood to support the baby's system, and lowered blood volume is thought to be the cause of respiratory problems. However, if the cord is left uncut, the baby can become overtransfused, which puts stress on all the vital organs.

Physiological third stage

The alternative to 'active management' is the 'physiological third stage'. This is the best way to prevent postpartum haemorrhage in mothers who have had normal labours (i.e. without induced or instrumental deliveries). If the mother puts her baby to the breast immediately after birth, oxytocin is released into her system as a natural reflex, which helps the placenta to separate naturally.

The newborn baby

Midwives and medical staff have a good idea of the condition of the baby at birth from the way the labour has progressed and through monitoring the heartbeat of the baby. If there is meconium present (i.e. baby has opened its bowels in utero) or the fetal heart rate has dropped, a paediatrician may be called to the delivery to assess the baby and give oxygen as required.

How the baby is assessed at the birth

A baby is assessed at birth by the Apgar score. For each vital organ the baby is given a score of 2, 1 or 0 points. A total Apgar score of 8 or 10 indicates that the baby is in good condition. A score of 4–7 indicates moderate birth asphyxia. A score of 2–4 indicates severe birth asphyxia and a need for urgent resuscitation. The Apgar score is reassessed after 5 minutes; most healthy babies have an Apgar score of 9.

Resuscitation

It can be very distressing for the mother to have her baby taken for resuscitation at birth, but midwives do their best to ease her fears. There is a resuscitation machine in every delivery room where the baby will be placed and given oxygen via a mask. Some suction may be used to clear the airways. If the baby's condition is serious, it will be taken to the hospital's special care unit.

Normal procedure

Before the mother is transferred to the main ward, a routine general examination of the newborn will be made. The baby will be weighed, a clamp will be placed on the cord and name-tapes will be attached.

Vitamin K

Administering vitamin K to the newborn is mentioned specifically in this chapter because women frequently ask me whether it is necessary or not. Much has been published about the possible risks. Vitamin K is necessary for the production of red blood clotting factors, and vitamin K prophylaxis was first introduced in the 1950s. There was little debate about the practice until the 1980s, when evidence was gathered to show that without vitamin K the baby has a risk of dying or of being permanently brain damaged by vitamin K deficiency. Then in May 1998 the *Daily Mail* reported that vitamin K injections were linked to child cancers. The Department of Health considered the matter and decided that the risk of haemorrhagic disease was certain but that the risk of cancer was not. It therefore concluded that oral vitamin K should be given to all newborn babies. It is likely this trend will continue until more research is available; however, hospitals have varying policies. Some babies (especially those who have had difficult births or caesarean sections) will be given the vitamin either orally or by intramuscular injection.

Role of the midwife

There are a number of tasks that the midwife must carry out following birth:

- ensure that the uterus is well contracted, to reduce the amount of blood loss to the mother
- examine the perineum for any tears or lacerations, and examine the vagina to decide whether sutures are needed, and if so to perform suturing
- examine the placenta and membranes to ensure that they are complete and nothing is left inside
- estimate the amount of blood the mother has lost, normally from 100 to 300 ml (Levy & Moone 1985). Loss of more than 500 ml is excessive
- care for the newborn baby.

The midwife is also responsible for the immediate care of the mother and her newborn baby. Routine observations are made of the mother's pulse and blood pressure, and the midwife will feel the uterus to check that it is well contracted.

The midwife will weigh the baby and affix labels to identify it in the hospital. She will observe its colour and breathing habits, and ensure that it stays warm.

Stitching up

Following delivery, the midwife will examine the woman and look at the perineum to assess whether sutures (stitches) are required. She will usually apply them herself. This takes 40 minutes to an hour, and the patient will be given a form of anaesthetic to numb the area prior to suturing. A synthetic material (usually Dexon) is used to suture because it dissolves after healing. A continuous stitch is used because it promotes better healing and causes less discomfort. If it is a bad tear, it is wise to insist that a registrar or senior midwife performs the suture.

The acupuncturist's role

Following delivery, the main weaknesses are going to be deficiency of Blood and Qi, because of the typical stresses and events of labour and birth. The acupuncturist can also give treatment as a general tonic. Third, acupuncture may be used to help expel a retained placenta.

Acupuncture treatment in the third stage of labour

Chinese viewpoints

According to Giovanni Maciocia (1998), Kidney Essence, known by the Chinese word Jing or simply as the Essence, nourishes the embryo and fetus during pregnancy and is dependent itself on nourishment derived from the mother's Kidneys. 'Preheaven' Essence is the only Essence present in the fetus and is what determines each person's constitutional type; that is, it represents a person's inherent constitutional weaknesses and strengths. 'Postheaven' Essence is refined from food and fluids from the baby's Stomach and Spleen following birth. In Western terms, as discussed earlier, the first breath sparks off a series of changes in the baby system. In Chinese terms, by breathing and eating, the Lungs, Stomach and Spleen start to function and to produce Qi from air, food and fluids. The Essences refined in this way are known collectively as the Postheaven Essence.

The Essence, derived from Preheaven and Postheaven Essences together, is called Kidney Essence because it is stored in the Kidneys. It circulates throughout the other meridians determining growth, reproduction and development.

Original Qi is a type of qi related to the Essence (Jing) in Qi form, again having its origin in the Kidneys. Original Qi relies on its nourishment from the Postheaven Essence and is derived from Preheaven Essence. As with everything in the newborn, Qi is the dynamic motive force that activates all the organs. It circulates around the body. Original Qi is the basis of Kidney Qi and related to the functional activities of the Kidneys. According to the classics, original Qi dwells between the two Kidneys below the umbilicus at the Gate of Vitality. Original Qi is closely related to the Gate of Vitality, and it shares a role of providing heat so that all the body functions can operate.

General treatment

In Chinese terms the vessels are depleted of Blood following delivery and are therefore prone to invasion of external pathogenic factors and Wind. Always keep the mother warm, therefore. Very often she is exposed to the air whilst feeding the baby or while she is being sutured following delivery.

Sometimes there is excessive blood loss (more than 500 ml) and in such cases treatment should be given to build up the Blood. Very often, however, minimal treatment is required and the importance of simple rest cannot be overemphasised. It is good to let the mother have a rest period and to be alone with her partner and her new baby. In hospital she will be given tea and a light snack.

POINTS TO TREAT FOLLOWING THE BIRTH

- **After 30 minutes or so, I tonify BL-17 and 20 as a general tonic. BL-17 is the influential point for Blood and can be combined with BL-18 or 20 for the production of Blood (Liver and Spleen respectively). From a practical point of view, these points offer easy access on the back and the mother will not want too much trouble immediately following the birth.**
- **If your patient is in shock, HT-7 is effective for disturbance of the spirit.**

Retained placenta

I have never had to use acupuncture for a retained placenta, but it would offer the obvious advantages of avoiding the general anaesthetic required for manual removal. This is particularly the case following a normal delivery, especially as the importance and pleasure of the mother's immediate bonding relationship with her baby should be so highly valued.

POINTS TO TREAT

- **My first choice would be CV-4, stimulated strongly, to help to regulate the uterus and to move the Blood. You can use this only when you have easy access to the point but, as the mother would in most cases be lying on the bed, it should be simple to locate.**
- **Other points to use are GB-21, which is the empirical point for treating the placenta, combined with BL-60 to help downward movement, stimulated strongly.**
- **LI-4 and LR-3 or SP-6 stimulated strongly again help to expel the placenta.**

Bear in mind that the mother may be tired and weak and not able to tolerate stimulation of many points.

Problems that may be experienced

Postpartum haemorrhage

This is the most serious condition following delivery. It is identified by excess bleeding from the genital tract following the birth of the baby. Primary postpartum haemorrhage occurs within 24 hours of the birth. Secondary postpartum haemorrhage occurs after 24 hours and up to 6 weeks following the birth.

Causes

Women at high risk should be identified antenatally, so that during labour careful management can reduce the likelihood of the occurrence of postpartum haemorrhage. Women at risk will have an intravenous cannula, from which a sample of blood is removed for cross-matching in case of the need for a transfusion. The cannula will provide instant access to the vein for drugs to be used to stop bleeding if the emergency arises.

Those at risk include women:

- whose uterus fails to contract
- who have had a previous postpartum haemorrhage
- who have had three or more children
- suffering from anaemia
- with an antepartum haemorrhage

- with a prolonged labour
- with a retained placenta
- with fibroids.

Traumatic postpartum haemorrhage

This will occur as a result of lacerations following delivery. These can be deep into the vaginal walls. Suturing is the only way to deal with these tears.

Prolonged third stage

The placenta and membranes normally come away within 10 minutes of the birth. A third stage is considered prolonged when it takes longer than 30 minutes. There can be many causes, including the uterus failing to contract, a full bladder, mismanagement or abnormality of the placenta.

Management

The dangers of postpartum haemorrhage are increased when the placenta is retained. The placenta will be removed manually under anaesthetic.

Nutrition

The role of specific nutrients, together with their food sources, was detailed in Chapter 3. Those that are particularly beneficial in aiding recovery after labour, and those that benefit the newborn, will be discussed in Chapter 15.

Summary

- Problems in the third stage of labour include: overlong labour, haemorrhage, consequences of perineal tearing, retention of the placenta and membranes, exhaustion and deficiency of Blood and Qi, and problems of the newborn baby including low heart rate, asphyxia and vitamin K deficiency.
- Acupuncture points used during the third stage of labour include:
  - *general tonic:* BL-17 and 18 or 20
  - *shock:* HT-7
  - *retained placenta:* CV-4 or CV-3 and BL-60, with LI-4 and LR-3 or SP-6.

References

Levy V, Moone J 1985 The midwife's management of the third stage of labour. Nursing Times 81(39): 47–50

Maciocia G 1998 Obstetrics and gynecology in Chinese medicine. Churchill Livingstone, New York

Sweet BR (ed.) 1997 Mayes' midwifery, 12th edn. Baillière Tindall, New York

15

Postnatal period: the fourth trimester

Chapter outline

A mother is normally expected to make her recovery in the 6 weeks after the birth of her baby. In medical terms, this period (starting as soon as the placenta is expelled) is called the puerperium, meaning 'the period belonging to the child'. During this time the mother's reproductive organs return to their pre-pregnant state.

Nevertheless, giving birth is a real shock to the new mother's system and the experience can affect every part of her life. A woman who has had a difficult or traumatic delivery, or for whom things have been badly managed, may have problems in the postnatal period that last for a long time. She may suffer problems for at least 3 months and full recovery can take longer still.

At 6 weeks she will have her routine check with the doctor and by this point it is expected that everything will have returned to normal. Very often, however, problems can become apparent much later. In my experience, many women have difficulties for up to 6 months after giving birth and yet they get professional support from doctors and health visitors only for the first 6 weeks. After that they are on their own.

In addition, although I do believe things are improving, the 6-week check-up is mainly concerned with the woman's physical well-being, making sure she is 'back to normal', has resumed sexual relations, etc. The odd question may be asked about her emotional health, but very often she is left feeling alone, isolated and not really listened to.

As an acupuncturist, I feel there is a great deal more that can be done during this period to help the mother and baby.

Physiological changes taking place during the first 10 days

Fundal height

After delivery, the uterus reduces and returns to its pre-pregnant state. The medical term for this process is involution. At the end of labour the uterus will have reduced in size to the level of the umbilicus or belly button. One week after labour it will be at the level of the symphysis pubis or pubic bone.

Lochia

Following delivery, the lining of the womb or uterus and blood from the placental site come away as a bloody discharge called the lochia. The amount of lochia lost varies from woman to woman.

Lochia rubra. Days 1–4: is red and consists mainly of blood.

Lochia serosa. Days 5–9: is a clear browny discharge that contains less blood and more serum.

Lochia alba. Days 10–15: is a creamy colour.

Persistent lochia. Lochia should stop after about 2 weeks, but sometimes it persists longer.

Breasts

The secretion of prolactin from the anterior pituitary initiates lactation. Breast milk contains proteins, carbohydrates, fats, minerals, salts, vitamins and hormones. It is without doubt the best food a baby can have, ideally suited to the infant digestive system and full of antibodies to help the immature immune system and protect him against allergies. The colostrum produced by the breasts in the first few days after childbirth has no substitute.

Urinary tract

There is a marked increase in output of urine following delivery. This lasts 2–3 days and results from high blood volume, which increased during pregnancy and is now returning to pre-pregnant levels.

Some women experience urinary problems following the birth. The strain of labour may also affect the kidneys, causing retention of urine. This is common if a woman has a urinary catheter following a caesarean section. After the catheter is removed, some women still experience problems passing urine.

Circulatory system

The blood volume decreases to the normal pre-pregnancy state.

Musculoskeletal system

Pelvic joints and ligaments will have softened during pregnancy in anticipation of the physical stresses of childbirth. They gradually return to normal over a period of about 3 months.

Complications of the puerperium

Many women experience discomfort during this stage. For most this is minor but for a few it can be more serious. Minor discomforts include the following.

- **Afterpains.** These occur during the first 2–3 days and are caused by the contracting uterus. They are more common in women who have had more than one baby and are worse when breastfeeding.
- **Perineal soreness.** Most women experience some degree of discomfort, particularly if they have had an episiotomy.
- **Haemorrhoids.** See the section on ailments of pregnancy in the second trimester (Ch. 13).
- **Puerperal infection.**

Mental and emotional problems

In the first trimester of pregnancy, as many as 15% of women may suffer mental and emotional problems, although only a third of these will have had any previous psychiatric history (Sweet 1997). The number drops to around 5% in the second and third trimesters. However, the risk of mental illness is known to increase significantly during the postnatal period. Following delivery, as many as 16% of mothers will develop problems. The risk of becoming mentally ill during this period is greater than at any other time in a woman's life.

Causes

The causes of postnatal depression are probably a combination of biological, psychological and social factors.

The biological reasons include: exhaustion, genetic make-up, gynaecological and obstetric problems, a woman's age, short gaps between pregnancies, hormonal changes associated with the early puerperium and the health, behaviour and appearance of her baby.

The psychological reasons include: a woman's early relationship with her parents, her personality type, her previous psychiatric history, her ability to accept dependence, her acceptance of her sexuality and anxious or obsessional traits in her personality.

Social factors include: stressful life events, such as poor housing or family problems, a lack of social support, an unsupportive or absent partner, low socio-economic status and tiredness, loneliness and an inability to cope.

Types of depression

There are basically five categories of depression after childbirth, any of which can merge together: the 'baby blues', postnatal exhaustion, postdelivery stress, severe postnatal depression and puerperal psychosis.

'Baby blues'

These usually kick in 3–5 days after delivery, at around the time that the milk comes in. They are experienced by 80% of women (Swyer 1985) and are probably linked to abrupt changes in hormone levels. They usually manifest as lots of tears and conflicting emotions, with unexplained bouts of crying.

Mild depression and postnatal exhaustion

This is often the result of exhaustion, hormonal changes and a natural reaction to the emotional intensity of giving birth. In the first 3 days after delivery, a woman is generally in a state of euphoria. She may find it difficult to rest sufficiently during the day and she may have problems sleeping at night. As a result she will end up doing too much and become overtired, suffering both mental and physical exhaustion. Lethargy is often a dominant feature. She may have problems concentrating, her memory may be poor and she will feel an endless yearning for sleep, never feeling able to get enough.

Postdelivery stress

It is now becoming recognised by the medical profession that women are sometimes left confused, frightened and traumatised as a result of their experience of delivery. Birth traumas have many causes. Each woman is an individual who brings her own unique profile into the delivery room. This includes the memory of experiences in her early life and her expectations of what is about to happen to her.

Whatever the reason for a woman's distress and whatever her perception of the birth experience, it should be recognised and acknowledged that women can be traumatised for a number of reasons, including: severe pain and inadequate analgesia, exhaustion, demoralisation, being left alone and unsupported and an emergency situation such as a caesarean section.

Severe postnatal depression

This is a non-psychotic depressive disorder, which develops during the first year following childbirth and varies in its severity, with symptoms including exhaustion, irritability, difficulty sleeping and physical 'flu-like symptoms. It occurs in 10–15% of new mothers and often begins within 2 weeks of delivery (Kendell 1985). It is often unrecognised or misdiagnosed, though the majority of women recover spontaneously with time.

The Western treatment of postnatal depression usually involves counselling and medication with antidepressant drugs. Care must be taken to monitor side-effects on both mother and baby, if the woman is continuing to breastfeed.

Puerperal psychosis

This is an acute psychiatric illness that requires prompt treatment, affecting about one woman in every 1000 (Kendell 1985). Occasionally severe episodes of the blues can lead to postnatal depression and untreated depression can develop into a major depressive psychosis.

Management after the birth

Breastfeeding and its problems

Ideally the baby should feed in the first hour after birth, when the rooting reflex is at its most powerful. A successful first feed can have a positive effect on the mother's confidence.

Correct positioning of the baby on the breast is one of the most important factors in successful breastfeeding. The baby has a natural sucking reflex, which in turn stimulates the mother's milk production. For this to be effective, the baby has to 'latch on' correctly, sucking on the whole nipple and surrounding areola, pulling it in towards the back of the mouth. The mother should support her back with pillows and lift the baby to the breast rather than bending over, putting a cushion under the baby if that helps. This will help to prevent sore nipples as well as upper back, neck and shoulder problems.

Engorged breasts

Breast milk takes 2–4 days after delivery to 'come in', encouraged by the stimulus of the baby's sucking. Initially the 'supply and demand' nature of milk production is not very efficient and the breasts may become engorged, overfull and painful, due to the increased blood supply to the breasts. This is a physiological process that will pass, but it can leave the mother feeling hot and bothered. It is very important to encourage the mother to continue breastfeeding through this period. Stopping feeding will only make matters worse.

Lack of milk

Unrestricted feeding in the first few weeks is by far the most important way to establish breastfeeding. It is also important that the mother allows herself time to rest as much as possible and not let herself get overtired.

Cracked and sore nipples

The nipples may well feel tender during the first few days of breastfeeding but this does improve as time goes on. The mother should be closely supervised during the early days to ensure that the baby is properly 'latched on'. A comfortable nursing bra is important, though sore nipples heal quicker if exposed to the air.

Creams such as Camillosan, calendula or Bach Rescue Remedy cream can be applied, though it is important to wash or wipe these off the nipples before the baby sucks. However, too much washing of the nipples, particularly using soap, is counterproductive as it will dry the nipples out further. You could suggest steeping two camomile tea bags in boiling water, cooling them and applying them to the nipples inside a bra.

Blocked ducts

Occasionally the milk becomes blocked, owing to pressure. The area will become reddened and, if not relieved, this could lead to mastitis, infection or even a breast abscess. Again, it is very important to continue feeding to relieve the pressure.

Mastitis

Mastitis can be non-infective or infective.

Non-infective

Non-infective mastitis usually occurs when a blocked duct prevents the flow of milk from one area of the breast. If this is not relieved or cleared, the pressure from the blockage forces the milk into the adjacent tissue, which activates the mother's immune system, causing the mother to complain of 'flu-like symptoms. Her breast becomes red and sore and she starts to sweat. The symptoms come on very quickly indeed and the patient can feel very ill.

Infective

Infective mastitis occurs when bacteria enter the breast. A cracked nipple is a frequent route for such infection. The organism that causes this is usually one called *Staphylococcus aureus* and can lead to a breast abscess if left untreated. With correct positioning of the baby, the mother should continue to breastfeed and antibiotic therapy is usually prescribed. If a breast abscess does form, surgical intervention is needed to drain the abscess and this can be very painful indeed.

The role of the midwife

For many women, the midwife will be the first port of call after the birth for support, information and advice. The midwife is well placed to: monitor the physical and mental well-being of both mother and baby, help with the establishment of feeding, whether breast or bottle, help give the new mother confidence, offer general health education and ensure that the mother's recovery is progressing well.

The midwife will make daily observations, which will include assessing whether the mother is getting adequate sleep and rest. This is considered a priority, as lack of sleep can quickly lead to anxiety and depression.

Other observations she makes will include:

- checking the perineum, to ensure there are no signs of infection and that healing is progressing well; the midwife will check this area daily and advise the mother on hygiene and healing
- caesarean section: to check healing of the scar and make sure that the woman is getting up and moving about sufficiently
- fundal height (see below)
- lochia (see below)
- checking that the mother is passing urine and opening her bowels regularly
- breasts and nipples: the midwife checks the mother's breasts, which are generally soft for the first couple of days after the delivery until the milk comes in, for signs of engorgement, mastitis, soreness or cracking
- breastfeeding: to make sure the baby is latching on correctly
- helping with any pain relief the mother may require
- blood pressure, pulse and temperature: these should all be recorded
- haemoglobin levels: a simple blood test should be taken to measure the haemoglobin and ensure the mother is not anaemic.

Fundal height assessment

Assessing the fundal height allows the midwife or health professional to gauge how well the mother is progressing and to spot any potential puerperal problems that may be occurring.

Part of the daily observation is to palpate the uterus abdominally to ensure that it is well contracted (it should feel like a cricket ball). The descent of the uterus can also be measured in centimetres to check that it is fitting in with normal patterns. Any deviation may mean that part of the placenta is still attached or there may be a possible infection. The fundus should descend by approximately 1 cm a day.

Assessment of lochia

The colour, consistency and quantity of lochia are important indications to the midwife that everything is going well. Any sudden increase in quantity, fresh blood or clots would be cause for concern and an offensive smell might suggest an infection.

Stitches

The midwife will check any stitches daily for 10 days. For the first 5–6 days, the degree of discomfort will depend on the amount of stitches. The worst pains usually occur a couple of days after delivery, when the area may have developed swelling and bruising. The experience of new mothers ranges from feeling sore to a throbbing bruised sensation or acute but brief pain when sitting down or going to the toilet. Occasionally a woman might feel a stitch pulling. The midwife may remove this to make her more comfortable.

In most cases stitches should heal well, but occasionally they can get infected. There are a variety of organisms found in and around the vagina, which cause no problems when the body is in a balanced state. After delivery the balance is upset and infection can occur in damaged tissues.

Good hygiene is essential:

- sanitary pads should be changed frequently
- the area should be cleaned thoroughly, especially after the bowels have opened
- the area should be dried properly – bacteria flourish in a moist environment.

The midwife will be able to tell if the area is getting infected, as it will become very red and tender. She may take a swab to see what bacteria are growing and an antibiotic may be prescribed.

Most infections can be treated with antibiotics. A very severe infection may cause the breakdown of the wound completely and need resuturing, but this is rare. A good diet will help to promote wound healing and prevent infection; guidance on good nutrition and other general advice to help healing is given at the end of the chapter.

Whether a woman delivers at home or in hospital, midwives and health visitors will support her for the first 10 days after the birth. Advice on all health and baby issues will be given routinely. If necessary, she will be visited at home and certain observations (see list above) on her physical and mental health will be made and fed back to other health professionals.

Role of the acupuncturist

There is much an acupuncturist can do to enhance the mother's well-being. The practice of 'mother roasting' with moxa aids recovery. Many postnatal problems such as persistent lochia, breastfeeding problems, puerperal complications, urinary problems and common patterns of disharmony can all be aided with acupuncture.

Acupuncture treatment after the birth

Mother roasting

'Mother roasting' is a general term to describe practices of warming the mother to aid recovery, which take different forms in various cultures.

In Malaysia, the mother is given a massage a week or so after giving birth, with a special stone that is heated on the fire, wrapped in a cloth and placed on the abdomen. In South East Asia, new mothers are encouraged to sit next to the open fire. In Thailand, newly delivered women are sometimes placed in a special bed above a fire.

Using moxa techniques that apply heat, I have practised mother roasting on a number of women and feel that heat really has something to offer. However, it is not suitable for every woman and it is important for the acupuncturist to judge each patient individually.

Contraindications

- Be cautious if there are any signs of infection, because moxa or heat could exacerbate this.
- Be wary of the effect of heat on scars and infection if the woman has had a caesarean section.
- Never use heat if there is a TCM (traditional Chinese medicine) diagnosis of Yin deficiency.

How to do it

For mother roasting, a moxa stick is required. It should not be attempted until approximately 1 week following the birth of the baby. Feel the Lower Chou. If it feels cool, this is a strong indication to use the moxa stick.

POINTS TO TREAT

- **With the mother lying on her back, I pass the stick close to the skin from CV-2 to 8, up and down for about 10 minutes.**
- **With the mother lying on her tummy, I then pass the moxa stick from GV-2 to 8.**

Persistent lochia

In Chinese terms, this is a result of Qi deficiency following a long labour, or Blood stasis. The amount, smell, colour and consistency of lochia will indicate to the practitioner whether this is a deficiency, heat or stagnation pattern.

Blood deficiency

The following are indications of Blood deficiency:

- smell: no smell
- colour: red
- consistency: profuse
- pain: bearing-down pain.

POINTS TO TREAT

- **Tonify the Spleen: SP-6, ST-36 CV-12 and BL-20 all tonify the Spleen.**
- **SP-1 with moxa cones, using an even technique.**
- **BL-17 with moxa: tonify to strengthen the Blood.**

Blood heat

The following are indications of Blood heat:

- smell: foul
- colour: dark red
- pain: abdominal.

POINTS TO TREAT

- **Use points SP-1 without moxa and LI-11, SP-10 and LR-3 to cool the Blood. Use even technique and leave needles in.**

Blood stasis

The following are indications of Blood stasis:

- colour: dark purple clots
- pain: abdominal, relieved by passing clots.

POINTS TO TREAT

- **To clear Blood stasis: SP-1, no moxa, even technique to move the Blood; BL-17, even technique; LI-11, SP-10.**

Other useful points include:

- **to raise the Qi: GV-20, tonification**
- **to stop uterine bleeding: SP-8, even technique**
- **to strengthen the Uterus: CV-4 tonification.**

Breastfeeding problems

Engorged breasts

POINTS TO TREAT

- **CV-17, with the needle left in for 30 minutes; although ST-18 is the local point to use for the breast, I am not keen to put the needle into breast tissue, especially if it is lumpy.**
- **GB-41: this is good for removing obstruction from the breast.**

Lack of milk

Heavy blood loss following delivery will lead to deficiency of Blood, which in Chinese terms is the source of breast milk. A long drawn-out labour leads to depletion of Qi, which may also result in insufficient milk. Worry or frustration also blocks the flow of milk.

POINTS TO TREAT

For Blood and Qi deficiency, I would suggest that you tonify Blood and Qi with ST-36 and SP-6. An empirical point that I have used a great deal for women who are having problems producing milk is SI-1. BL-17 and 20 also tonify Blood and Qi. I find that women who have had IVF pregnancies have great problems producing milk. Acupuncture points such as BL-23 will help them, with moxa if the mother is deficient, plus the above points.

Blocked ducts

I find acupuncture very useful for this, placing needles very superficially around the area of redness and leaving them in place for about 20 minutes.

Mastitis

From the Chinese viewpoint, mastitis is due to the effects of heat and toxins (see Importance of Blood below).

POINTS TO TREAT

- **LI-11 clears heat, using even method and no moxa.**
- **ST-44 for Stomach heat, using even technique.**
- **LR-2 if caused by Liver heat, using even technique.**

It also helps to use the needles superficially in a ring around the red area.

Urinary problems

Labour depletes the mother's Qi, especially if it has been long and drawn out. The Spleen will be affected and will be unable to raise the Qi sufficiently, resulting in sinking of the Bladder Qi. This will cause continuous flow and incontinence.

POINTS TO TREAT

This is not something I treat commonly but I have found CV-3 to work well, inserting the needle and using the reinforcing method. Other effective acupuncture points include:

- **BL-22: promotes the excretion of fluids in the Lower Burner.**
- **BL-28: tonifies the Bladder, in conjunction with CV-3, Back Transporting and Front Collecting points; tonify with moxa.**
- **BL-63 even technique: this can be used if there is a lot of pain.**
- **If there is a lot of pain and there is blood present in the urine, it can be a sign of heat. BL-63, SP-10 and KI-2 clear heat, all with even technique.**

Afterpains

In Chinese terms the pain is always a result of a deficiency or a condition of excess.

Manifestations of *deficiency* are: the pain is better for pressure, better for heat and will be mild.

POINTS TO TREAT

- **CV-4 and 6: tonify; use moxa.**
- **ST-36 tonifies Qi and Blood.**
- **CV-6 tonifies Qi generally and moves Qi in the abdomen.**

Manifestations of *excess* are: the pain is worse with pressure and is a fixed stabbing pain.

POINTS TO TREAT

- **SP-10 moves Blood in the Uterus: even technique.**
- **BL-17 moves the Blood.**
- **ST-29 is good for abdominal pain. Use of the Acu-TENS on ST-29 can also give great relief.**

Perineal soreness

I have found by far the most successful treatment has been lying the woman down on her side with a cushion between her knees, inserting a needle in GV-1 and leaving it in place for 30–40 minutes. This can bring great relief.

For other remedies that will help, see the section on the perineum (Ch. 10).

Other patterns of disharmony: the Chinese viewpoint on the importance of Blood following the birth

Blood is very important in a woman's physiology and pathology. Pre-existing conditions can affect a woman even before she becomes pregnant (see Ch. 8). The four most common patterns that occur following delivery are listed below, but also refer to the section on patterns of disharmony in Chapter 12, as this will also help you to assess your treatments.

1. Blood and Qi deficiency due to loss of Blood
2. Invasion of pathogenic factors
3. Blood stasis
4. Mental and emotional problems

Most conditions following delivery are connected to disorders of the Blood. In Chinese terms, the Heart houses the Mind/Shen and governs the Blood. If the Blood is deficient, it cannot house the Mind/Shen. Blood deficiency eventually turns to Yin deficiency and Empty-Heat to Blood stasis.

If a woman's Heart Blood is strong, her Mind will be healthy and she will be able to think clearly. Her memory will be good and she will sleep well. If the Mind is affected, her thoughts will be muddled, her memory will be poor and her sleep restless.

Although the Heart plays a pivotal role in mental and emotional activities, very often pre-existing conditions will come into their own in pregnancy. If Heart Blood is deficient, it is likely that Liver Blood will also be deficient, as the Liver is closely linked to the Heart and houses the Ethereal Soul. Liver Yin deficiency will follow, resulting in: a lack of sense of direction, insomnia, fear, restless sleep and waking exhausted from dreaming.

Blood and Qi deficiency

This can occur as a result of heavy blood loss (more than 300 ml) at delivery or a postpartum haemorrhage (more than 500 ml) or following a caesarean section.

Treatment

Assessing the type of delivery will give a good guide to what treatment can be used.

Length of labour. If labour was long and drawn out, the patient will be exhausted and Qi deficient.

Type of labour. If progress was very speedy, the patient may be in shock.

Forceps or any other kind of medical intervention. This may lead to blood loss, bruising and Qi deficiency.

Tears. If there was heavy blood loss, the Blood and Qi will need nourishing and additional help will be needed for a painful perineum.

Type of drugs administered in labour. These can deplete a mother, making her very tired and exhausted.

Mental and emotional state of the mother during labour. Every woman is different and enters the delivery suite with a different set of emotions, depending on her expectations and past experiences. Some may be very fearful as a result of abuse in the past.

Short staffing levels on the unit. This can give the woman added anxiety that she may not get the help she requires. She could also feel insecure about not having a medical term explained or worried that there is a problem with her baby.

Lack of support. Some women feel unable to cope with the pain. Others are unable to cope if an emergency arises or are mortified if they feel they have been angry with the staff.

POINTS TO TREAT

- **I tonify HT-7 soon after the birth, which helps settle the mother; it is especially useful in cases of shock.**
- **I use a lot of Blood points to build up the Blood, placing 2–3 small moxa cones on each point (if the mother is deficient).**
- **I use BL-15 and CV-14 to tonify Heart Qi.**
- **I use SP-6 and ST-36 with moxa to nourish the Blood.**

Sweating following delivery

As a midwife, I had never appreciated this as a problem. However, when I had my own children I would wake in the night sweating profusely and I had no idea why. From my treatment of other mothers, it seems to be very common and, I consider, indicates some kind of Yin deficiency.

According to Maciocia (1989), daytime sweating is due to Qi deficiency and night sweats to Yin deficiency. He explains this by the type of fluid lost in the day, which is different from that lost at night. During the day it is the defensive Qi that leaks out, but at night it is the Yin essence and this is more serious as it is on a deeper level.

POINTS TO TREAT

- **Qi deficiency: for sweating during the day, use LI-4 with even technique and KI-7 with tonification.**
- **Yin deficiency: for night sweats, use HT-6 with even technique and tonification.**

Invasion of pathogenic factors

The sheer energy used up in delivery affects not only the Blood but also the mother's Qi generally, weakening the Directing and Penetrating Vessels and channels and leaving the woman prone to the invasion of external pathogenic factors.

Insufficient rest following labour can also lead to weakness, allowing pathogenic factors to enter between the skin and muscles. This will happen as a result of Blood and Qi deficiency.

External invasion of Wind-Heat

Yet another predisposing factor is if a woman's body has been left uncovered during delivery or if after delivery, her lower half is exposed while she awaits stitches or examination. The mother's Qi is generally weakened by being exposed and Wind can enter, causing fever. Heavy blood loss will have a similar effect, as it can cause exhaustion of Blood and Yin.

Clinical manifestations include: feeling shivery, headaches and stiff neck.

POINTS TO TREAT

- **LI-4 and TE-5 expel Wind, even technique.**
- **BL-12 and 13 expel Wind, even technique.**
- **BL-17 with moxa if deficient; tonification nourishes the Blood.**

External invasion of toxins

If the mother's Qi is generally weak, her resistance becomes lowered, allowing toxins to invade. It is more likely to happen if she has had a long labour, a heavy blood loss or is anaemic.

In Western medicine, this corresponds to a bacterial infection. Any infection occurring after delivery is called a puerperal infection. The placental site is a large unhealed vascular area, which is warm and moist and an ideal breeding ground for bacteria. If laceration has occurred anywhere in the genital tract, it can become infected. Such problems generally manifest themselves a couple of days after delivery, possibly as the result of an infection from the uterus, stitches, a wound or a breast infection.

Factors that contribute are: poor nutrition, a long labour, frequent vaginal examinations, caesarean section and internal retention of small fragments of the placenta (known as retained products of conception). Usually the midwife who delivered the baby will have noted that the placenta may have been incomplete. The mother may also notice that her blood loss is smelly or that she is passing clots. She may develop a fever.

Clinical manifestations include: high fever, smelly discharge, general malaise and high temperature.

The Western treatment would be to take a swab from the site of the infection in order to see what bacteria are growing. The woman would then be started on antibiotics.

POINTS TO TREAT

- **LI-11 to clear heat.**
- **GV-14 to clear heat.**
- **LR-3 and KI-2 to cool the Blood.**
- **CV-3 to get rid of retained products.**

Needles should be left in for between 30 and 40 minutes.

Blood stasis

This is usually the result of a pre-existing condition of stasis. Because the Heart governs the Blood and houses the Mind, stagnant Blood can obstruct the Mind. The condition is likely to manifest as unreasonable or aggressive behaviour, hallucinations, destructive thoughts and failure to bond with the baby.

Mental and emotional problems

In Chinese terms, postnatal depression is centred on the Blood. If a woman is Blood deficient, her Heart will be affected, as the Heart houses the Shen and governs the Blood. If Heart Blood is deficient, the mother will become depressed and anxious.

Heart Blood deficiency

Heart Blood deficiency symptoms will include: anxiety, insomnia, exhaustion, tearfulness, resentment, anger, poor memory, palpitations and inability to cope.

If the condition is left untreated, Yin deficiency and Empty-Heat will follow. Heart Blood deficiency always involves Liver Blood deficiency, so treatment is based on nourishing the Blood and the Yin and calming the Mind.

POINTS TO TREAT

- **HT-7, CV-14 and 15: to tonify the Heart.**
- **GV-20: tonify to lift the mood.**
- **PC-6: even technique to calm the Mind.**

Heart Yin deficiency

Heart Yin deficiency will manifest as: waking up frequently at night, restlessness, exhaustion, heat and night sweats.

POINTS TO TREAT

- **HT-7 and 5: to tonify the Heart.**
- **SP-6: to nourish Yin.**

Heart Blood stasis

Heart Blood stasis will manifest as: aggressive behaviour, hallucinations and destructive behaviour.

POINTS TO TREAT

- **BL-17 and SP-10: to move the Blood.**
- **BL-15: to clear the Heart and calm the Mind.**
- **SP-4 and PC-6: to invigorate the Blood.**

CASE STUDY 15.1

During her second pregnancy, Mary was convinced her baby was not lying correctly. Despite reassurance from the medical staff that everything was OK, she felt all the way through her pregnancy that something was wrong. A very long labour ended in an emergency caesarean section – because the baby was not lying the correct way. She was haunted by this after delivery, became very depressed and was finally diagnosed as having posttraumatic stress syndrome. When she became pregnant again, she continued anxious and depressed, finally coming for acupuncture during her third trimester. She went on to have a normal delivery.

CASE STUDY 15.2

Anne came to me for treatment for anxiety during her second pregnancy. During her first labour she had needed an epidural, a process during which the patient is gently held by the midwife as the anaesthetist inserts the needle into her back. However, this experience had unlocked for Anne repressed memories of being raped at the age of 6. She became hysterical when she felt she was being forced down and had to be restrained. She subsequently received counselling but when she came to me for acupuncture, she was full of fear and anxiety about what would happen in her next labour. Together, we wrote a long letter to explain to the midwifery staff what had happened to her and why it had happened, asking that she be treated with care and understanding. This letter was put in an envelope and placed in her hospital notes so that only the medical staff would see it. (This can be done on behalf of any patient.) The staff were very understanding and Anne went on to have a normal delivery with no complications.

Care of the woman who has had a caesarean section

It is important to remember that a caesarean section is major abdominal surgery and that a mother who has undergone such an operation has not only to make her recovery, but also to deal with a newborn baby. If the operation was performed as an emergency, the emotional and mental stresses caused by it are also going to be very significant indeed. In hospital, a postcaesarean patient is usually put in a side room to have some peace and quiet. During the first 24 hours frequent observations are made. Her abdominal wound will be checked and pain relief and intravenous infusions will be given. Urine will be passed via a catheter.

Pain management is an important part of hospital care for caesarean sections and is usually managed well. However, I find that I can give additional help using my electroacupuncture machine (Fig. 15.1). In the first 24 hours in particular, four pads either side of the scar can help enormously with the pain.

The role of nutrition following delivery

The general role of individual nutrients, together with their food sources, was discussed in Chapter 3. The following are particularly beneficial in aiding recovery from labour and will also benefit the newborn.

Copper and zinc

After delivery, most women will have a high copper level and a low zinc level. Copper levels rise during pregnancy and reach a peak immediately after the birth.

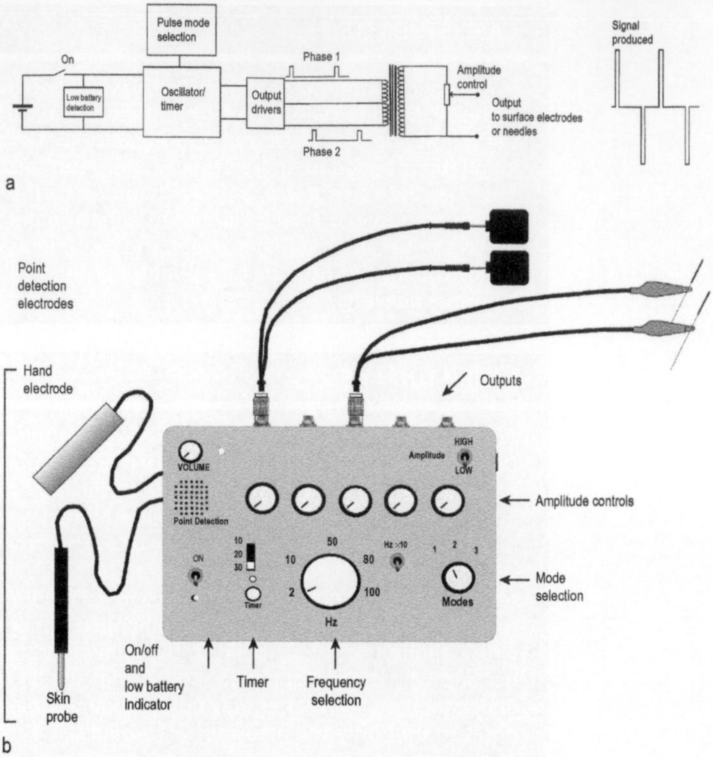

Figure 15.1 A typical electroacupuncture stimulator. (Courtesy of Riccardo Cuminetti.)

This can be kept in hand by maintaining a good zinc status but many women are depleted of zinc, especially if they have been on the contraceptive pill prior to conception. Copper levels will rise as further amounts of zinc are lost because of abrasions following the birth – a vicious circle.

The placenta is an exceedingly rich form of zinc, which is why most animal mothers eat their placenta after birth. I am not suggesting this, but it *is* important to remember that copper and zinc imbalance can lead to a hormonal imbalance, which is connected with postnatal depression. Zinc is also vital for wound healing (see Ch. 3, p. 42).

Manganese, zinc and chromium

These together are an important factor in blood sugar metabolism and deficiency can lead to blood sugar swings.

Good food sources include nuts, leafy and green vegetables (such as broccoli, chard, etc.), wholegrains, barley, liver, ginger and brewer's yeast, molasses, butter.

Iron

Iron is needed to make haemoglobin, which carries oxygen in the blood, and so is needed for the supply of oxygen to the muscles. A shortage reduces the capacity to supply the muscle around the perineum with oxygen to aid healing. Iron also helps to resist postnatal infection. If there has been heavy blood loss at the birth, it is particularly important to replenish stocks of iron. But giving iron as a supplement on its own will cause loss of other essential minerals. (For food sources see Ch. 1, p. 10.)

Vitamin C

Vitamin C helps to form collagen and capillaries, so is very important in the wound-healing process, particularly if a woman has torn at delivery. It strengthens the immune system and helps fight postnatal infections. It also helps the body's absorption of iron, preventing anaemia. (For food sources see Ch. 1, p. 9.)

Extra vitamin C is required for breastfeeding.

Vitamin B

Vitamin B is important for lactation and to help prevent blood sugar problems. (For food sources see Ch. 1, p. 9.)

Vitamin F (EFAs)

Essential fatty acids are vital for the baby's brain development so should be included in the diet of breastfeeding women. (For food sources see Ch. 1, p. 9.)

Fluids

The mother should be encouraged to drink plenty of fluids (water, herb teas and diluted fruit juices rather than drinks containing caffeine) to encourage milk flow.

General advice to help healing in the postnatal period

The midwife can advise what to take for pain relief after delivery. An obstetric physiotherapist is available on the wards and will be able to treat the perineum with ultrasound or pulsed electromagnetic energy, called megapulse. This helps both to relieve the pain and to reduce oedema (swelling). There are also many self-help remedies to aid comfort.

When feeding her baby, the woman should sit with a pillow under each buttock to relieve the pressure on the perineum, or lie on her side on a pillow with another pillow between the knees. When resting, she should lie on her back, with a pillow under her bottom and shoulders, or on her tummy.

Pain can be eased by the application of ice. It can be flaked or crushed and put inside a polythene bag or gauze and placed on the perineum for 10 minutes. It should not be left on any longer, as it might delay healing by restricting blood circulation to the area.

Pelvic floor exercises (see Ch. 10) help to relieve the pressure on the perineum by contracting and relaxing the muscles. They also help to improve the local circulation, which aids healing.

Bathing the area is very therapeutic, using either a bidet or a bath. The area should always be dried well after bathing to prevent the risk of infection.

There are many products available on the market, many of them based on traditional remedies. They include the following.

- Witch-hazel is an astringent that helps with bruising and inflammation; it can be bought either in the form of an ointment or as a tincture to add to the bath.
- An old favourite is to add salt to the bath; salt is not harmful but research has not shown any overall benefit.
- Arnica is recommended by many midwives to be taken orally prior to delivery, to help with traumatised tissues; it can also be bought as a lotion but

it should not be used on open wounds (in such cases calendula can be used instead). It has anti-inflammatory properties and will help with skin healing.

Summary

- Problems after the birth include: persistent lochia, breastfeeding problems, urinary problems, afterpains, perineal soreness, haemorrhoids, puerperal infection and mental and emotional problems.
- Acupuncture points used in the postnatal period include:
  - *mother roasting:* moxa on CV-2 to 8, then GV-2 to 8
  - *Blood deficiency:* SP-6, ST-36, CV-12 and BL-20; plus moxa on SP-1 and BL-17
  - *Blood Heat:* SP-10 and 6, LI-11 and LR-3
  - *Blood stasis:* SP-1, BL-17 and LI-11
  - *to raise the Qi:* GV-20
  - *uterine bleeding:* SP-1
  - *to strengthen the uterus:* CV-4
  - *engorged breasts:* CV-17 and GB-41
  - *lack of milk:* ST-36 and SP-6, SP-1, also BL-17, 20 and 23, with moxa if the mother is deficient
  - *blocked ducts:* needles placed superficially around the area of redness
  - *mastitis:* LI-11, ST-44 and LR-2
  - *urinary problems:* CV-3, with BL-22, 28 or 63; plus BL-63, SP-10 and KI-2 (for extensive pain and blood in urine)
  - *afterpains:* (deficiency) CV-4 and 6 and ST-36; (excess) SP-10, BL-17 and ST-29
  - *perineal soreness:* GV-1
  - *Blood and Qi deficiency:* HT-7, BL-15, CV-14, SP-6, with moxa if deficient, and ST-36
  - *sweating following delivery:* (Qi deficiency) LI-4 and KI-7; (Yin deficiency) HE-6
  - *external invasion of Wind-Heat:* LI-4 and TE-5, BL-12 and 13, BL-17
  - *external invasion of toxins:* LI-11 and GV-14 (to clear heat), LR-3 and KI-2 (to clear the Blood); plus CV-3 (for retained products)
  - *Heart Blood deficiency:* HT-7, CV-14 and 15, GV-20 and PC-6
  - *Heart Yin deficiency:* HT-7 and 5 and SP-6
  - *Heart Blood stasis:* BL-17 and SP-10, BL-15 and SP-4 and PC-6

References

Kendell RE 1985 Emotional and physical factors in the genesis of puerperal mental disorders. Journal of Psychosomatic Research 29(1): 3–11

Maciocia G 1989 The foundations of Chinese medicine. Churchill Livingstone, New York

Sweet BR (ed.) 1997 Mayes' midwifery, 12th edn. Baillière Tindall, New York

Swyer G 1985 Postnatal mental disturbance. British Medical Journal 20: 1232–1233

Tiran D, Mack S 1995 Complementary therapies for pregnancy and childbirth. W B Saunders, London

16 Classical Five Element acupuncture and its use in postnatal depression

Gerad Kite

Chapter outline

The term 'postnatal depression' describes a period of 'mental illness' the mother may experience after the birth of her child. This label is used in a way that often suggests that all mothers will experience the same symptoms to a greater or lesser degree and the cause will come from the same emotional and physical experience of pregnancy. In reality, the only link many mothers will experience is that this period of illness comes after the birth of a child, yet the experience will differ greatly from person to person. Obviously, we are looking at a situation that arises as a result of childbirth, but is that the actual cause of the problem or simply an event that triggers something on a deeper level?

For many mothers the experience of pregnancy and giving birth is very traumatic. Not only does the mother have to cope with massive physical changes but she also has to adapt to her new role in life through her own perception as well as that of others. Postnatal depression is the most well-known form of mental illness connected with pregnancy; however, many women experience depression during the pregnancy, although this does not seem to be as recognised or as well documented as that in the postnatal period. This probably has something to do with our expectation of a mother's joy at giving birth and when she responds in any way contrary to this, we see it as 'wrong'.

Classical Five Element acupuncture seeks to isolate the true source of the problem and eradicate it for all time, rather than simply dealing with a presenting symptom and clearing the problem for that moment. I am not suggesting that all postnatal depression is old, deep-rooted psychological baggage rising to the surface; rather that any extreme experience in life, be it good or bad, can throw us off our natural cycle, and the apparent cause (childbirth in this case) may not actually be the cause but simply the trigger.

Five Element theory

The Chinese recognised that there was a natural flow of energy that moved through everything in the universe. They observed it in everything around them and particularly the seasons. They saw there was a precise order and relationship between the different phases of this energy which generated and controlled, maintaining a perfect balance, which in turn nourished and supported everything around them.

It is important to remember that this flow of energy or life force is one continuous flow, having no beginning or end. The Chinese recognised that the energy had five major movements, which corresponded with the seasons, and so they named these phases the Five Elements. For our purposes, it is easier to break things down so that we can look at them singly with greater clarity, but we must always remember we are looking at a part of the whole and in separation have only a small part of the picture. Postnatal depression is a small snapshot of the patient's life. It tells us where she is right now but little else, and so to diagnose or treat with such minimal information would be illogical.

The Five Elements are apparent in everything we experience and see in ourselves and the world around us. In any situation or event in life we can see this movement of energy leading the way and pregnancy is no different. If we look at the creation of new human life from conception to birth in relation to the Five Elements, we can see how the natural flow of the universe steers and supports the generation of our species.

Conception – the Water Element

Winter is the season of the Water Element. The energy at this time of year has descended deep within ourselves and the earth, and symbolises a time of resting and quiet contemplation. It is the time when we build our reserves, much like the wells of the earth filling as the winter rain descends deep into the ground. It is a time of year when the nights are long and we retreat from the cold and conserve what we have. The sperm and the egg formed deep within the body represent the true essence of ourselves. It is the manifest part of us that carries all information about our identity and the blueprint to produce new life. It is from the deepest part of us that a new and expansive life force will emerge. The winter is the most contracted time of the year and the energy is at its most Yin. By virtue of their extreme Yin nature, winter and Water have no choice but to turn from Yin to Yang and emerge as the spring, the Wood phase of the energetic cycle. The joining of the egg and the sperm gives rise to new life, opening and creating, driven by the pure power and force of the Water.

For couples planning to try and conceive, the 3 months prior to conception could be considered the 'Water' period, as it is at this time that they need to conserve their energy, eat well, drink plenty of fluids and generally build their reserves to ensure the quality of the egg and the sperm is optimum and that they have the resources to cope with everything that will follow.

This obviously is paramount for the mother who will have to carry and feed the new life for the following 9 months. The concept of preconceptual care is largely overlooked, particularly in the case of men in whom in recent years sperm counts have fallen dramatically. If the mother is at all weak at this stage, the future will be so much more difficult, not only physically but also emotionally. The cause of some postnatal depression may have its roots at this stage.

Growth/gestation – the Wood Element

Spring is the time of the Wood element. This phase of this cycle is full of promise and growth. The energy yawns and stretches from the deep sleep of winter. It opens and the hidden potential of the seed within is realised by its expanding nature. This is the time for the development of the fetus to the fully formed child. The natural laws and plans of nature combine with the inherent knowledge of the seed to create the new life and take it all the way through to maturity at the point of birth. For the mother, this is a time where nature takes over and she is simply required to follow her natural instincts to maintain her health and provide the optimum space for the baby to flourish and grow. This is the time when we talk of a mother 'blooming'.

The forces of nature surge through her, ensuring health and vitality for mother and baby. As we all well know, this is not true for all pregnant women and in fact pregnancy can be a very difficult, draining time. Why is this? This surely must make us question the health of this part of the energetic cycle for these women.

Maturity/birth – the Fire Element

Summer is the time of the Fire Element. It is the point of maturity, the apex of the cycle, the high point, the point of arrival. The flowers are in full bloom and nature boasts its success by displaying the bright result of its previous plans and hard work.

The birth of the child is the same. The long-awaited child appears in the world for all to see. The mother has succeeded in producing the new life and for the first time in almost a year, is able to sit back and 'be'. There is a stillness in this maturity – not the stillness of water but a relaxed, satisfied feeling knowing the work has been done. The focus shifts from the mother to the child and the survival of the newborn is dependent on its outside support. This can be a huge relief for the mother as she now is able to share the responsibility with others. This can also be a difficult time as the attention she may have grown used to during the pregnancy will shift to the newborn child.

Nourishment/separation – the Earth Element

The mother for the first time since conception is separated from the child. Much like the flower that turns into the fruit that will fall from the tree to create the next new life, the mother will see the child as separate from her and start to experience the partial loss of that innate connection. The child will take from the mother, by suckling and soaking up her love, but the intention of the hungry baby is to feed and grow to be eventually independent of her. This relationship is not equal. The mother must be able to give to the child with generosity whilst holding on to her own centre. For some women the experience of pregnancy can be so fulfilling, they actually feel empty once the child is born. Rather than giving from the centre of their being to the child, the child becomes their centre and for this brief period of time during pregnancy, they feel for the first time complete and happy. This emptiness is often there long before the pregnancy but having felt complete and the resulting contentment, the refound emptiness can cause extreme depression.

Letting go/preparing for the new – the Metal Element

Autumn is the time of the Metal Element. It is the time of letting go of that which is no longer useful and clearing the way to prepare for the new. It is also the time of objectively seeing the value of all that has been achieved. Whereas the Earth Element is the time for the mother to see herself as one and separate from the newborn child, the Metal Element re-establishes the mother's independence, as the body, mind and spirit reconnect with the individuality of the mother whilst naturally maintaining the nurturing link of motherhood. Physically the body rids itself of anything no longer needed to support the child and the mother starts to feel as she was prior to pregnancy.

This part of the cycle is as important as any of the others as in order to regain strength and rebuild, the body, mind and spirit must be able to shed before returning to the resting phase. Often postnatal depression is simply linked with this period. Obviously, chronologically we can place the event at this time and the process of letting go evokes the emotion of grief, which we often associate with depression; however, this is often not the case.

Diagnosis of the true cause

So if it is true that the cause can come from any of these stages, what does this mean exactly? Do we mean the cause originates at a particular phase of the pregnancy and is then experienced after the birth? This could be true but to understand the method of diagnosis fully, we have to look at the theory of classical Five Element acupuncture, not just in the context of pregnancy or postnatal depression but in the general concept of an underlying causative factor that will lead to illness or disharmony in any individual.

The theory of the 'causative factor' as taught in Five Element acupuncture simply states that within every person's energetic make-up there is a weakness, or a part that is weaker than the rest, and if disease is going to enter this person's body, mind or spirit it will be through this window of weakness. Why this weakness exists is of no consequence as we simply need to be able to make a diagnosis in order to treat and support it. This underlying weakness is not necessarily an obvious tangible weakness that can be observed through symptoms, and a history of the patient's traumas and troubles will not give us the cause. This 'causative factor' will only be seen by the struggling aspect of the person's energetic system sending out alarm signals for practitioners to experience through their senses.

The way we are able to differentiate the area of distress is to see the greater flow of energy and break it down into five major groups. These are the Five Elements: five phases of one continuous flow of energy. As the energy moves and changes its vibration and function, it takes on a different form we can identify as separate. Our senses can detect the different phases, through smell, vision, hearing and our ability to feel emotion. The energy of Wood, for example, is doing exactly the same thing when we 'see' green in the face, 'hear' shout in the voice, 'smell' rancid in the air, and 'feel' the anger in the person. We are simply witnessing the same thing but experiencing it through our different senses. When we witness in a patient the overwhelming presence of this part of the energetic cycle, it is probable that it is calling for help as it dominates over the other phases. This clear message nature gives us directs us to the true cause of distress. The power of the 'causative factor' cannot be ignored because there is no mystery to unravel; it calls for our help and as long as we can see, smell, hear and feel the call, we know where to go to help.

An example: postnatal depression

How does the above help us with postnatal depression? If this theory is true for any illness then postnatal depression will be no different. The experience of pregnancy and childbirth as stated before can be extremely taxing and traumatic. It may not be an unpleasant experience but nevertheless it is exhausting and, by virtue of that, any weakness in the person may be exposed. If we imagine we have a mother with a 'causative factor' in the Fire Element, her natural weakness may be to feel a little vulnerable, finding it hard to communicate at times – experiences associated with the Fire Element. As pregnancy takes its toll on her, this weakness may be further exposed as this part of her energetic system is stressed even further than normal. By the time she has given birth and fulfilled her role of bringing new life into the world, she may be left feeling raw and even more exposed, leading to a form of depression.

CASE STUDY 16.1

A woman in her late 30s was pregnant for the third time. Her previous two pregnancies had been difficult both physically and emotionally and she had suffered severe postnatal depression after both births. She had felt very nauseous and irritable throughout the pregnancy. She had felt low and very isolated and felt she was 'being taken over' by the pregnancy.

The birth was relatively straightforward, but almost immediately after the birth she felt very depressed and at times suicidal. She felt hopeless and couldn't imagine how she would cope. Her main feeling was that she was trapped in an impossible situation that no one could help her with, and felt angry but was unable to express anything externally. Six months after the first two births she started to feel much better and eventually felt her normal self again. She came for treatment mainly to help with the morning sickness at the early stages of her third pregnancy.

Her diagnosis was that she had a causative factor in the Wood Element (Liver and Gall Bladder) and treatment was given based on this diagnosis, not because of the presenting physical symptom. She initially came weekly for 6 weeks and then monthly. Her sickness reduced dramatically but, more importantly for her, emotionally she felt completely different from the first two pregnancies. She felt calm and in control of herself and after the birth maintained an equilibrium not experienced before.

CASE STUDY 16.2

A woman in her mid-20s had just given birth for the first time. She had recently married and had never lived away from her parents before. The pregnancy had been perfect in every way, giving her wonderful energy and a feeling of absolute joy she had never experienced before. However, 3 weeks after the birth she started to worry about the health of the baby. She was reassured that everything was perfect, but she found it impossible not to imagine something was wrong. A week after this she started to imagine she had breast cancer and stopped breastfeeding and also started to reject the child, passing all mothering responsibilities to her husband. As soon as she was given a clear bill of health for breast cancer, she convinced herself she had ovarian cancer. She was not depressed but rather obsessed, spending most of the day reading medical journals and researching everything she could on cancer. She was diagnosed as having a causative factor in the Earth Element (Stomach and Spleen) and was treated on this element twice a week for 1 month. Initially her anxiety and fear of illness increased but after 2 weeks very suddenly she took back her responsibilities as a mother and no longer mentioned her imagined personal illnesses.

CASE STUDY 16.3

A woman in her mid-30s gave birth to twins, her first pregnancy. The pregnancy had been without incident although the birth was traumatic, with a 30-hour labour ending with a caesarean section. The mother recovered well physically but emotionally became very withdrawn, having previously been very extrovert and fun loving. She talked of feeling 'fat and ugly' and felt sexually rejected by her partner even though he claimed to enjoy sex with her. Even after 3 months she still felt as bad, resenting the twins for 'taking away her figure' and negating the role of a mother, seeing it as a 'worthless occupation'. She had very black moods and fought daily with her husband, who was at a complete loss with her behaviour, not understanding the dramatic change in her. When she came for treatment she was diagnosed with a causative factor in Metal (Lung and Large Intestine) and was treated on this Element weekly for 3 months. She noticed a dramatic improvement almost immediately, feeling lighter, less angry and as if she had been 'living a nightmare' for the past 3 months. She also realised she had felt very similar during her teen years until she met her current husband in her early 20s.

The beauty of this system is that we do not need to use our heads to discover the source of the problem. A woman experiencing postnatal depression is likely to be exhausted and probably incapable of articulating why she feels so awful. By using our senses and reading the distress call, we can treat the area in need of support with little or no help from the mother, who at this stage may just need to rest and recuperate, whilst being supported energetically with treatment.

Even better than treating the mother after the birth would be to treat her in advance so that she is able to cope and survive the experience without collapsing at the end. This is the most extraordinary aspect of this type of diagnosis and treatment. By reading the signals of the person's energetic make-up, we are able to support in advance of illness or trauma the 'Achilles heel' and in turn strengthen the whole system.

Obviously the hardest part of this system of medicine is our ability to rediscover our senses and fine-tune them enough that we can clearly read the distress call. This is something we cannot learn from a book or study with someone else. We simply have to allow our senses to awaken and try and put our clever minds out of the picture.

Although it is interesting to look at the different emotional experiences and how they relate to the Five Elements, it should be stressed that the case studies here could all have been diagnosed with each other's causative factor. It is true we can often see a direct relation to the issues we associate with the elements and in the above three case studies this is somewhat true, but a diagnosis can never be made on what someone says or feels, but only by observing the distressed Element or causative factor by colour, sound, odour and emotion.

Treatment

This chapter is not intended as a 'how to' section for practitioners of different acupuncture backgrounds or training. Therefore I am not suggesting a treatment protocol or a selection of points that may be useful. The Five Element style of acupuncture requires a full training to be able to diagnose correctly and apply the appropriate treatment. This is meant as an introduction to a style that I believe to be most useful in the treatment of postnatal depression.

Summary

- The stages of pregnancy and birth in terms of Five Element theory are: conception (Water Element), growth/gestation (Wood Element), maturity/birth (Fire Element), nourishment/separation (Earth Element) and letting go/preparing for the new (Metal Element).
- Five Element theory helps the diagnosis of physical and psychological problems in pregnancy by revealing the woman's energetic make-up and the associated weaknesses.
- The emphasis of Five Element diagnosis is to find the true cause of distress within the body, mind and spirit of the person.
- Using the term 'postnatal depression' for any mother who feels low or depressed after childbirth seems useless and misleading as it implies that this emotional state has its own form and pattern, which it does not. Similarities may be found in many case studies of postnatally depressed mothers but the cause is never *simply* the result of giving birth.
- By using the Five Element model to diagnose and treat, the practitioner can be sure the true cause has been tackled and feel certain that whatever may have happened during the period of pregnancy and childbirth that may have adversely affected the mother will be helped and supported by addressing the true 'causative factor' in that person.

Appendix

Standard international nomenclature for the 14 meridians

Name or meridian	Alphabetic code	
	Agreed	Former
Lung	LU	Lu, P
Large Intestine	LI	CO, Co, IC
Stomach	ST	S, St, E, M
Spleen	SP	Sp, LP
Heart	HT	H, C, Ht, He
Small Intestine	SI	Si, IT
Bladder	BL	B, Bi, UB
Kidney	KI	Ki, R, Rn
Pericardium	PC	P, Pe, HC
Triple Energizer	TE	T, TW, SJ, 3H, TB
Gallbladder	GB	G, VB, VF
Liver	LR	Liv, LV, H
Governor Vessel	GV	Du, Du Go, Gv, TM
Conception Vessel	CV	Co, Cv, J, REN, Ren

Bibliography

Balen A, Jacobs HS 2003 Infertility in practice, 2nd edn. Churchill Livingstone, Edinburgh

Barker DJP 1998 Mothers, babies and health in later life. Churchill Livingstone, Edinburgh

Betts D 2006 The essential guide to acupuncture in childbirth. Journal of Chinese Medicine, Hove

Dooley M 2006 Fit for fertility. Hodder and Stoughton, London

Glenville M 2000 Natural solutions to infertility. Piatkus, London

Jin Y 1998 Obstetrics and gynecology in Chinese medicine. Eastland Press, Seattle

Liang L 2003 Acupuncture and IVF. Blue Poppy Press, Boulder

Lyttleton J 2004 Treatment of infertility with Chinese medicine. Churchill Livingstone, Edinburgh

Morgan JB, Dickerson JWT 2002 Nutrition in early life. Wiley, New York

Reagan L 2005 Your pregnancy week by week. Dorling Kindersley, London

Ross J 1995 Acupuncture point combinations – the key to clinical success. Churchill Livingstone, Edinburgh

Sher G, Marriage Davis V, Stoess J 2005 In vitro fertilization. The A.R.T. of making babies, 3rd edn. Checkmark Books, New York

West Z 2001 Natural pregnancy. Dorling Kindersley, London.

West Z 2003 Fertility and conception. Dorling Kindersley, London

West Z 2005 Guide to getting pregnant. Harper Thorsons, London

West Z 2006 Babycare before birth. Dorling Kindersley, London

Western medical glossary

Abruptio placentae:

early separation of the placenta. Occurs in the late stage of a pregnancy: the woman presents with uterine pain and vaginal bleeding.

Afterpains:

these occur during the first 2–3 days after birth and are caused by the contracting uterus. They are more common in women who have had more than one baby and are worse when breastfeeding.

Alpha-fetoprotein (AFP):

routine blood test offered in pregnancy. The concentration of AFP in the blood can be accurately assessed between weeks 16 and 18, in conjunction with an ultrasound scan. A high level of AFP may indicate that the pregnancy is more advanced, a multiple pregnancy, a spinal tube defect such as spina bifida, or death of the baby. A low level of AFP might indicate the pregnancy is less advanced or possibly Down's syndrome.

Amniocentesis:

a test in which a specially designed needle is inserted through the abdominal wall to take a sample of the amniotic fluid. It is safest when performed between 14 and 16 weeks. Reasons for carrying out this test include: suspicion of an abnormality following AFP, family history of congenital illness, maternal age over 37. There is a 1 in 150/200 of miscarriage following amniocentesis.

Anoxia, fetal:

this is starvation of oxygen to the fetus, which can occur due to cord prolapse, the placenta not functioning properly, the placenta coming away from the uterine wall, diabetes, infection or traumatic delivery. It can be the cause of still birth.

Antepartum haemorrhage:

bleeding after 24 weeks of pregnancy; this is a serious complication, which can result in death of the mother and baby.

Antiphospholipid antibodies:

antibodies to the chemical substances which coat the placenta as it grows in the wall of the uterus.

Apgar score:

the evaluation of the newborn baby's physical condition, usually performed at 1 and 5 minutes after birth. It is based on five factors: respiratory effort, heart rate, muscle tone, colour and reflex irritability. Each factor is given a score of 2, 1 or 0 points. An Apgar score of 8–10 indicates a healthy baby.

Bart's test:

a blood test, usually taken at 16 weeks, which checks levels of AFP and the hormones oestriol and human chorionic gonadotrophin. It can show increased risk of spina bifida or Down's syndrome.

Braxton-Hicks contractions:

painless, irregular uterine contractions, usually occurring in late pregnancy.

Caesarean section:

a surgical operation for delivering a baby through the abdominal wall.

Cardiotocograph (CTG):

a machine that monitors the baby's heartbeat. It is attached on to the mother's abdomen in two places, one to monitor the contractions and one to monitor the baby's heartbeat.

Cephalopelvic disproportion (CPD):

a misfit between the baby's head and the mother's pelvis.

Cervical dilation:

opening of the cervix.

Cervix:

the opening to the uterus, found at the top of the vagina.

Chorionic villus sampling:

antenatal test for chromosomal and/or genetic disorders, usually given between 8 and 12 weeks. It is often recommended in women over 35 or if there is a family history of genetic disorder. It carries a 2% risk of spontaneous miscarriage.

Crowning:

when the full diameter of the baby's head has emerged under the pubic arch, during labour.

Diabetes:

a medical condition in which the pancreas fails to produce sufficient insulin.

Doppler device:

a sonic listening device used by a midwife to listen to the baby's heartbeat.

Ectopic pregnancy:

a pregnancy that occurs outside the uterus, generally in the fallopian tubes. The pregnancy is usually not viable and may become a medical emergency.

Engagement, fetal head:

this is when the baby drops into the pelvic cavity in the late stage of pregnancy.

Epidural:

a form of pain relief used during labour in which anaesthesia is inserted via a catheter into the epidural space around the spinal cord in the lower back.

Episiotomy:

a surgical incision into the woman's perineum during labour to enlarge the opening of the vagina in a controlled manner, so as to make delivery easier.

Forceps delivery:

specially designed forceps are used to expedite the baby's delivery.

Fundus:

the top of the uterus, the part furthest away from the cervix.

Hydatidiform mole:

where the placenta cells grow abnormally in the absence of a fetus. There will be large quantities of human chorionic gonadotrophin (HCG) which give the positive pregnancy test. The ultrasound will show absence of an embryo and the uterus will contain tiny cysts. The high levels of HCG will cause severe sickness and abdominal swelling. Treatment will involve hospitalisation to remove the mole.

Hyperemesis gravidaram:

severe morning sickness.

Induction:

the deliberate attempt by artificial means to pre-empt the spontaneous and natural start of labour.

Lochia:

the discharge that comes away from the vagina following birth.

Mastitis:

inflammation of the breast, usually caused by a bacterial infection from damaged nipples or a blocked milk duct.

Meconium:

a black sticky substance which, if present in the amniotic fluid, indicates that the baby has opened its bowels and may be in distress.

Multiparous:

a term used for a woman having her second or subsequent baby.

Nuchal ultrasound scan:

antenatal test performed between 11 and 13 weeks. The scan results are compared with the woman's age to calculate the risk of Down's syndrome and other chromosomal abnormalities.

Obstetric cholestasis:

a medical condition that occurs in pregnancy caused by an overflow of bile passing through the placenta. It is toxic to the fetus and if untreated may result in still birth. The symptoms are severe itching in the third trimester and it is diagnosed by a blood test and liver function test.

Placenta:

an organ within the uterus by which the embryo is attached to the uterine wall. Its main function is to provide the embryo with nourishment, eliminate waste and exchange respiratory gases. It also functions as a gland, secreting human chorionic gonadotrophin, progesterone and oestrogens, which help regulate and maintain the pregnancy.

Placenta previa:

a placenta which is situated wholly or partially in the lower and non-contractile part of the uterus.

Pre-eclampsia (pregnancy-induced hypertension):

high blood pressure developing during pregnancy in a woman whose blood pressure was previously normal. It is often accompanied by excessive fluid retention and protein in the urine. It is a potentially serious complication and the treatment is bedrest, relaxation and intravenous medication to prevent eclampsia occurring. **Eclampsia** manifests with convulsions; it can lead to coma and labour may be induced or emergency caesarean section performed.

Primigravida:

a term used for a woman having her first baby.

Puerperal psychosis:

this is an acute severe depression that requires prompt treatment, affecting one woman in 1000, following childbirth.

Scalp electrode diagram:

used in late labour; when the baby's head is visible, it is possible to monitor the baby with an electrode attached to the scalp. This technique is used if the baby is diagnosed as being at risk, particularly if the heart rate is dropping.

Still birth:

a baby who has been born after 24 weeks of pregnancy but did not breathe or show any signs of life.

Trophoblast:

cells of the blastocyst which attach the embryo to the uterine wall and form the placenta.

Umbilical cord:

the strand of tissue connecting the fetus to the placenta. It contains two arteries that carry blood to the placenta and one vein that returns it to the fetus.

Uterus:

the womb; the pear-shaped organ of the female reproductive tract that is specialised to allow the embryo to implant and to nourish the growing fetus from the mother's blood. The uterus has an inner mucous lining (the endometrium) and a thick wall of smooth muscle (the myometrium).

Ventouse (vacuum extraction):

this is an alternative method of instrumental delivery that might be preferred in certain circumstances, such as where the cord is prolapsed and the cervix is dilated. The instrument consists of a suction cap made of metal or rubber. It is placed on the baby's head and suction is applied through an attached tube and vacuum pump. The baby can then be gently pulled out.

Index

Page numbers in *italics* refer to figures; those in **bold** to tables or boxes.

T

U

V

W

Y

Z

Printed and bound by CPI Group (UK) Ltd, Croydon, CR0 4YY
03/10/2024
01040366-0013